Biomass Processing Technologies

Biomass Processing Technologies

Edited by
Vladimir Strezov
Tim J. Evans

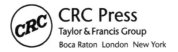

CRC Press
Taylor & Francis Group
Boca Raton London New York

CRC Press is an imprint of the
Taylor & Francis Group, an **informa** business

CRC Press
Taylor & Francis Group
6000 Broken Sound Parkway NW, Suite 300
Boca Raton, FL 33487-2742

First issued in paperback 2020

ISBN-13: 978-1-4665-6616-3 (hbk)
ISBN-13: 978-0-367-51954-4 (pbk)

Library of Congress Cataloging-in-Publication Data

Biomass processing technologies / [edited by] Vladimir Strezov and Tim J. Evans.
  pages cm
  Includes bibliographical references and index.
  ISBN 978-1-4665-6616-3 (alk. paper)
  1. Biomass conversion. 2. Plant biomass. 3. Plant products--Biotechnology. 4. Biomass energy. I. Strezov, Vladimir. II. Evans, Tim J.

TP248.27.M53B563 2014
662'.88--dc23   2014000454

Visit the Taylor & Francis Web site at
http://www.taylorandfrancis.com

and the CRC Press Web site at
http://www.crcpress.com

Contents

Preface

Most of the environmental and sustainability challenges of modern life are associated with energy generation. These challenges are largely related to the use of fossil fuels for providing human society's energy needs. Fossil fuels are natural products that are readily available for use with minor preparation requirements, and that are high in energy and mass density. Fossil fuel–based technologies are well-developed and mature. They are the main drivers of the global economy, with the central economical parameters being based on the price of fossil fuels or their derivatives. Although fossil fuels are products with amazing properties, their large and widespread use over the past centuries has left a legacy to the environment that now needs to be addressed. The main environmental consideration of our current civilisation is the challenge we face with the ever-growing greenhouse gas emissions. The scientific community provides stronger connections among the use of fossil fuels, atmospheric greenhouse gas concentrations and their effect on the climate. Fossil fuels are also associated with emissions of priority pollutants to the atmosphere, the acidic gases of SO_x and NO_x, particulate matter (both fine and coarse particles), CO and heavy metals. These pollutants then contribute to regional air quality through photochemical reactions or acidic deposition. Emissions of trace metals from coal-fired power stations, particularly mercury, are now being recognised as another emerging environmental challenge that has global environmental considerations due to the long atmospheric lifetime of elemental mercury. Management of power station and coal mine wastes poses additional risks due to the potential leaching of toxic metals from ash dams.

Fossil fuels, as amazing or as troublesome as they are, have limited supplies. They are being depleted and, eventually, humanity will reach a generation that will not have the same opportunity of our current luxury to comfortably spend these natural products at rates set to satisfy the needs of the present generation. A question of philosophical interest to the editors of this book is 'Are the sustainability and environmental problems that we are facing today from power generation due to the intrinsic nature of the fossil fuels, or are they because of the rates of their use?' It is inevitable that we need to use alternative energy sources that will reduce the current rates of use of fossil fuels and further contribute to meeting the increase in demand for energy in the future.

Biomass is positioned as one of the most promising alternative energy sources because it is a carbon-based renewable fuel that can be utilised in current fossil fuel–based technologies either directly or through primary processing. Biomass is generally low in sulphur and ash, and when used for energy, has low to zero net atmospheric greenhouse gas contributions on a full life-cycle basis. Biomass is also the only renewable energy source that can be used to produce alternative solutions to liquid transportation fossil fuels. Biomass exists as a by-product or waste in many industrial activities, and has been traditionally discarded in dams or burnt in the field; hence, its use as an energy source contributes to the effective management of these wastes. The aim of this book is to provide a comprehensive overview of all the technologies that have been developed and can be applied to processing the biomass into fuels.

Editors

Vladimir Strezov is an associate professor and environmental science program director at the Faculty of Science, Macquarie University, Australia. He earned his PhD in chemical engineering at the University of Newcastle, Australia, where he worked jointly with the pyrometallurgy research team of BHP Research Laboratories. Before joining Macquarie University in 2003, he was a research associate and laboratory manager at the University of Newcastle. Dr. Strezov's current research projects are concerned with the improvement of energy efficiency and the reduction of emissions in minerals processing, electricity generation and production of biofuels. He has established close links with several primary industries leading to successful joint projects in the field of energy and sustainability. He currently manages a laboratory for thermal and environmental processing funded in collaboration with the Rio Tinto Group.

Tim J. Evans is an adjunct professor at the Faculty of Science, Macquarie University and principal engineer at Rio Tinto. He has a long association with Australian primary industries such as BHP Billiton, HIsmelt and Rio Tinto. He earned a PhD in chemical engineering from the University of Newcastle. Dr. Evans' expertise is in energy transformation and mineral processing, specifically high-temperature industrial processing.

Contributors

Annette Evans
Department of Environment and
    Geography
Graduate School of the Environment
Macquarie University
New South Wales, Australia

Tim J. Evans
Department of Environment and
    Geography
Graduate School of the Environment
Macquarie University
New South Wales, Australia

Tao Kan
Department of Environment and
    Geography
Graduate School of the Environment
Macquarie University
New South Wales, Australia

Gary Leung
Department of Environment and
    Geography
Graduate School of the Environment
Macquarie University
New South Wales, Australia

Cara J. Mulligan
Department of Environment and
    Geography
Graduate School of the Environment
Macquarie University
New South Wales, Australia

Les Strezov
The Crucible Group
New South Wales, Australia

Vladimir Strezov
Department of Environment and
    Geography
Graduate School of the Environment
Macquarie University
New South Wales, Australia

Katrin Thommes
Department of Environment and
    Geography
Graduate School of the Environment
Macquarie University
New South Wales, Australia

1

Properties of Biomass Fuels

Vladimir Strezov

CONTENTS

1.1 Introduction

Biomass is a ubiquitous and readily available energy source. Biomass encompasses any renewable material sourced from a biological origin and includes anthropogenically modified material including products, by-products, residues and waste from agriculture, industry and the municipality (McKendry 2002). Solar energy is transformed and stored in plants through the process of photosynthesis:

$$CO_2 + H_2O + hv \rightarrow \{CH_2O\} + O_2$$

where hv is the energy from the sun, and $\{CH_2O\}$ is the organic plant material with the basic form accepted to be that of glucose $C_6H_{12}O_6$.

The discovery of energy release from wood through fire more than 1 million years BC transformed humanity and civilisation. This early form of biomass use was, essentially, combustion, used to fulfill the basic human needs for cooking, heating and protection. The early forms of basic application of carbon for energy have engraved the long-lasting human admiration and dependency on combustion.

The industrial revolution brought about a change of living conditions and technology, and by the mid-19th century, technological advancements introduced power stations and the internal combustion engine, requiring a major shift in fuel sources as energy demand increased (Rosillo-Calle et al. 2007). During the 19th century, the human population became more densely clustered, and the sources of biomass around these populations were becoming less economically viable as more proximate sources were depleted, contributing to the amount of energy that was required to be invested in transporting the fuel. As the popularity of fossil fuels increased, the role of biomass decreased to an extent that biomass is now no longer the primary fuel source.

The dominance of fossil fuels for energy generation in our increasingly energy-intensive society brings a number of challenges associated with greenhouse gas emissions – emissions of atmospheric pollutants (SO_2, NO_x, particles, trace metals), management of the fly ash waste, water pollution from coal mine activities, depletion of fossil fuels (specifically oil and natural gas) and uneven geographical distribution of some fossil fuel types, such as oil – drawing fears of energy insecurity, which is reflected in political and social instabilities. For these reasons, biomass is gaining new attention in energy research and development, bringing major advantages that can address the growing challenges in energy generation.

Biomass is a renewable energy source that has no contribution to atmospheric greenhouse gas emissions, because the CO_2 released during biomass combustion is the same as the CO_2 fixed through photosynthesis during the lifetime of the plant. Most plants have, generally, short lifetimes, especially when deliberately cultivated for food or energy; hence, the CO_2 cycle of fixation and release is short. It is only when long-lived biomass sources (such as some old trees) are harvested for energy that the CO_2 cycle closure has a long life span, and the atmospheric CO_2 emissions may need to be accounted for. Some trees are known to be several hundreds or even thousands of years old. Although CO_2 closure may be possible through replanting of the same tree species if they are used for energy, it takes a long time for these species to grow to the point at which their photosynthetic activity reaches the same levels.

Natural biomass has a very low sulphur content, hence very low SO_2 emissions when utilised for energy. However, the nitrogen content in biomass is large, and nitrogen needs to be monitored closely. Biomass utilisation also produces waste; but in most processing technologies, this waste is beneficial for agricultural applications because of the large quantities of N, P and K nutrients present in the biomass post-processing residues. Industrial contamination of the biomass (sewage sludge, painted wood, algae used to remediate industrial wastewater, etc.) limits the use of the post-processing residues. Biomass does not require mining; however, in many cases, it requires agricultural activities. Because it is renewable and can be deliberately cultivated with species that are geographically suitable and process-specific, biomass may play a major role in enhancing the energy security of individual countries.

1.2 Current Biomass Applications and Trends

Currently, biomass constitutes 10% of the worldwide primary energy production, as shown in Figure 1.1, equating to 1.277 Gt oil equivalent (Gtoe) (53.47 EJ) of primary energy consumption of total biomass in 2012 (International Energy Agency [IEA] 2013). The contribution of fossil fuels to energy production amounted to more than 80% of the primary energy production.

In 2011, 337 TWh of electricity was produced from combustible renewable energy sources and waste generation. Table 1.1 presents the production of electricity from biomass for 2011 for the largest producing countries in the world, based on electricity production per capita and percentage of the

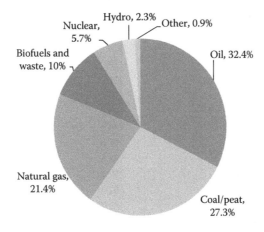

FIGURE 1.1
Total world primary energy according to the energy source. (From International Energy Agency, Biofuels and Waste, 2013. http://www.iea.org/stats/defs/sources/renew.asp.)

TABLE 1.1

Electricity Production from Biomass for 2011 per Capita and as a Percentage of the Total Electricity Production from Renewables and Waste

Country	kWh per capita	%
Finland	1949	3.14
Sweden	1241	3.52
Denmark	870	1.45
Austria	745	1.88
Estonia	609	0.23
Belgium	535	1.77
Germany	531	12.90
Netherlands	523	2.60
Uruguay	338	0.33
Portugal	306	0.96
Switzerland	305	0.73
Czech Republic	256	0.80
United Kingdom	235	4.41
Singapore	227	0.36
United States	220	20.60
Italy	220	3.97
Poland	205	2.35
Chile	205	1.01
Hungary	194	0.57
Canada	182	1.89
Japan	182	6.87
Brazil	176	10.10
Guatemala	169	0.77
Taiwan	160	1.11
Australia	153	1.05
New Zealand	136	0.18
Slovakia	127	0.20
Spain	111	1.55
France	108	2.11
Norway	95.4	0.14
Ireland	74.6	0.10
Nicaragua	67.0	0.12
Thailand	55.4	1.08
Argentina	52.4	0.62
Malaysia	52.4	0.46
Cuba	41.2	0.14
Ecuador	31.1	0.14
Peru	26.6	0.24

(continued)

TABLE 1.1 (Continued)

Electricity Production from Biomass for 2011 per
Capita and as a Percentage of the Total Electricity
Production from Renewables and Waste

Country	kWh per capita	%
South Korea	24.2	0.36
Russia	19.8	0.84
Colombia	10.7	0.15
China	9.88	3.97
Mexico	8.16	0.27
Turkey	5.96	0.13
India	1.75	0.63

Source: Euromonitor International, 2012. http://www.
euromonitor.com (Accessed December 10, 2012).

countries' contribution to the total electricity production from biomass. The United States (20.6%), Germany (12.9%), Brazil (10.1%), Japan (6.9%) and the United Kingdom (4.4%) are the largest producers of electricity from biomass and waste on a total production scale. Considering electricity production per capita, the Northern European countries, Finland, Sweden and Denmark have the largest production rates of electricity from biomass and waste.

Table 1.2 shows biofuel production for individual countries for 2011, according to Euromonitor (2012). Statistically, biofuels are divided into biodiesel, biogasoline and other liquid biofuels. Biodiesel includes methylester, dimethylether, Fischer–Tropsch produced from biomass syngas, cold-pressed bio-oil and all other liquid biofuels that are added to, blended with or used straight as transport diesel (IEA 2013). Biogasoline includes bioethanol, biomethanol, bio-ETBE (ethyl-tertio-butyl-ether) and bio-MTBE (methyl-tertio-butyl-ether). Other liquid biofuels include those not reported in either biogasoline or biodiesels. The United States and Brazil are the largest biofuel-producing countries in the world. The main feedstock for biodiesel production in the United States, Brazil and the other American countries is soybean oil. Corn is the main feedstock used for ethanol production in the United States, whereas Brazil uses sugarcane (Food and Agricultural Policy Research Institute [FAPRI] 2013). Other biomass feedstocks used for ethanol production include sugar beet, wheat and barley, which are mainly used by European countries. Biodiesel is also produced from rapeseed oil and sunflower oil in Europe, palm oil in Asian countries and other fats and waste oils, which are now increasingly applied for biodiesel production.

Figure 1.2 illustrates the emphasis placed on new investments in renewable energy and specifically biomass energy. The investments in renewable energy increased by 33% from 2009 to 2010, equating to US$211 billion

TABLE 1.2

Biofuel Production for 2011 Expressed in Million Tonnes of Oil Equivalent

Country	Total Biofuels (Mtoe)	Biodiesel (Mtoe)	Biogasoline (Mtoe)	Other Liquid Biofuels (Mtoe)
United States	29,626	2807	26,721	99
Brazil	17,629	2427	4540	10,662
Germany	4224	2499	367	1358
Argentina	2543	2543		
France	1921	1494	428	
China	1359	194	1165	
Italy	1246	554	145	547
Spain	844	609	235	
Canada	839		839	
Thailand	808	588	222	
Sweden	638	233	213	192
Indonesia	524	524		
Netherlands	441	434		6.8
Poland	436	262	97	76
Belgium	378	285	50	42
Portugal	323	319		3.5
Australia	320	62	259	
Austria	309	178	49	83
South Korea	294	294		
United Kingdom	279	136	143	
Cuba	235		235	
Czech Republic	221	186	35	
India	201		201	
Slovakia	176	123	53	
Finland	176	176		
Philippines	156	148	8	
Hungary	142	127	15	
Lithuania	142	111	30	
Malaysia	118	118		
Greece	93	93		
Romania	69	15	54	
Denmark	69	68		0.90
Paraguay	67		67	
Latvia	61	49	12	
Belarus	45	45		
Ireland	41	41		
Colombia	31	21	9.2	
Bulgaria	21	21		
Croatia	17			17

(continued)

TABLE 1.2 (Continued)

Biofuel Production for 2011 Expressed in Million Tonnes of Oil Equivalent

Country	Total Biofuels (Mtoe)	Biodiesel (Mtoe)	Biogasoline (Mtoe)	Other Liquid Biofuels (Mtoe)
Turkey	6.2	6.2		
New Zealand	6	1.9	4.1	
Switzerland	5.4	5.4		
Cyprus	5.2	5.2		
Macedonia	1.8	1.8		

Source: Euromonitor International, 2012. http://www.euromonitor.com (Accessed December 10, 2012).

(McCrone et al. 2011). As a subset of renewable energy, new investments on infrastructure, research and development on biofuels and biomass were flatlining in 2010, amounting to US$5.5 billion and US$11 billion, respectively, although there is still continual annual growth of new investments over the 2004 to 2010 period, as seen in Figure 1.2 (McCrone et al. 2011).

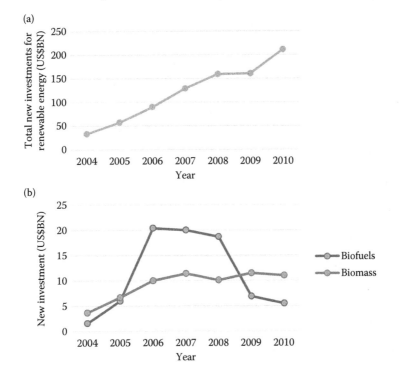

FIGURE 1.2

Historical trends in investments in (a) renewable energy and (b) biomass and biofuels. (From McCrone, A. et al., Global Trends in Renewable Energy Investment 2011: Analysis of Trends and Issues in the Financing of Renewable Energy. United Nations Environment Programme, 2011.)

1.3 Classification of Biomass

Table 1.3 lists various biomass classifications derived from the literature. There is no generic agreement for international standard classification of biomass, and the classification does not discriminate between the properties of the biomass and the way the biomass was produced. Therefore, two-dimensional classification of the biomass fuels is essential, accounting for the biological origin of the biomass and the biomass production conditions, as shown in Table 1.4.

TABLE 1.3

Summary of Classifications of Biomass

Categories	Reference
Woody plants, herbaceous plants and grasses, aquatic plants, manure	McKendry 2002
Wood, short-rotation woody crops, short-rotation herbaceous species, bagasse, biosolids, grass, aquatic plants and a host of other materials, agricultural wastes, wood wastes, sawdust, industrial residues, waste paper, municipal solid waste, animal wastes, waste from food processing	Demirbas 2004
Woody biomass (trees, shrubs and scrub, bushes, sweepings from forest floor, bamboo, palms), nonwoody biomass (energy crops, cereal straw, cotton/cassava/tobacco stems and roots, grass, bananas/plantains, soft stems, swamp and water plants), processed waste (cereal husks and cobs, bagasse, wastes from fruits, nuts, plant oil cake, sawmill residues, industrial wood bark and logging wastes, black liquor, municipal waste), processed fuels (charcoal, briquette/densified biomass, methanol/alcohol, plant oils, producer gas, biogas)	IEA 1998
Wood and wood, herbaceous and agricultural, aquatic, human and animal wastes, contaminated and industrial waste, mixture	Vassilev et al. 2010
Production on surplus agricultural land, surplus degraded land, biomaterials, agricultural residue, forest residues, animal manure, organic waste (including municipal) and primary, secondary and tertiary residues	Hoogwijk et al. 2003
Natural forests/woodlands, forest plantations, agroindustrial plantations, trees outside forests and woodlands, agricultural crops, crop residues, processed residues, animal wastes	Rosillo-Calle et al. 2007
Wood from natural forests and woodlands, forestry plantations, sugar and grain for fermentation, grains and oil seeds for transesterification, forestry residues, agricultural residues, black liquor from paper manufacturing, sewerage wastes	Fletcher et al. 1999
Energy crops, agricultural waste, refuse	Fowler et al. 2009
Virgin wood, energy crops, agricultural residues, food waste, industrial waste and coproducts	Biomass Energy Centre 2011

The biological origin (plant, animal or human origin) essentially determines the physicochemical properties of the biomass. Although traditionally the biomass is considered to consist of various plant materials, animal waste (tallow and manure) and human sewage are now emerging as sources of biomass fuels. Plant biomass can be divided into terrestrial and aquatic.

TABLE 1.4

Biomass Classification and Characteristics

Biological origin	Plants	Terrestrial	Wood	Roots		
				Trunk		
				Leaves		
			Nonwood	Herbaceous plants		
				Grasses		
			Fruit	Soft fruit		
				Seeds		
				Hard shells		
		Aquatic	Freshwater algae			
			Saltwater	Microalgae		
				Macroalgae		
	Animals	Tallow				
		Manure				
	Human	Sewage				
Biomass production route	Accidental (wastes and residues)	Weeds				
		Agricultural wastes				
		Forest wastes				
		Industrial and commercial wastes				
	Deliberately cultivated (energy crops)	Cultivation conditions	Soil	Biomass cultivated on agricultural soils		
				Biomass cultivated on marginal soils and degraded land		
			Water	Freshwater	Natural (creeks, rivers, lakes, sea, ocean)	Photobioreactor
				Saltwater		
		Edible properties	Edible (food crops)			
			Nonedible			
	Natural biomass	Biomass replanted after harvesting	Short regrowth rates			
			Long regrowth rates			
		Biomass not replaced after harvesting	Biomass regenerated naturally			
			Biomass regeneration suppressed by other plants and weeds			

Terrestrial biomass is based on woody biomass, nonwoody biomass and fruits. Aquatic biomass is generally composed of microalgae and macroalgae species from fresh or saltwater environments.

The biomass production route determines the sustainability of biomass utilisation and will affect the full life-cycle analysis of the environmental and greenhouse gas effects of biomass utilisation. It is highly important to distinguish between biomass produced as a waste and residues from biomass deliberately cultivated for energy use, or whether it was naturally occurring biomass before it was removed for energy use. In the case of energy crops, the competition of energy with food for agricultural soils or for products (food converted to energy products) has not only sustainability but also considerable ethical implications. The removal of naturally occurring biomass (deforestation, algae removal, etc.) for energy applications needs to be weighed against the long-term effects on the environment and the ability of the ecosystem to self-balance through natural or human-induced regrowth of the biomass.

The end-use processing pathways of the biomass fuels depend on the physicochemical properties. These properties are composed of the following:

1. Biochemical composition
   a. Wood chemistry
      i. Cellulose
      ii. Hemicellulose
      iii. Lignin
   b. Non-wood chemistry
      i. Saccharides
      ii. Lipids
      iii. Proteins
2. Moisture content
   a. Intrinsic moisture
   b. Extrinsic water
3. Mineral matter content
   a. Major elements
   b. Trace elements
   c. Nutrients
   d. Salts
4. Elemental composition of organic matter (C, H, N, S, O)
5. Physical properties
   a. Density
   b. Grindability

The biomass should have a high organic fraction, should be low in ash, moisture, O and S and should have high density and favourable grinding properties.

1.4 Quality of the Biomass Fuels

1.4.1 Woody Biochemical Compounds

Woody biomass is composed of the three main constituents: cellulose, hemicellulose and lignin. Cellulose is the main constituent of plants and contributes 40% to 45% of the dry wood weight. It has the role of maintaining the plant's structure but is also found as a component of the cell walls in bacteria, fungi, some algae and can even be found in some animals (O'Sullivan 1997). Cellulose is a water-insoluble biopolymer, a polysaccharide composed of a large (~10,000 in wood and ~15,000 in cotton cellulose) number of glucose units linked by β-(1-4)-glycosidic bonds (Kögel-Knabner 2002). Cellulose chains with regular arrangements of the hydroxyl groups lead to the formation of microfibril structure with crystalline properties. The cellulose elementary microfibril structure is associated with hemicellulose and lignin, as presented by a simplified Fengel model shown in Figure 1.3 (O'Sullivan 1997). The model suggests that cellulose elementary microfibrils are bound with a hemicellulose monolayer forming the cellulose fibrils, which are also bound with several layers of hemicellulose. Lignin is the surrounding layer of one whole microfibral system.

There are four major types of cellulose comprising six different polymorphs (I, II, III_1, III_{11}, IV_1 and IV_{11}). Cellulose I is the only naturally occurring cellulose and is largely unstable. It is now believed that cellulose I is

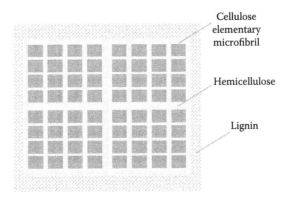

Cellulose elementary microfibril

Hemicellulose

Lignin

FIGURE 1.3
Ultrastructural organisation of woody cell wall according. (Adapted from O'Sullivan, A., *Cellulose* 4, 173–207, 1997.)

a mixture of two polymorphs (Iα and Iβ) (O'Sullivan 1997). Cellulose II is derived from cellulose I through the processes of regeneration or mercerisation. These processes involve chemical interactions between cellulose I and solvent or sodium hydroxide. Celluloses III_1 and III_{11} are formed from celluloses I and II by their treatment with amine solutions such as liquid ammonia. Celluloses IV_1 and IV_{11} are prepared by heating celluloses III_1 and III_{11}, respectively, to 206°C in glycerol.

Hemicelluloses are chemically heterogeneous polysaccaharides consisting of polymers of pentoses (xylose, arabinose), hexoses (mannose, glucose, galactose) and sugar acids (Saha 2003). Hemicelluloses can be classified into four major types: xylans, xyloglucans, mannans (glucomannans and galactomannans) and mixed linkage β-glucans (Schädel 2009). Xylans are the most abundant hemicelluloses and are the major component of hardwoods. Xyloglucans are the main hemicellulose types found in higher plants. Mannans are the main hemicelluloses in the tissues of conifers, whereas mixed linkage β-glucans are components of grass species.

Lignin is a highly complex aromatic polymer, commonly found in the cell walls of vascular plants, ferns and club mosses. It has the role of filling the cell walls and acting as a protective coating from microbial attacks for the polysaccharide constituents of the plant (Kenney et al. 1990). Lignin consists of a number of phenyl propane units with the primary building units being composed of coumaryl alcohol, coniferyl alcohol and sinapyl alcohol (Kögel-Knabner 2002). There are three general classification groups of lignin based on the chemical structure of their monomer units: softwood lignin, hardwood lignin and grass lignin (Higuchi 1990).

The proportion between the major wood constituents is of significant importance for biomass utilisation. Table 1.5 provides the generic contents of cellulose, hemicellulose, lignin and proteins of selected biomass groups. Although cellulose and hemicellulose composition in the wood can be processed through biochemical processing, lignin has very low biodegradation properties. Hence, for the production of ethanol or methane through biochemical processing, a low lignin content is preferred. For this reason, thermochemical processing routes are favourable options for high lignin content – biomass fuels.

1.4.2 Non-Woody Biochemical Compounds

1.4.2.1 Saccharides

Saccharides, also known as sugars or carbohydrates, are the most abundant biological molecules and are some of the most useful biomass compounds for biofuel production because they can be converted to alcohols through biochemical processing. Saccharides are polyhydroxylated aldehydes with only three elements: carbon, hydrogen and oxygen, representing a generic formula $(C·H_2O)_n$ where $n \geq 3$ (Voet et al. 2006). Saccharides in the living

TABLE 1.5

Cellulose, Hemicelluose, Lignin and Extractives in Selected Biomass Groups

Biomass	Cellulose (%)	Hemicellulose (%)	Lignin (%)	Extractives (%)
Hardwood	45–50	20–25	20–25	2–4
Softwood	35–40	20–25	27–30	1–10
Lignin-containing crop residues (corn stover, wheatstraw)	38	26–29	15–19	5
Lignin-free crop residues (soybean, rye straw, barley straw)	31–42	15–25	—	3–7
Lignin-containing warm season grasses (switchgrass, mischantus, big bluestem)	37–43	24–29	18–19	3–6
Lignin-free warm season grasses	35–40	30–33	—	0–3
Cool season grasses	25–35	30–35	—	3–15

Source: Sjostrom, E. *Wood Chemistry. Fundamentals and Applications.* 292, 2nd ed., San Diego: Academic Press, 1993; McKendry, P., *Bioresource Technology* 83(1): 37–46, 2002; Lee, D. et al., Composition of Herbaceous Biomass Feedstock. Report SGINC1-07, South Dakota State University, 2007.

organisms act as sources of energy and as structural material blocks, but they are also key code molecules in biological communication events that control egg fertilisation, microbial infection, inflammation and cancer-growth processes (Davis and Fairbanks 2002). Generically, the saccharides can be grouped into the number of individual sugar units as monosaccharides, disaccharides and polysaccharides. Table 1.6 presents the most common types of saccharides (Ophardt 2003). Monosaccharides are the simplest forms of carbohydrates, with glucose being the most abundant monosaccharide. There are two major groups of monosaccharides: aldoses and ketoses. Disaccharides have two monosaccharides bound together, whereas

TABLE 1.6

Common Types of Carbohydrates

Monosaccharides	Disaccharides	Polysaccharides
Glucose	Sucrose	Starch
Galactose	Maltose	Glycogen
Fructose	Lactose	Cellulose
Ribose		
Glyceraldehyde		

polysaccharides are complex carbohydrates with more than three bonded monosaccharides.

1.4.2.2 Lipids

Lipids are the major organic compounds naturally found in plants and animals, which can be used for the direct production of biodiesel. They are organic substances grouped according to their single common physical characteristics of being insoluble in water but soluble in nonaqueous solvents such as chloroform, hydrocarbons or alcohol (Kögel-Knabner 2002). Lipids are a heterogeneous group of organic compounds that are not necessarily chemically related to each other. The lipids are constituted of various fats, waxes and oils, nonpolymeric in structure, which have the major role in biological life as energy storage, as component materials of biological membranes and as chemical messengers for intracellular and intercellular signal transduction (Voet et al. 2006). Because of the vast difference in the chemical compounds that fall into the lipid category, their classification is still not standardised. Fahy et al. (2005) provide lipid classification according to the distinct hydrophobic and hydrophilic elements that constitute the lipid, as shown in Table 1.7. Fatty acyls are the major building blocks of lipids and are the most abundant lipids in plants and animals. Glycerolipids function mainly as energy reservoirs in animals and plants. Glycerophospholipids, sphingolipids and sterols are the major lipid components in biological membranes, with sphingolipids having distinctive structural features. Saccharolipids were described by Fahy et al. (2005) as compounds by which the fatty acids are linked directly to a sugar backbone.

1.4.2.3 Proteins

Proteins are molecules consisting of amino acids that the biological cells need for functioning. There are 20 types of amino acids (Table 1.8) that can form the structure of the protein. Proteins can have any of these 20 types of amino acids, which makes for a very large number of possible protein molecules. Although the types and number of amino acid molecules define the primary structure of the protein, the local spatial arrangement and the three-dimensional structure of the molecule make the secondary and tertiary structure of the proteins, with some even exhibiting quaternary structures (Voet et al. 2006).

In biofuel processing technologies, proteins are not used in fuel synthesis because of the difficulties of deaminating protein hydrolysates (Huo et al. 2011). In fermentation-based biofuel production, proteins are a by-product, rich in nitrogen, often used as animal feed or as fertilisers in land applications. In thermal processing technologies, the amine groups in the proteins have adverse effects on the process because part of the nitrogen evolves as

TABLE 1.7

Lipid Classification Categories

Fatty acyls	Fatty acids
	Fatty alcohols
	Fatty aldehydes
	Fatty esters
	Fatty amides
	Fatty nitriles
	Fatty ethers
	Hydrocarbons
Glycerolipids	Monoradylglycerols
	Diradylglycerols
	Triradylglycerols
Glycerophospholipids	Phosphatic acid
	Phosphatidylethanolamine
	Phosphatidylcholine
	Phosphatidylserine
	Phosphatidylglycerol
	Diphosphatidylglycerol
Sphingolipids	Sphingoid bases
	Ceramides
	Phosphosphingolipids
	Phosphonosphingolipids
	Neutral glycosphingolipids
	Acid glycosphingolypids
	Basic glycosphingolypids
	Amphoteric glycosphingolipids
	Arsenosphingolipids
Sterol lipids	Sterols
	Cholesterol
	Steroids
	Secosteroids
	Bile acids
	Steroid conjugates
	Hopanoids
Prenol lipids	Isoprenoids
	Quinones and hydroquinones
	Polyprenols
Saccharolipids	Acylaminosugars
	Acylaminosugar glycans
	Acyltrehaloses
	Acyltrehalose glycans
Polyketides	Macrolide polyketides
	Aromatic polyketides
	Nonribosmal peptides/polyketide hybrids

Source: Fahy, E. et al., *Journal of Lipid Research* 46, 839–861, 2005; Voet, D., Voet, J.G. and Pratt, C.W.: *Fundamentals of Biochemistry.* 2006. Copyright Wiley-VCH Verlag GmbH & Co. KGaA. Reproduced with permission.

TABLE 1.8

Common Amino Acids of the Proteins

Name	Average Occurrence in Proteins (%)	Formula
Amino Acids with Nonpolar Structure		
Glycine	7.2	$C_2H_5NO_2$
Alanine	7.8	$C_3H_7NO_2$
Valine	6.6	$C_5H_{11}NO_2$
Leucine	9.1	$C_6H_{13}NO_2(HO_2CCH(NH_2)CH_2CH(CH_3)_2)$
Isoleucine	5.3	$C_6H_{13}NO_2(HO_2CCH(NH_2)CH(CH_3)CH_2CH_3)$
Methionine	2.2	$C_5H_{11}NO_2S$
Proline	5.2	$C_5H_9NO_2$
Phenylalanine	3.9	$C_9H_{11}NO_2$
Tryptophan	1.4	$C_{11}H_{12}N_2O_2$
Amino Acids with Uncharged Polar Side Chains		
Serine	6.8	$C_3H_7NO_3$
Threonine	5.9	$C_4H_9NO_3$
Asparagine	4.3	$C_4H_8N_2O_3$
Glutamine	4.3	$C_5H_{10}N_2O_3$
Tyrosine	3.2	$C_9H_{11}NO_3$
Cystine	1.9	$C_6H_{12}N_2O_4S_2$
Amino Acids with Charged Polar Side Chains		
Lysine	5.9	$C_6H_{12}N_2O_2$
Arginine	5.1	$C_6H_{14}N_4O_2$
Histidine	2.3	$C_6H_9N_3O_2$
Aspartic acid	5.3	$C_4H_7NO_4$
Glutamic acid	6.3	$C_5H_9NO_4$

Source: Voet, D., Voet, J.G. and Pratt, C.W.: *Fundamentals of Biochemistry*. 2006. Copyright Wiley-VCH Verlag GmbH & Co. KGaA. Reproduced with permission.

acidic gas and acts as one of the primary pollutants during biomass pyrolysis, gasification or combustion and also is corrosive to infrastructures.

Table 1.9 gives a list of oil-rich crops, carbohydrate-rich crops, grasses and microalgae with their moisture-free protein, lipid, carbohydrate, fibre and ash contents. The oil-rich crops with lipid to carbohydrate (L/C) ratio greater than 0.5 are suitable for biodiesel production, with African oil palm showing the largest L/C fraction. The carbohydrate crops with higher carbohydrate to fibre (C/F) ratios may indicate suitability for fermentation applications.

1.4.3 Moisture Content

The moisture content in the biomass may be considered as one of the critical parameters that will determine the applicability of a specific biomass

TABLE 1.9

Protein, Lipids, Carbohydrate, Fibre and Ash Content in Selected Range of Oil-Rich Crops, Carbohydrate-Rich Crops, Grasses and Microalgae

Common Name	Botanical Name	Moisture	Protein	Lipids	Moisture Free Carbohydrates	Fibre	Ash	L/C	C/F
Oil Crops (Seeds)									
African oil palm	*Elaeis guineensis*	26.2	2.6	79.1	16.9	4.3	1.4	4.7	3.9
Coconut	*Cocos nucifera* L.	36.3	7.1	65.3	20.4	5.7	1.6	3.2	3.6
Cotton seed	*Gossypium hirsutum* L.	7.3	24.9	24.7	46.6	18.2	3.8	0.5	2.6
Flax seed	*Linum usitatissimum* L.	6.45	20.5	38.1	37.8	7.3	3.6	1.0	5.2
Jatropha	*Jatropha curcas* L.	6.6	19.5	40.7	35.9	16.6	4.8	1.1	2.2
Jojoba	*Simmondsia chinensis*	4.45	15.7	54.4	28.1	4.0	1.6	1.9	7.0
Mustard seeds	*Brassica juncea*	24.6	32.6	47.1	37.7	10.6	7.0	1.3	3.6
Niger seed	*Guizotia abyssinica*	7	19.7	35.1	39.7	14.5	5.5	0.9	2.7
Peanut	*Arachis hypogaea* L.	8.5	31.4	49.2	16.9	3.0	2.7	2.9	5.6
Rapeseed (canola)	*Brassica napus* L.		23.3	43.9	25.9	15.1	6.9	1.7	1.7
Soybean	*Glycine max*	68.2	40.9	17.9	35.8	6.0	5.3	0.5	6.0
Sunflower	*Helianthus annuus* L.	4.8	25.2	49.7	20.4	4.0	4.2	2.4	5.1
Carbohydrate Crops (Soft Fruits)									
Barley	*Hordeum vulgare* L.	11.8	10.6	1.8	85.4	15.6	1.9	0.02	5.5
Corn	*Zea mays* L.	72.7	12.8	3.7	81.0	2.6	2.6	0.05	31.6
Date palm	*Phoenix dactylifera* L.	15.3	3.0	0.5	94.1	4.6	2.5	0.01	20.4
Grape	*Vitis vinifera* L.	82.7	3.5	2.3	91.3	11.6	2.9	0.03	7.9
Job's tears	*Coix lacryma jobi* L.	11.2	17.3	7.0	73.5	0.9	2.1	0.09	81.6
Oat	*Avena sativa* L.	11	14.7	6.9	75.7	6.5	2.7	0.09	11.6

(continued)

TABLE 1.9 (Continued)

Protein, Lipids, Carbohydrate, Fibre and Ash Content in Selected Range of Oil-Rich Crops, Carbohydrate-Rich Crops, Grasses and Microalgae

| Common Name | Botanical Name | Moisture | Protein | Lipids | Moisture Free | | | | |
					Carbohydrates	Fibre	Ash	L/C	C/F
Carbohydrate Crops (Soft Fruits)									
Peach palm	*Bactris gasipaes*	50.5	5.3	8.9	84.2	2.0	1.6	0.11	41.7
Potato	*Solanum tuberosum* L.	78.75	10.6	0.7	84.7	2.4	5.9	0.01	36.0
Rye	*Secale cereale* L.		13.2	2.5	82.5	2.2	1.9	0.03	37.5
Sorghum	*Sorghum bicolor*	12	11.4	4.2	82.6	2.3	1.7	0.05	36.7
Sugar beet	*Beta vulgaris* L.	76.6	4.7	0.4	87.2	4.7	3.0	0.00	18.5
Sugarcane	*Saccharum officinarum* L.	82.5	3.4	0.6	94.3	17.7	1.7	0.01	5.3
Sweet birch	*Betula lenta* L.		28.1	8.6	55.6	16.9	7.7	0.15	3.3
Sweetpotato	*Ipomoea batatas*	69.15	4.4	1.0	91.7	2.8	2.8	0.01	33.3
Turnip	*Brassica campestris* L.	91.5	11.8	2.4	77.6	10.6	8.2	0.03	7.3
Wheat	*Triticum aestivum* L.	12.8	13.4	2.5	82.9	14.9	1.9	0.03	5.6
Energy Crops (Perennial Grasses)									
Alfalfa	*Medicago sativa* L.	82.7	34.7	2.3	54.9	17.9	8.1	0.04	3.1
Bahia grass	*Paspalum notatum*	69.4	8.5	1.6	79.7	31.6	10.2	0.02	2.5
Barnyard grass	*Echinochloa crusgalli*		13.7	2.9	72.2	22	11.2	0.04	3.3
Bermuda grass	*Cynodon dactylon*		11.6	2.1	75.9	25.9	10.4	0.03	2.9
Buffel grass	*Cenchrus ciliaris* L.		11	2.6	73.2	31.9	13.2	0.04	2.3
Diaz bluestem	*Dichanthium annulatum*	25	10.4	1.7	75.8	34.9	12.1	0.02	2.2
Elephant grass	*Pennisetum purpureum*	10.9	9.2	2.0	77.0	38.2	23.0	0.03	2.0
Guinea grass	*Panicum maximum*	75	5.9	1.6	81	35.7	10.6	0.02	2.3
Johnson grass	*Sorghum halepense*		12.3	2.6	39.6	27.7	15.9	0.07	1.4

Common name	Scientific name								
Meadow foxtail	Alopecurus pratensis L.	73.9	17.2	4.6	67.5	21.5	10.7	0.07	3.1
Molasses grass	Melinis minutiflora	74.5	6.75	1.55	77	35.6	14.7	0.02	2.2
Orchardgrass	Dactylis glomerata L.		13.8	4.3	72.7	27.9	9.2	0.06	2.6
Pangola grass	Digitaria decumbens	28.6	10.8	2	74.4	29.8	9.8	0.03	2.5
Perennial ryegrass	Lolium perenne L.	73.4	11.3	4.9	74.8	25.2	9.0	0.07	3.0
Red clover	Trifolium pratense L.	81	21.1	3.7	64.7	13.7	10.5	0.06	4.7
Reed	Phragmites australis		10.6	2.1	72.7	31.9	14.6	0.03	2.3
Reed canarygrass	Phalaris arundinacea L.		8.8	2.2	81.8	34.3	7.2	0.03	2.4
Rhodes grass	Chloris gayana	71.8	8.9	1	84.1	37.9	6	0.01	2.2
Russian thistle	Salsola kali L.	60.6	12.3	1.8	70.7	31.7	15.2	0.03	2.2
Smooth bromegrass	Bromus inermis Leyss.	10.3	12.3	2.6	76.3	31.7	8.8	0.03	2.4
Sudan grass	Sorghum sudanense	11.1	12.7	2.2	75.5	28.9	9.6	0.03	2.6
Timothy grass	Phleum pratense L.	76.1	19.7	3.8	65.7	19.2	10.9	0.06	3.4
Weeping lovegrass	Eragrostis curvula		13.1	2.1	78.8	31.5	6	0.03	2.5
Microalgae									
	Anabaena cylindrica		43–56	4–7	25–30				
	Aphanizomenon flos-aqua		62	3	23				
	Arthrospira maxima		60–71	6–7	13–16				
	Botryococcus braunii		4	86	20				
	Chlamydomonas rheinhardii		48	21	17				
	Chlorella ellipsoidea		5	84	16				
	Chlorella pyrenoidosa		57	2	26				
	Chlorella vulgaris		51–58	14–22	12–17				
	Dunaliella bioculata		49	8	4				
	Dunaliella salina		57	6	32				
	Euglena gracilis		39–61	14–20	14–18				

(continued)

TABLE 1.9 (Continued)

Protein, Lipids, Carbohydrate, Fibre and Ash Content in Selected Range of Oil-Rich Crops, Carbohydrate-Rich Crops, Grasses and Microalgae

Common Name	Botanical Name	Moisture	Moisture Free						
			Protein	Lipids	Carbohydrates	Fibre	Ash	L/C	C/F
Microalgae									
	Porphyridium cruentum		28–39	9–14	40–57				
	Prymnesium parvum		28–45	22–38	25–33				
	Scenedesmus dimorphus		8–18	16–40	21–52				
	Scenedesmus obliquus		50–56	12–14	10–17				
	Scenedesmus quadricauda		47	1.9	—				
	Spirogyra sp.		6–20	11–21	33–64				
	Spirulina maxima		60–71	6–7	13–16				
	Spirulina platensis		46–63	4–9	8–14				
	Synechoccus sp.		63	11	15				
	Tetraselmis maculata		52	3	15				

Source: Duke, J.A. Handbook of Energy Crops, New Crop Resource Online Program, Purdue University, 1983; Becker, E.W. *Microalgae: Biotechnology and Microbiology.* Cambridge University Press, 1994; Gebruers, K. et al., *Journal of Agricultural and Food Chemistry* 56(21), 9740–9749, 2008; Khalaf, G., and Mohamed, A-G., *Egyptian Journal of Histology* 31(2), 245–255, 2008; Edwards, M. *Green Algae Strategy.* CreateSpace Independent Publishing Platform, 2008; Arif, M. et al., ARPN *Journal of Agricultural and Biological Science* 7(9), 730–734, 2012.

Note: C/F is carbohydrate to fibre ratio; L/C is lipid to carbohydrate ratio.

processing technology. The biochemical processing technologies (fermentation and digestion) typically favour high-moisture saturated biomass feedstocks, whereas the thermal processing technologies, such as combustion, gasification and pyrolysis, can only accept low-moisture content biomass fuels of less than 40% (Kenney et al. 1990). To address the applicability of high-moisture content biomass fuels for thermal processing, hydrothermal processing technologies are now being developed.

The moisture content in the biomass can be separated between intrinsic and extrinsic moisture (McKendry 2002). Intrinsic moisture is the moisture that the plant naturally contains, whereas extrinsic moisture is the moisture that the biomass absorbs from weather during harvesting and storage. The water content also has adverse economic effects as the transportation costs increase with increased moisture content (Lewandowski and Kicherer 1997).

1.4.4 Mineral Matter

Biomass mineral matter is mostly naturally present inorganic compounds; but sometimes, it can originate from chemically contaminated biomass from industrial processes and applications. The mineral matter deposits in the biomass post-processing residues and the type and concentration of inorganic matter present in the post-processing residue can determine its potential further applications. The concentration of mineral matter in the biomass is highly variable, from less than 1 to 3 wt% for wood and sawmill residues, to 20 wt% in case of straw and husks, up to more than 50 wt% in case of sewage sludge, manure and black liquor (Table 1.10). The heating value of the biomass is dependent on the mineral matter present.

Generally, the main constituents of the biomass minerals are Si, Ca, K, Na and Mg, with smaller amounts of S, P, Fe, Mn and Al (Raveendran et al. 1995). The alkali metals of biomass (Na, K, Mg, P and Ca) are important for thermochemical processing because they react with the silica to produce a sticky liquid phase that leads to blocked airways in furnaces and boilers (McKendry 2002). Silica in the biomass also traps the carbon particles, making the carbon unavailable for conversion (Raveendran et al. 1995). K and Ca in the biomass lower its ash melting point, which is generally lower than coal's ash melting point (Lewandowski and Kicherer 1997). Ash melting produces slag, which impedes heat transfer and requires frequent removal.

Chloride (Cl) has a significant effect on biomass processing performance. Cl is present in large concentrations in straw and cereals as well as in marine algae. Chloride forms dioxins during thermochemical processing at a temperature range of 250°C to 450°C (Lewandowski and Kicherer 1997) and requires strict control due to the highly toxic nature of these chemicals. Cl is highly reactive and forms various salts and acids that are responsible for the corrosion of the boiler. The salts also cause deactivation of the $deNO_x$ catalytic converter and suppress the formation of tars (Raveendran et al. 1995).

TABLE 1.10

Range of Mineral Matter for Various Biomass Materials

	Minimum	Maximum	Average
Sawmill residues	0.1	2	1
Wood trees	0.1	6	2
Nut shells	0.4	6	3
Fruit waste	0.5	16	5
Energy crops (grasses)	1.1	17	6
Bagasse	1.9	13	6
Bio-oil postproduction cake	2.2	16	6
Sweepings	1.3	15	6
Cereal straw	1.3	20	7
Cereal husks	1.0	20	9
Shrubs and bushes	0.7	30	10
Freshwater algae	3.7	22	13
Saltwater algae	2.9	37	21
Manure	11	62	25
Black liquor	21	76	34
Sewage	21	74	49

Mineral matter is the major constituent of the biomass post-processing residues. Depending on the initial composition and elemental concentration of the mineral matter, the end-use application of the biomass post-processing residues can be planned. High nutrient (N, P, K) concentration in the post-processing residues would mean their application as fertilisers. However, the presence of toxic metals in the post-processing residues and ashes is a major limiting factor for the further use of these residues.

1.4.5 Elemental Composition of Organic Matter

The elemental composition of organic matter is determined through proximate (volatile matter and fixed carbon contents) and ultimate analysis (C, H, N, S and O). Proximate analysis is a standard test developed for the coal industry and applied to biomass fuels in which volatiles, excluding free moisture, are evolved by heating the biomass in an inert atmosphere up to 950°C. The fixed carbon is the mass of the residue left after heating the biomass. The volatile matter and fixed carbon determine the ignition and thermochemical conversion potential of the biomass.

Ultimate analysis of the fuels is used to determine the elemental composition of volatile matter and fixed carbon. The major elements determined through ultimate analysis are C, H, N and S, with O determined by the difference. N and S are important constituents because they often determine the environmental quality of the fuels. High N and S are unfavourable because

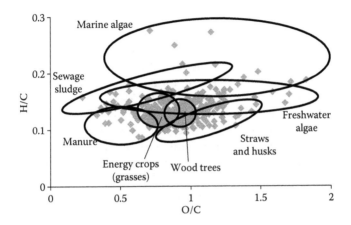

FIGURE 1.4
H/C to O/C diagram of biomass fuels.

they produce acidic gases during thermochemical conversion and malodours during biochemical conversion. Biomass has very low concentrations of S, from trace amounts up to 1% in case of husks, rapeseed and chicken manure. It is only in the case of sewage sludge, black liquor and some marine algae species wherein S content is more than 1% (black liquor) and can reach up to 6% (or even higher in the case of some sewage sludge samples). Nitrogen content, on the other hand, is much higher in biomass than in coal, with N reaching as high as 10% to 12% for some algae species (*Spirulina platensis* and *Synechococcus*), sewage sludges and some seeds and seed cakes.

C and H content in the fuels determine the calorific value and biofuel conversion potential. O is associated with losses and greater CO_2 emission during processing. In case of thermochemical conversion, carbon–carbon bonds contain greater energy than carbon–oxygen and carbon–hydrogen bonds (McKendry 2002). The Van Krevelen atomic H/C to O/C diagram for 400 different biomass species found in the literature are shown in Figure 1.4. The diagram shows that marine algae species have the greatest H/C ratios although dispersed over a wide O/C range. Freshwater algae exhibit lower H/C ratios but similarly wide O/C ratios as the marine algae species. The wood and energy crop species have very similar and uniform H/C to O/C ratios. Manures and sewage sludge have the lowest O/C ratios with manure, straws and husks exhibiting the lowest H/C ratios.

1.4.6 Physical Properties

One of the disadvantages of biomass fuels over coal is the low physical density of the biomass, which means that it attracts larger transportation costs; hence, utilisation of biomass closer to the biomass production site is required for its economical processing. Alternatively, preprocessing steps may be required to increase the density of the biomass. These steps may be physical, through compaction, or thermal, through torrefaction (mild heating of biomass to 300°C). Straws have the lowest density, reportedly being as low as 18 kg/m³ for wheatstraw, 80 kg/m³ for flaxstraw and barley straw, 180 kg/m³ for sawdust, 170 kg/m³ for soybean hulls, 240 kg/m³ for oat hulls and 275 kg/m³ for corn cobs; on the other hand, hardwoods have the highest density at 330 kg/m³ (Wilén et al. 1996; Clarke and Preto 2011).

Size reduction is a form of pretreatment of biomass for energy conversion as part of the densification process (Mani et al. 2004). Particle size reduction increases the pore size of the biomass and its total surface area. Some of the thermochemical processing technologies, such as combustion and gasification, require crushing and grinding of the biomass to a fine particle size. It is known that some types of biomass are difficult to grind (Arias et al. 2008). Although there is no standard measurement to determine the grindability of biomass, one option may be the energy required to grind biomass to a specific particle size range. Mani et al. (2004) presented variations in energy required to grind four biomass samples to various different particle size ranges, and determined corn stover as the least energy-intensive biomass species to grind, followed by straws. Switchgrass was the most energy-intensive biomass species for grinding.

1.5 Technologies for Biomass Processing

There is a range of different biomass processing technologies (Table 1.11), which can be classified into three categories: thermochemical, biochemical and physicochemical processing. Thermochemical processes have some advantages: offering faster conversion rates and, in case of combustion and gasification, can utilise already existing fossil fuel–based technologies. The conversion efficiency rates in the combustion of biomass are approximately in the range of 20% to 40% (Caputo et al. 2005). Most of the current research trends are focused on co-combustion of biomass and fossil fuels in existing coal-fired power plants (Baxter 2005). Conversion rate efficiencies are higher in the case of co-combustion rather than when biomass is combusted alone. The ratio of biomass combusted in blends with coal currently ranges between 2% and 20%, mainly depending on the differences in international commitments and policies.

Gasification is one of the most feasible biomass-based processing technologies. A number of commercial biomass gasification plants have been built recently, which are generally small in capacity (5–300 MW) and are located closer to the biomass producing and agricultural sites (Maniatis and Millich 1998; Leung et al. 2004). During gasification, biomass is thermally treated in

TABLE 1.11

Processing of Biomass Materials

Thermochemical processing	Combustion	Heat
		Steam
		Electricity
	Gasification	Steam
		Heat
		Electricity
		Methane
		Hydrogen
	Pyrolysis	Charcoal/biochar
		Biogas
		Bio-oil
	Hydrothermal processing	Charcoal
		Biogas
		Bio-oil
Biochemical processing	Anaerobic digestion	Biogas
		Digestate
	Fermentation	Ethanol fermentate
Physicochemical processing	Esterification	Biodiesel

a supersaturated steam or CO_2 atmosphere converting the material to combustible products (methane, hydrogen or CO), which can be further combusted to produce heat for electrical power generation. With the emerging integrated gasification combined cycle (IGCC) technologies, the biomass to energy conversion efficiency rates can be significantly higher and may reach up to 50% (Caputo et al. 2005).

Pyrolysis is the process in which biomass materials are heated and decomposed under inert atmospheric conditions. Pyrolysis processes convert biomass materials to gaseous and liquid products and create carbon-rich charcoal residue. Pyrolysis also occurs as an intermediate step in combustion and gasification. Liquefaction is a thermal process similar to pyrolysis in which biomass materials are heated under hydrogen or methane atmosphere aiming to convert the lignocellulosic materials to higher molecular weight hydrocarbons.

The biochemical processes involve anaerobic digestion, in which biomass materials are converted through anaerobic bacterial action in the absence of air. The solid products of compost are marketed as fertilisers, whereas biogas is recovered as an energy product. Fermentation is another biochemical process in which the biomass sugar composition is converted to alcoholic fuels through microbial action and distillation.

Physicochemical processing primarily comprises mechanical or solvent extraction of the lipids from the biomass materials, followed by a process known as transesterification. This process also involves the conversion of waste cooking oils, grease and animal fats to biodiesel (Van Gerpen 2005).

Depending on the type of final product, biomass technologies can be divided into those that convert biomass directly to energy (heat, steam, electricity) or to higher calorific value biofuels (charcoal, biogas, ethanol, methane, hydrogen, bio-oil, etc.). Direct energy conversion is more suitable for combustion or gasification plants located near the major biomass production and agricultural sites, thereby overcoming the necessity for preprocessing, briquetting and transportation. Technologies offering the conversion of biomass to higher calorific value fuels are applied to increase the energy density and hence reduce biomass transportation costs, or to convert it to the different fuel forms required by the energy utilisation processes. The biofuel products can be used as energy carriers, providing more sustainable fuel options for energy generation, cooking, transportation or industrial processes.

1.6 Different Generations of Biofuels

Biomass can be used to produce electricity and liquid biofuels suitable for use as transportation fuels. The conversion of biomass to liquid biofuels is currently at its first-generation biofuel stage, with the second-generation biofuels emerging from their current position at the research and development stage.

1.6.1 First Generation of Biofuels

The first generation of biofuels consists of the conversion of high saccharide content and high lipid content biomass to ethanol and biodiesel through the processes of esterification and fermentation/distillation. The high saccharide content biomass sources consist of a wide range of biomass types, including sugarcane, sugar beet, corn, potatoes, wheat, etc. The biomass sources high in lipids are sunflower, canola, soybean, tallow, palm, etc. The first generation of biofuels utilises well-known and established biomass sources and technologies applicable for food production. Because the input material for the first-generation biofuel production is, essentially, edible biomass, this poses significant challenges to sustainability due to competition with food.

Figure 1.5 illustrates biofuel production in 2012, showing that 88.2% of biodiesel and 99.93% of ethanol production in 2012 were derived from the first generation of biofuels. Rapeseed makes the largest feedstock for biodiesel production, followed by soybean. Ethanol production is largely produced from sugarcane, with corn also having considerable input.

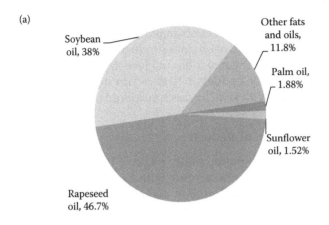

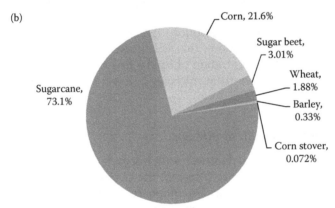

FIGURE 1.5
Biofuel production in 2012: (a) biodiesel production, (b) ethanol production. (From Food and Agricultural Policy Research Institute, 2011. http://www.fapri.iastate.edu/tools/outlook.aspx.)

1.6.2 Second Generation of Biofuels

The second generation of biofuels consists of the utilisation of lignocellulosic biomass for the production of liquid biofuels. The lignocellulosic biomass is non-edible and can be sourced from a range of industrial and agricultural technologies as a by-product or waste. The conversion of lignocellulosic biomass to biofuels requires an intermediate technology based either on the biochemical or thermochemical route. The biochemical route requires engineering of dedicated enzymes and microorganisms, which can convert the complex polysaccharides, cellulose and hemicellulose, to simpler saccharides that can be then processed to ethanol. The thermochemical route involves either pyrolysis of the lignicellulosic biomass to biogas, bio-oils and biochar, and then upgrading of the bio-oils to biodiesel through hydrothermal processing, or gasification of the biomass to syngas and then synthesising the syngas to biodiesel through the Fischer–Tropsch synthesis route. The second generation of biofuels have only contributed to 11.8% of the biodiesel production in 2012 and less than 1% of ethanol production (see Figure 1.4). Cooking oil waste and tallow are the major biofuel feedstocks that fall into the category of second-generation biofuels, whereas corn stover is the only representative in this category, with switchgrass considered to have an emerging role.

1.6.3 Third Generation of Biofuels

The third generation of biofuels mainly involves the use of microalgae as an energy crop. Microalgae do not compete with food crops for agricultural soil; they consist of high lipid and protein contents and have very fast growth rates. Microalgae can also be cultivated in soils unsuitable for agricultural purposes using wastewater, hence reducing the environmental effect from soil and water pollution. The processing routes for the production of biofuels may be composed of all of the options listed in Table 1.11. Current research investigates microalgae strains that can grow at very fast rates and can produce the largest concentration of lipids. It is expected that the biodiesel production rates per acre from microalgae have far greater potential than terrestrial crops.

1.6.4 Fourth Generation of Biofuels

The fourth generation of biofuels will integrate biofuel production with carbon sequestration potential, so that the overall life cycle of the carbon footprint is negative. This may be composed of lignicellulosic or high lipid content biofuels with integrated oxy-firing combustion, followed by carbon capture and storage or pyrolysis during which solid, carbon-rich biochar is produced and then stored in soils. Figure 1.6 shows an example of the fourth generation of biofuels with the carbon sequestration pathway. This figure shows a self-sustaining pyrolysis process during which biomass is converted to biogas, bio-oils and biochar. The biogas is combusted to produce heat to drive the pyrolysis process. The bio-oil is further upgraded to biodiesel and petrochemicals, whereas the biochar, rich in carbon and nutrients, is used for storage in soils, improving soil properties and sequestering carbon.

1.6.5 Beyond Fourth Generation Biofuels

The ultimate goal of the biofuel industry is to design an industry that is founded on the principles of industrial ecology and sustainability. This involves not just zero or negative carbon emissions but also developing a system in which the biofuel industry resolves a multitude of environmental problems. The system solution may involve, for instance, the cultivation of salt-resistant energy crops on saline soils. These crops will help reduce the need for water, which is the leading cause for the salinisation of the soils, and

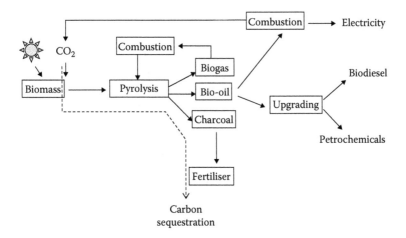

FIGURE 1.6
Fourth generation of biofuels based on pyrolysis of biomass and production of biofuels, while sequestering carbon.

thus, help gradually reduce soil salinity. Energy crops can then be harvested and processed through second-generation biofuel technologies with CO_2 capture or production of biochar, used as fertilisers to sequester the carbon and further improve the quality of the saline soils to their full rehabilitation. Another option may be to use algae for industrial wastewater decontamination and then process the algae in a technology that can enable metal and contaminant recovery whilst producing liquid biofuels.

References

Arias, B., Pevida, C., Fermoso, J., Plaza, M.G., Rubiera, F. and Pis, J.J. Influence of torrefaction on the grindability and reactivity of woody biomass. *Fuel Processing Technology* 89(2), 169–175, 2008.

Arif, M., Masdoon, T. and Shah, S.S. Evaluation of oil seeds for their potential nutrients. *ARPN Journal of Agricultural and Biological Science* 7(9), 730–734, 2012.

Baxter, L. Biomass-coal co-combustion: Opportunity for affordable renewable energy. *Fuel* 84, 1295–1302, 2005.

Becker, E.W. *Microalgae: Biotechnology and Microbiology*. Cambridge University Press, 1994.

Biomass Energy Centre. Sources of biomass, 2011. http://www.biomassenergycentre.org.uk/portal/page?_pageid=75,15174&_dad=portal&_schema=PORTAL (Accessed February 2013).

Caputo, A.C., Palumbo, M., Pelagagge, P.M. and Scacchia, F. Economics of biomass energy utilization in combustion and gasification plants: Effects of logistic variables. *Biomass and Bioenergy* 28, 35–51, 2005.

Clarke, S., and Preto, F. Biomass Densification for Energy Production, Factsheet, AGDEX 737/120, 2011.

Davis, B.G., and Fairbanks, A.J. *Carbohydrate Chemistry.* Oxford University Press, UK, 2002.

Demirbas, A. Combustion characteristics of different biomass fuels. *Progress in Energy and Combustion Science* 30(2), 219–230, 2004.

Duke, J.A. Handbook of Energy Crops, New Crop Resource Online Program, Purdue University, 1983.

Edwards, M. *Green Algae Strategy.* CreateSpace Independent Publishing Platform, 2008.

Euromonitor International, 2012. http://www.euromonitor.com (Accessed on December 10, 2012).

Fahy, E. et al. A comprehensive classification system for lipids. *Journal of Lipid Research* 46, 839–861, 2005.

Fletcher, S., O'Mara, K. and Rayner, M. *Biomass.* Australian Institute of Energy, Surrey Hills, 1999.

Food and Agricultural Policy Research Institute (FAPRI), 2011. http://www.fapri.iastate.edu/tools/outlook.aspx (Accessed on May 09, 2013).

Fowler, P., Krajačić, G., Lončar, D. and Duić, N. Modeling the energy potential of biomass—H2RES. *International Journal of Hydrogen Energy* 34(16), 7027–7040, 2009.

Gebruers, K., Dornez, E., Boros, D., Fraś, A., Dynkowska, W., Bedo, Z., Rakszegi, M., Delcour, J.A. and Courtin, C.M. Variation in the content of dietary fiber and components thereof in wheats in the HEALTHGRAIN Diversity Screen. *Journal of Agricultural and Food Chemistry* 56(21), 9740–9749, 2008.

Higuchi, T. Lignin biochemistry: Biosynthesis and biodegradation. *Wood Science and Technology* 24, 23–63, 1990.

Hoogwijk, M., Faaij, A., van den Broek, R., Berndes, G., Gielen, D. and Turkenburg, W. Exploration of the ranges of the global potential of biomass for energy. *Biomass and Bioenergy* 25(2), 119–133, 2003.

Huo, Y-X., Cho, K.M., Rivera, J.G.L., Monte, E., Shen, C.R., Yan, Y. and Liao, J.C. Conversion of proteins into biofuels by engineering nitrogen flux. *Nature Biotechnology* 29, 346–351, 2011.

International Energy Agency (IEA). Biomass Energy: Data, Analysis and Trends. IEA, Paris, 1998.

International Energy Agency (IEA). Biofuels and Waste, 2013. http://www.iea.org/stats/defs/sources/renew.asp.

Kenney, W.A., Sennerby-Forsse, L. and Layton, P. A review of biomass quality research relevant to the use of poplar and willow for energy conversion. *Biomass* 21, 163–188, 1990.

Khalaf, G., and Mohamed, A.-G. Effect of barley (*Hordeum vulgare*) on the liver of diabetic rats: Historical and biochemical study. *Egyptian Journal of Histology* 31(2), 245–255, 2008.

Kögel-Knabner, I. The macromolecular organic composition of plant and microbial residues as inputs to soil organic matter. *Soil Biology & Biochemistry* 34, 139–162, 2002.

Lee, D., Owens, V.N., Boe, A. and Jeranyama, P. Compostion of Herbaceous Biomass Feedstock. Report SGINC1-07, South Dakota State University, 2007.

Leung, D.Y.C., Yin, X.L. and Wu, C.Z. A review on the development and commercialization of biomass gasification technologies in China. *Renewable and Sustainable Energy Reviews* 8, 565–580, 2004.

Lewandowski, I. and Kicherer, A. Combustion quality of biomass: Practical relevance and experiments to modify the biomass quality of *Mischanthus x giganteus*. *European Journal of Agronomy* 6, 163–177, 1997.

Mani, S., Tabil, L.G. and Sokhansanj, S. Grinding performance and physical properties of wheat and barley straws, corn stover and switchgrass. *Biomass and Bioenergy* 27, 339–352, 2004.

Maniatis, K., and Millich, E. Energy from biomass and waste: The contribution of utility scale biomass gasification plants. *Biomass and Bioenergy* 15, 195–200, 1998.

McCrone, A., Usher, E., Sonntag-O'Brien, V., Moslener, U., Andreas, J.G. and Gruning, C. Global Trends in Renewable Energy Investment 2011: Analysis of Trends and Issues in the Financing of Renewable Energy. United Nations Environment Programme, 2011.

McKendry, P. Energy production from biomass (part 1): Overview of biomass. *Bioresource Technology* 83(1), 37–46, 2002.

O'Sullivan, A. Cellulose: The structure slowly unravels. *Cellulose* 4, 173–207, 1997.

Ophardt, C.E. Virtual Chembook, Elmhurst College, 2003. http://www.elmhurst.edu/~chm/vchembook/545polycarbo.html (Accessed May 2013).

Raveendran, K., Ganesh, A. and Khilar, K.C. Influence of mineral matter on biomass pyrolysis characteristics. *Fuel* 74, 1812–1822, 1995.

Rosillo-Calle, F., de Groot, P., Hemstock, S.L. and Woods, J. *Biomass Assessment Handbook—Bioenergy for a Sustainable Environment*. London, Earthscan, 2007.

Saha, B.C. Hemicellulose bioconversion. *Journal of Industrial Microbiology and Biotechnology* 30, 279–291, 2003.

Schädel, C. Cell-Wall Hemicelluloses as Mobile Carbon Stores in Plants. PhD Thesis, University of Basel, 2009.

Sjostrom, E. *Wood Chemistry. Fundamentals and Applications*. 2nd ed., San Diego: Academic Press, 292, 1993.

Van Gerpen, J. Biodiesel processing and production. *Fuel Processing Technology* 86, 1097–1107, 2005.

Vassilev, S.V., Baxter, D., Andersen, L.K. and Vassileva, C.G. An overview of the chemical composition of biomass. *Fuel* 89(5), 913–933, 2010.

Voet, D., Voet, J.G. and Pratt, C.W. *Fundamentals of Biochemistry*. John Wiley & Sons, 2006.

Wilén, C., Moilanen, A. and Kurkela, E. *Biomass Feedstock Analyses*. VTT Publications 282, Technical Research Centre of Finland, 1996.

2

Sustainability Considerations for Electricity Generation from Biomass

Annette Evans, Vladimir Strezov and Tim J. Evans

CONTENTS

2.1 Introduction

There are three primary technology categories used for the thermal-based conversion of biomass into electricity. Each category has undergone significant development, and therefore, many different methods are available.

Pyrolysis is the thermal destruction of biomass in an anaerobic environment, without the addition of steam or air, to produce gases and condensable vapours (Bain et al. 1998). Combustion of these gases occurs in a gas turbine, typically a combined-cycle gas turbine (Ganesh and Banerjee 2001).

In gasification, biomass is partly oxidised by controlling oxygen with the addition of steam to produce combustible gases that have a high calorific value (Bain et al. 1998). Product gases are fed into a combined-cycle gas turbine power plant (Department of Trade and Industry 1998).

Direct combustion is the complete oxidation of biomass in excess air to produce carbon dioxide and water. Hot flue gases are used to heat-process water to steam, which drives a turbine, typically via a Rankine cycle (Bain et al. 1998). Direct combustion is the oldest and simplest, but most inefficient, technology. Gasification and pyrolysis have higher efficiencies but require significantly more process control and investment.

2.2 Biomass Types

There are many biomass types available for the production of energy, as shown in Chapter 1. This discussion is limited to biomass residues and dedicated energy crops, as listed in Table 2.1. Residues are waste products after a higher value product has been obtained. In the case of bagasse, it is the sugarcane residue once sugar and molasses have been extracted. It can also be the tops and leaves of the sugarcane. Dedicated energy crops are grown exclusively for the purpose of energy production.

2.2.1 Residues

2.2.1.1 Bagasse

Bagasse electricity generation is a proven process, taking the waste products generated on-site and reusing them directly. Waste heat after power

TABLE 2.1

Biomass Types

Residues
Agricultural crop and process residues
Bagasse
Other
Forestry residues
Wood wastes
Dedicated Energy Crops
Food competitive
Short rotation croppice
Arid/unusable land
Mallee

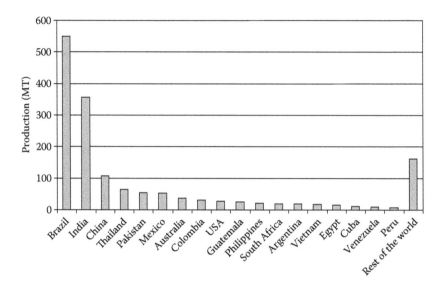

FIGURE 2.1
Sugarcane production by country, 2007. (From Food and Agriculture Organization of the United Nations (FAO). Food and Agricultural Commodities Production, 2009. Available at http://faostat.fao.org/site/339/default.aspx, accessed 1/9/2009.)

generation is typically applied to sugar refining. In this way, costs and transportation are minimal. The inherent linkage provides one of the most sustainable methods of electricity generation available. However, the seasonality of sugarcane harvesting may limit the applicability of bagasse as a stand-alone product. This limitation does not exist when used solely in conjunction with sugar production, because no electricity is required when sugarcane is unavailable.

Sugarcane is produced in more than 100 countries worldwide. The main sugar-producing countries are shown in Figure 2.1 (Food and Agriculture Organization of the United Nations [FAO] 2009). Brazil is by far the most dominant sugar-producing country, accounting for nearly 35% of the global production in 2007, followed by India at more than 22%. All other countries produce much less, but with many countries such as China, Thailand and Australia still producing considerable amounts. In 2005, more than 10^{15} tonnes of bagasse were consumed for power production (FAO 2009).

2.2.1.2 Forest and Non-Bagasse Agricultural Residues

There are many benefits of using residues for energy production, including redirecting a waste product from landfill that can be obtained at little or no cost. Available wastes include large amounts of leftover material such as stalks, prunings, skins, shells and off-cuts from rice, grain, cotton, vegetables and fruit that are not used as agricultural products. However, residues are a low-density and low-value fuel where transportation costs per unit of energy are high. Additionally, agricultural wastes have limited quantities, they are location-specific and are not always of the ideal quality for power generation (Thornley 2006).

2.2.2 Dedicated Energy Crops

For biomass to play a significant role in the world's energy future, dedicated energy crops are essential. Short-rotation energy crops are gaining popularity internationally. Typical crops include poplar, willow, eucalyptus and non-woody perennial grasses such as *Miscanthus*. Crop rotation periods are usually 3 to 10 years for woody crops such as willow and poplar (Goor et al. 2001). Important issues to be addressed in dedicated energy crops are the depletion of soil nutrients, organic matter and moisture-holding capacity.

Ideal biomass characteristics are high-yield, low-input energy, low-cost, a composition with the least amount of contaminants and low-nutrient, water, pesticide and fertiliser requirements. Essential biomass properties are moisture content, calorific value, percentage of fixed carbon and volatiles, ash/residue content, alkali metal content, cellulose to lignin ratio and bulk density (McKendry 2002).

Crops grown solely for their energy content should give good crop yields. Switchgrass and wood from short-rotation forestry, such as poplar and willow, are ideally suited as energy crops (Tampier et al. 2004). Crops such as wheat and corn require applications of fertiliser, take up prime agricultural land and give low crop yields, making them unsuitable energy crops.

One of the key concerns regarding bioenergy crops is the loss of biodiversity. This concern is due to monocultures being less stable than forests and requiring increased energy inputs, such as pesticides and fertilisers, to maintain productivity (Abbasi and Abbasi 2000). To mitigate this issue, patches/riparian corridors of natural vegetation should be maintained as well as native vegetation be re-established.

Biomass feedstock yields vary considerably according to climatic and soil conditions, and agriculture and silviculture practices. The competitiveness of biomass is essentially dependent on the development of short-rotation coppice and enhanced yields without great cost increases (McCarl et al. 2000). Heller et al. (2003) found that willow biomass crops are sustainable from an energy balance perspective and contribute environmental benefits.

The Clean Energy Council (CEC 2008a) found that, unless stationary energy prices and CO_2 taxes increase significantly, dedicated energy crops are unlikely to be economically viable. The CEC (2002) also state that dedicated energy crops only make sense in the medium term for combating salinity, land erosion and loss of biodiversity. Dedicated energy crops are less viable than crops with multiple economic benefits. Strezov et al. (2008) and Hoogwijk et al. (2009) believe that the production of energy crops on abandoned agricultural land and land at rest may allow for large amounts of biomass to be produced at a reasonable cost. Koh and Hoi (2003) claim that there is insufficient surplus agricultural land for dedicated energy crops to meet demand.

2.3 Sustainability Assessment

To conduct this assessment, several key sustainability indicators were identified: the price to produce electricity, efficiency of energy conversion, total carbon dioxide emissions, availability, limitations, water use and social issues. All indicators are assessed over the entire life cycle on a per kilowatt-hour basis.

Biomass conversion processes include thermal conversion technologies in which biomass energy is converted to electricity via combustion. Power production from methane emitted due to decomposing landfill and sewage are also considered biomass combustion-based electricity.

Significant amounts of biomass are used in co-combustion with coal, typically up to around 15% biomass. Overall, this is not a renewable process and the co-combustion with coal is excluded from discussion in this work.

The most common types of biomass used for electricity production and analysed in this work are agricultural residues, forest residues and dedicated energy crops. Other biomass sources include landfill gas and animal and human waste. However, as plant material is the most common form of biomass used for electricity generation, these other sources will not be discussed in this work.

The sustainability assessed here considers the entire life cycle, from biomass growth, collection and transportation to power production and waste disposal. Power plant lifetimes are assumed as 20 years.

2.3.1 Price

2.3.1.1 Total Cost of Electricity Production

Variability in feed materials and processing technologies results in large biomass price variations, as shown in Table 2.2 (Evans et al. 2010). The lowest values are seen for waste materials with little or no cost and minimal transportation requirements. Due to the low energy density (energy yield per hectare) of most biomass and the high costs of transport from the gathering site, any transportation significantly affects the resulting feedstock cost (Hamelinck et al. 2005). A high biomass density is therefore essential to profitability. Biomass quantities and costs vary with fluctuating harvests, increased utilisation by competitors and transportation (Junginger 2001).

TABLE 2.2

Cost for Biomass Power Production

Author/s	Year	c/kWh (US)	Technology	Size (MW)	Fuel
Ganesh and Banerjee	2001	3.8–10.2	Pyrolysis	5	Energy Crops
Bridgwater et al.	2002	9.4	Pyrolysis	20	Wood chip
Elliot	1993	7.8	Gasifier	25	Low cost plantation
Bridgwater	1995	6	Gasifier	60	Wood
Craig and Mann	1996	6.5–8.2	Gasifier	56–132	Wood
Faaij et al.	1997	−7.5–+9.6	Gasifier	30	Wastes and residues
Faaij et al.	1998	7.7	Gasifier	30	Willow
McKendry	2002	16.4	Gasifier	7.5	Energy Crops
Hamelinck et al.	2005	4.2	Gasifier	300	Wood
Gan and Smith	2006	5	Gasifier	10+	Poplar
Braunbeck et al.	1999	4.5–7.1	Combustion	Large	Bagasse
van den Broek et al.	2000	4.9	Combustion	23.4	Bagasse
van den Broek et al.	2001	9.1	Combustion	24	Wood
van den Broek et al.	2002	7.5	Combustion	13.5	Energy Crops
Fung et al.	2002	2.8–8.5	Combustion	10	Wood
Bain and Overend	2002	8–12	Combustion	20	Mixed
Gustavsson and Madlener	2003	4–6.5	Combustion	50–100	Logging residues
Gustavsson and Madlener	2003	3.9–6.9	Combustion	50–100	Logging residues
Kumar et al.	2003	6.3	Combustion	137	Forest harvest residues
Kumar et al.	2003	5	Combustion	450	Agricultural residues
Kumar et al.	2003	4.7	Combustion	450+	Whole forest harvesting
Bakos et al.	2008	12.7	Combustion	2+	Agricultural residues
Alonso-Pippo et al.	2008	6	Combustion	600	Bagasse
Blanco and Azqueta	2008	9.3–12.4	Combustion	25	Straw
Kumar et al.	2008	5.4–5.9	Combustion	240	Trees killed by pine beetle

Source: Evans, A. et al., *Renew Sust Energ Rev* 2010; 14: 1419–1427, 2010.

There is a wide debate on the cost-effectiveness and major influences on price. Bridgwater (1995) claims that the economics lie in low-cost waste or fiscal incentives regardless of scale, as opposed to Siewert et al. (2004), who state that 50 to 100 MW plants offer greater economy than smaller plants, without the need for financial support. According to Dornburg and Faaij

(2001), wood waste needs to be provided at zero cost to make profits from electricity generation possible. This agrees with the findings of Ganesh and Banerjee (2001), confirming that the largest influence on price is the fuel cost. This is in contrast with IEA Bioenergy (2002), which found that energy crops are typically low-value products and that profitability comes from low production costs.

The negative cost value given by Faaij et al. (1997) are for instances in which current waste disposal costs can serve as income for the facility. With prices ranging from –7.5 to 16.4 c/kWh and an average price of 6.9 c/kWh, biomass power production is not currently cost-effective where fossil fuel technologies are available for an average of 4.2 to 4.8 c/kWh. However, according to Sáez et al. (1998), when externalities, such as human health, soil erosion and others are included, the total price of biomass is cheaper than coal. Hatje and Ruhl (2000) state that biomass is the most profitable renewable energy source after hydropower, with respect to total energy and carbon-reduction costs. Compared with the median electricity costs of the remaining renewable electricity technologies shown by Evans et al. (2009), biomass is cheaper than photovoltaics (24 c/kWh), approximately equal with geothermal (6.8 c/kWh), but is more expensive than wind (6.6 c/kWh) and hydropower (5.1 c/kWh).

2.3.1.2 Investment Costs and Technology Choice

Investment costs for biomass to energy conversion exceed other thermal technologies by a factor of 3 to 4 due to higher processing volumes and increased handling requirements. The capital-intensive nature of biomass technology can deter investment. Also, financing biomass plant construction can be complicated because many conversion technologies are still in pilot scale (CEC 2008a).

When selecting between different technologies, combustion-based technologies are more profitable over their life cycle than gasification and pyrolysis, despite higher operating costs (Caputo et al. 2005). Capital costs for direct combustion are around \$1.9 to \$2.9/kW. For pyrolysis, costs are much higher at \$3.5 to \$4.5/kW, making it one of the most capital-intensive electricity generation technologies (Yoshida et al. 2003) comparable with nuclear.

2.3.1.3 Process versus Feedstock Price

Blanco and Azqueta (2008) found that the fuel cost comprised between 56% and 75% of the total price when using straw in Spain.

Gan and Smith (2006) found that the non-fuel costs of capital, maintenance and operation of biomass-fired electricity generation was nearly the same as the total electricity production cost of coal systems. They also found that the fuel accounted for approximately 50% of the total electricity cost for biomass gasification systems. Biomass procured from logging residues was more cost-effective than energy plantations.

Stucley et al. (2004) showed that fuel procurement costs can account for some 50% to 60% of the total bioelectricity production costs. The total delivered fuel cost is typically 25% for biomass production and 25% for transportation to the power plant, with harvesting accounting for the remaining 50% of the total delivered fuel cost. Accordingly, reductions in fuel costs will improve overall power supply prices.

McIlveen-Wright et al. (2001) found that dedicated forestry crop plants handling more than 500 dry tons per day could be economically viable. Plants handling more than 1000 dry tons per day would be competitive with coal if there is enough wood available. According to other authors, such as Koh and Hoi (2003), it is unlikely that there would be sufficient wood available to meet this target sustainably.

2.3.2 Efficiency

Efficiencies of energy conversion from biomass vary widely across different technologies. This is an area under intense development, with many new, highly efficient technologies emerging. Table 2.3 (Evans et al. 2010) summarises efficiencies found in literature. Combined cycle gasification processes show the greatest efficiencies of up to 43% (Gustavsson and Madlener 2003). The average efficiency of all technologies is 27%. There are diminishing returns from efficiency improvements because small improvements at low efficiencies significantly affect profit margins, whereas at high efficiencies, large improvements are necessary for the same gain (Elliott 1993).

As process efficiencies improve, greater attention will need to be given to efficiencies of cultivation (if applicable), collection and transportation of fuels. Improvements in this area will allow for significant price improvements.

2.3.3 Greenhouse Gas Emissions

Power production from biomass is often said to be carbon neutral. In some instances, it is claimed that carbon sequestration to plant and soil, along with non-invasive farming methods, make biomass electricity carbon negative, that is, less carbon is emitted than is removed from the atmosphere overall (IEA Bioenergy 2002). Many authors assert carbon neutrality, with emissions from combustion balanced by the carbon capture of the next crop (Sáez et al. 1998; Matthews 2001; Lettens et al. 2003; Matthews and Robertson 2005; Vande Walle et al. 2007). There is inevitably some fossil fuel usage not balanced by this equation resulting from fertilisers, cultivation, collection and transportation. According to some authors, harvest methods that remove vegetation at or above soil level (i.e. leaving roots in the soil), leave sufficient carbon to balance all other emissions and maintain carbon neutrality (Sáez et al. 1998; Matthews 2001; Lettens et al. 2003). Mann and Spath (2000) claim net carbon negativity because the combustion of biomass avoids anaerobic decomposition that results in methane emissions.

TABLE 2.3

Efficiency of Energy Conversion from Biomass to Electricity

Author/s	Year	% Efficiency	Comment
Craig and Mann	1996	35.4–39.7	Gasifier
Gustavsson	1997	36	Combustion
Faaij et al.	1997	35.4–40.3	Gasifier
Bain et al.	1998	35	
Stahl and Neergaard	1998	32	Gasifier
Chum and Overend	2001	17.2	Gasifier
Berndes et al.	2001	20–25	Combustion
Ganesh and Banerjee	2001	26	Combustion
Ganesh and Banerjee	2001	40	Combustion
Ganesh and Banerjee	2001	28	Gasifier
Ganesh and Banerjee	2001	31	Pyrolysis
Bain and Overend	2002	20	
IEA Bioenergy	2002	25	5–10 MW
McKendry	2002	30	Gasifier
Gustavsson and Madlener	2003	30	Combustion
Gustavsson and Madlener	2003	43	Combustion
la Cour Jansen	2003	24	
Yoshida et al.	2003	19–26	Combustion
Yoshida et al.	2003	16–30	Gasifier
Benetto et al.	2004	22	
Corti and Lombardi	2004	35	Gasifier
Siewert et al.	2004	35	Foster Wheeler high efficiency small to lg, depends steam temp wood to electricity
Franco and Giannini	2005	15–30	
Ahrenfeldt et al.	2006	25	
WEC	2007	20	

Source: Evans, A. et al., *Renew Sust Energ Rev* 2010; 14: 1419–1427, 2010.

In most cases, authors find that electricity generation from biomass produces low net carbon emissions, mostly in the form of carbon dioxide, as shown in Table 2.4 (Faaij et al. 1998; Norton 1999; Gustavsson and Madlener 2003; Chatzimouratidis and Pilavachi 2007; Styles and Jones 2007). Other greenhouse gases, such as methane and nitrous oxide, are emitted in smaller amounts (2% or less of total emissions [Wihersaari 2005]). Where emissions include methane and nitrous oxide, figures are reported as carbon dioxide equivalent, or CO_2eq. The average carbon emission in Table 2.4 is 62.5 g CO_2/ kWh. The highest emission, 132 g CO_2eq/kWh (Styles and Jones 2007) is less than one-third of the lowest natural gas and one-fifth of the current lowest coal fired-power station emissions proven.

TABLE 2.4

Full Life Cycle Carbon Dioxide Emissions from Biomass Power Production

Year	Author/s	Year	gCO$_2$/kWh	Comment
1998	Faaij et al.	1998	24	
1999	Norton	1999	30–40	
2003	Gustavsson and Madlener	2003	48	Steam turbine
2003	Gustavsson and Madlener	2003	37	CC
2007	Chatzimouratidis and Pilavachi	2007	58 eq[a]	
2007	Styles and Jones	2007	131 eq	Miscanthus
2007	Styles and Jones	2007	132 eq	SRC willow

[a] eq denotes CO$_2$ equivalent in these values.

Wihersaari (2005) calculated the minimum greenhouse gas reduction when substituting biomass in the place of fossil fuels at 74%, up to a maximum of 98%.

The calculation of carbon emissions can be complex, particularly when land clearing and soil carbon balances are included. If not produced sustainably, biomass-generated electricity can actually emit more carbon dioxide per kilowatt-hour than fossil fuels (IEA Bioenergy 2002). Biomass effects are negative when native vegetation is removed for plantation. The establishment of such biomass crops is not renewable as its use as a fuel results in significant net carbon dioxide emissions (Balat 2006). For this reason, carbon emissions must include land clearing, deforestation and soil emissions (Edmonds et al. 2007). Changing land use patterns can also affect greenhouse gas emissions. Highest emissions are seen where grassland and broadleaved forests are converted to arable cropland (St Clair et al. 2008).

In dedicated energy crop cultivation, crops that grow with the least maintenance requirements, in particular, little or no fertiliser and highest energy densities, give the lowest emissions. This is of particular importance because nitrous oxide has a much higher global warming potential (GWP) of 298 compared with carbon dioxide, with a GWP of 1 or methane with a GWP of 25 (Forster et al. 2007). Also, an important consideration in dedicated energy crops is the optimisation of harvesting time. Van Belle (2006) showed that an increase in the diameter of wood residues being chipped from 4 to 16 cm reduced the carbon emissions per megawatt-hour by a factor of seven.

The consideration of carbon storage in soils is also essential. There are more than 1200 Gt of carbon stored in the world's soils, in comparison with the 550 Gt carbon stored above ground (mostly in trees; Edmonds et al. 2007). Modern farming methods rely on carbon sequestration to soil in their carbon balance and take measures to prevent the loss of this carbon, such as using no-dig cultivation.

TABLE 2.5

Emissions from Alternative Fuels, Sources and Technologies

Fuel	CO_2eq/kJ
UK electricity grid 1996	160
Straw combustion	63
SRC woodchip combustion	21
FR woodchip combustion	19
SRC woodchip pyrolysis	14
FR woodchip pyrolysis	12
SRC woodchip gasification	9
FR woodchip gasification	8

Source: Galbraith, D. et al., Review of greenhouse gas life cycle emissions, air pollution impacts and economics of biomass production and consumption in Scotland. SEERAD project FF/05/08 final report 2006.

According to Tampier et al. (2004), crop yield is the largest influence on greenhouse gas emissions. Higher crop yields give larger carbon savings due to the carbon in the crops. Transportation does not add greatly to carbon emissions. Process emissions, although significant, are easily balanced by the fossil fuel displacement through biomass use. Dornburg et al. (2007) also found that increased crop yields reduce greenhouse gas emissions. In their study using different crops, the most greenhouse gas–friendly crop was found to be hemp grown in the Netherlands.

Technology choice affects emissions, with pyrolysis and gasification showing significantly lower emissions than direct combustion, and gasification showing slightly lower emissions than pyrolysis (Galbraith et al. 2006). This is highlighted in Table 2.5 (Galbraith et al. 2006), which also shows the difference in emissions from alternative fuel sources. Straw combustion shows the highest emissions, whereas emissions from forest residues (FR) are always lower than emissions from dedicated short-rotation energy crops. Although emissions from straw combustion are much higher than for other biofuels, they are still less than 40% of the standard UK grid emissions for 1996.

2.3.4 Water Use

Horticulture has significant water requirements (Abbasi and Abbasi 2000); therefore, biomass will have a higher overall water use than coal. There is also significant water pollution from the use of pesticides and fertilisers (Abbasi and Abbasi 2000). Significant amounts of water are used during the cultivation, harvesting, transportation and processing of biomass. Berndes et al. (2001) gives a net water use on lignocellulosic bioenergy crops of 50 Mg/GJ of energy in the crops.

Because the technology for processing is essentially the same, cooling water for biomass-based power plant operation requirements is similar to coal-based power plants at 78 kg water/kWh of electricity (Bain et al. 1998).

2.3.5 Availability

The sustainability of biomass resources is dependent on the rate of regeneration versus the rate of consumption, including nonenergy demands.

The availability of feedstock is problematic for large-scale generation. Crops are cheaper when waste products are used; however, significant demands on wastes outstrip supply, increase prices and traditional waste streams then become primary products. Due to resource constraints, many biomass plants operate for limited periods whilst feedstock is available. This severely limits the possible penetration of biomass technology. For example, Matsumura et al. (2005) explored the possibility of using Japan's main agricultural waste, rice straw and residue, to produce electricity and found that supplies would only be sufficient to operate a plant for two months per year.

Where dedicated energy products are grown, they compete with agriculture for space. Global overpopulation and starvation rates make this competition highly undesirable.

Novel ideas for feedstocks are continually under development. For example, the Northern Territory government is helping to establish a pilot plant producing electricity from the environmentally damaging mimosa weed (*Mimosa pigra*). The perceived benefits of this project are the control and eventual eradication of mimosa as well as remote area access to electricity (Australian Government Department of the Environment 2009).

It has been estimated by the IEA Bioenergy (2002) that there is a global potential for electricity production from biomass as high as 200 EJ/year. Kaygusuz (2002) gave an estimated potential of 270 EJ on a sustainability basis, significantly higher than the sustainable potential of 100 EJ/year given by Parikka (2004). It must be noted that even the lowest of these values, 100 EJ/year, still represents 30% of the global total energy consumption for 2004. There is significant room for increased utilisation of this resource. The CEC (2008a) calculated the long-term potential of bagasse at 7800 GW/year.

It is the opinion of the CEC (2008a) that biomass in stationary energy will almost always be from recovered wastes/by-products of higher value processes. Supply will be subject to the long-term viability of the primary product. Australia has a long-term potential of 50 TWh/year from agricultural wastes and 5 TWh/year from wood-related wastes (CEC 2008a). The long-term potential from grain crop residues, primarily cotton and wheat, is 47 TWh/year (CEC 2008b).

Fertilisation effects are a function of harvest intensity and short rotation periods. Ash fertilisation may alleviate nutrient losses. Protecting organic layers in soil from disturbance and compaction helps to reduce runoff that causes stream and waterbody contamination by soil and silt (IEA Bioenergy

2002). Poplar short-rotation forestry with a 2-year cycle yielded 16 dry Mg/ha per year with CO_2 emissions of 7330 kg/ha per year, mostly from diesel-fuelled machines. Fertilisers produce ammonia, methane and nitrous oxides emissions and groundwater pollution by acids and nitrates (Rafaschieri et al. 1999). Toonen (2005) studied *Miscanthus* and received yields of more than 20 tons/ha with a net energy of 17 GJ/ton produced. They found a long harvest window and low input of fertilisers and pesticides.

2.3.6 Limitations

Biomass use is resource and land-constrained. The most productive crop land is agricultural pasture, otherwise used to produce food. In areas where soils are less ideal, crop yields are lower, sometimes to the point where the energy density is too low to be economical.

Crops must also be able to grow with minimal maintenance, including watering, fertiliser and pest and disease control. High maintenance requirements reduce the environmental benefits and increase carbon emissions and costs.

Abbasi and Abbasi (2000) found that forest products have a higher economic value per kilojoule in their original form than when converted to heat or gaseous energy. This is an important consideration because it will affect the sustainability of the process.

The highly variable nature of the biomass feedstocks causes complications. A product such as coal is carefully monitored and maintained at steady calorific and ash levels, allowing for steady process control and minimising fouling. Biomass does not allow the same control; even when using the same crops, significant variations can be seen. The combustion of biomass also causes high levels of boiler fouling and corrosion (Bridgwater 1995).

Junfeng and Runqing (2003) concluded that biomass supply by energy crop cultivation cannot match full biomass demand, even if all feasible lands were developed.

2.3.7 Land Use

Land used for biomass growth will often compete with food crops, forest and urbanisation; however, in some situations, biomass growth can be used to rehabilitate degraded or marginal soil. For example, the mallee plantations in Western Australia are successfully helping to resolve salinity problems where other plants could not survive. A pilot plant is developing ideal conditions to produce electricity from this tree (Wu et al. 2007; Yu et al. 2008). Where environmental benefits are shared between several areas, economics should improve with respect to electricity price allocation. In the instance of mallee eucalypts, the cost of environmental rehabilitation of the site should be accounted separately from the electricity cost. The San Antonio sugar mill established eucalyptus plantations on degraded soils and on soils in which the cultivation of common agricultural crops would be uneconomic (van den Broek et al. 2001).

Fthenakis and Kim (2009) compared the land occupation of different electricity-generating technologies and found that electricity production from willow has significantly the highest land transformation of any technology, at more than 12,500 m^2/GWh, whereas all other technologies were less than 4500 m^2/GWh.

The allocation of valuable agricultural land and the destruction of natural forestry for energy crops growth is unsustainable. These situations should always be avoided and other alternatives should be sought.

2.3.8 Social Effects

There is a wide range of social effects arising from the production of electricity from biomass. The extent of the effect will depend on the type of crop, how and why it was cultivated, the technology used to produce the electricity and how that electricity is distributed.

Food competition is ultimately the key social issue to be addressed. In many cases, energy crops compete with food crops for valuable agricultural land. To avoid this competition, energy crops need to be grown only on agricultural land that is not used for food crops.

Along with agricultural land, forests are an essential site for biomass crop growth. The removal of wood waste from forests can be partially compensated for by returning wood ash, which is rich in mineral nutrients and counteracts acidification; however, nitrogen and organic matter are lost and the effects of stump harvesting and loss of biodiversity are not balanced (Møller 2006). Møller (2006) also recommends that deadwood of a large size should be left as habitat for wildlife. The loss of habitat and biodiversity are key influences on the lack of public acceptance and support for the use of native forest residues, which are the main available biomass resource (Raison 2006). There is a general public perception that biomass power is not environmentally friendly (Thornley 2006). Even scientific authors, such as Miranda and Hale (2001), conclude that natural gas shows more favourable combined economic and environmental costs than biomass technology. IEA Bioenergy (2002) concluded that the increased productivity of short-rotation crops over forestry creates a smaller physical footprint, which is an important consideration.

Direct labour inputs for wood biomass are two to three times greater per unit energy compared with coal (Abbasi and Abbasi 2000). There is also an increased labour requirement for construction, operation and maintenance. The employment generated by the production of electricity from fuel oil is 15 person-years/MW year, compared with 32 person-years/MW year for biomass (van den Broek et al. 2000). More occupational injuries and illnesses are associated with biomass in agriculture and forestry than with underground coal mining or oil and gas extraction. Agriculture has 25% more injuries per man day than all other private industries (McCarl et al. 2000). If the safety of the agricultural sector could be improved, this would become a lucrative employment opportunity.

Taking waste wood from poor communities may remove self-sufficiency in areas where wood fuel is their only source of heating. Efforts must be made when establishing biomass sources to ensure that competing users are not disadvantaged by biomass removal.

Comparing biomass with fuel oil, emissions of CO_2 and SO_2 equivalents are, respectively, 67 and 18 times lower (van den Broek et al. 2000). With adequate flue gas cleaning and particulate removal, biomass power generation could be a much cleaner option than alternative fossil fuel technologies in terms of all pollutants.

References

Abbasi, S. A., and Abbasi, N. Likely adverse environmental impacts of renewable energy sources. *Appl Energ* 2000; 65: 121–144.

Ahrenfeldt, J., Henriksen, U., Jensen, T. K., Gobel, B., Wiese, L., Kather, A. et al. Validation of a continuous combined heat and power (CHP) operation of a two-stage biomass gasifier. *Energ Fuel* 2006; 20: 2672–2680.

Alonso-Pippo, W., Luengo, C. A., Koehlinger, J., Garzone, P. and Cornacchia, G. Sugarcane energy use: The Cuban case. *Energ Policy* 2008; 36: 2163–2181.

Australian Government Department of the Environment, World Heritage and the Arts Renewable Energy Commercialisation Programme 2009. http://www.environment.gov.au/settlements/renewable/recp/projects.html (accessed 14/7/2009).

Bain, R. L., Overend, R. P. and Craig, K. R. Biomass-fired power generation. *Fuel Process Technol* 1998; 54: 1–16.

Bain, R. L., and Overend, R. P. Biomass for heat and power. *Forest Prod J* 2002; 52: 12–19.

Bakos, G. C., Tsioliaridou, E. and Potolias, C. Technoeconomic assessment and strategic analysis of heat and power co-generation (CHP) from biomass in Greece. *Biomass Bioenerg* 2008; 32: 558–567.

Balat, M. Electricity from worldwide energy sources. *Energ Source Part B* 2006; 1: 395–412.

Benetto, E., Popovici, E.-C., Rousseaux, P. and Blondin, J. Life cycle assessment of fossil CO_2 emissions reduction scenarios in coal-biomass based electricity production. *Energ Convers Manage* 2004; 45: 3053–3074.

Berndes, G., Azar, C., Kåberger, T. and Abrahamson, D. The feasibility of large-scale lignocellulose-based bioenergy production. *Biomass Bioenerg* 2001; 20: 371–383.

Blanco, M. I., and Azqueta, D. Can the environmental benefits of biomass support agriculture? The case of cereals for electricity and bioethanol production in Northern Spain. *Energ Policy* 2008; 36: 357–366.

Braunbeck, O., Bauen, A., Rosillo-Calle, F. and Cortez, L. Prospects for green cane harvesting and cane residue use in Brazil. *Biomass Bioenerg* 1999; 17: 495–506.

Bridgwater, A. V. The technical and economic-feasibility of biomass gasification for power-generation. *Fuel* 1995; 74: 631–653.

Bridgwater, A. V., Toft, A. J., Brammer, J. G. A techno-economic comparison of power production by biomass fast pyrolysis with gasification and combustion. *Renew Sust Energ Rev* 2002; 6: 181–248.

Caputo, A. C., Palumbo, M., Pelagagge, P. M. and Scacchia, F. Economics of biomass energy utilization in combustion and gasification plants: Effects of logistic variables. *Biomass Bioenerg* 2005; 28: 35–51.

Chatzimouratidis, A. I., and Pilavachi, P. A. Objective and subjective evaluation of power plants and their non-radioactive emissions using the analytic hierarchy process. *Energ Policy* 2007; 35: 4027–4038.

Chum, H. L., and Overend, R. P. Biomass and renewable fuels. *Fuel Process Technol* 2001; 71: 187–195.

Clean Energy Council (CEC). Biomass Resource Appraisal, 2002.

Clean Energy Council (CEC). Australian Bioenergy Roadmap: Setting the direction for biomass in stationary energy to 2020 and beyond, 2008a.

Clean Energy Council (CEC). Biomass Resource Appraisal, 2008b.

Corti, A., and Lombardi, L. Biomass integrated gasification combined cycle with reduced CO_2 emissions: Performance analysis and life cycle assessment (LCA). *Energy* 2004; 29: 2109–2124.

Craig, K. R., and Mann, M. K. *Cost and Performance Analysis of Biomass-Based Integrated Gasification Combined-Cycle (BIGCC) Power Systems*. National Renewable Energy Laboratory, Golden, Colorado, 1996.

Department of Trade and Industry. Gasification of Solid and Liquid Fuels For Power Generation. Cleaner Coal Technology Programme. Department of Trade and Industry 1998.

Dornburg, V., and Faaij, A. P. C. Efficiency and economy of wood-fired biomass energy systems in relation to scale regarding heat and power generation using combustion and gasification technologies. *Biomass Bioenerg* 2001; 21: 91–108.

Dornburg, V., van Dam, J. and Faaij, A. Estimating GHG emission mitigation supply curves of large-scale biomass use on a country level. *Biomass Bioenerg* 2007; 31: 46–65.

Edmonds, J., Wise, M., Dooley, J., Kim, S., Smith, S., Runci, P. et al. *Global Energy Technology Strategy—Addressing Climate Change*. Battelle Memorial Institute 2007.

Elliott, P. Biomass-energy overview in the context of Brazilian biomass-power demonstration. *Bioresource Technol* 1993; 46: 13–22.

Evans, A., Strezov, V. and Evans, T. J. Assessment of sustainability indicators for renewable energy technologies. *Renew Sust Energ Rev* 2009; 13: 1082–1088.

Evans, A., Strezov, V. and Evans, T. J. Sustainability considerations for electricity generation from biomass. *Renew Sust Energ Rev* 2010; 14: 1419–1427.

Faaij, A., van Ree, R., Waldheim, L., Olsson, E., Oudhuis, A., van Wijk, A. et al. Gasification of biomass wastes and residues for electricity production. *Biomass Bioenerg* 1997; 12: 387–407.

Faaij, A., Meuleman, B., Turkenburg, W., van Wijk, A., Bauen, A., Rosillo-Calle, F. et al. Externalities of biomass based electricity production compared with power generation from coal in the Netherlands. *Biomass Bioenerg* 1998; 14: 125–147.

Food and Agriculture Organization of the United Nations, (FAO) 2009. Food and Agricultural commodities production http://faostat.fao.org/site/339/default. aspx (accessed 1/9/2009).

Forster, P., Ramaswamy, V., Artaxo, P., Berntsen, T., Betts, R., Fahey, D.W. et al. Changes in Atmospheric Constituents and in Radiative Forcing. In: Climate Change 2007: The Physical Science Basis. Contribution of Working Group I to the Fourth Assessment Report of the Intergovernmental Panel on Climate Change, IPCC 2007. Available from http://www.ipcc.ch/pdf/assessment-report/ar4/wg1/ar4-wg1-chapter2.pdf.

Franco, A., and Giannini, N. Perspectives for the use of biomass as fuel in combined cycle power plants. *Int J Therm Sci* 2005; 44: 163–177.

Fthenakis, V., and Kim, H. C. Land use and electricity generation: A life-cycle analysis. *Renew Sust Energ Rev* 2009; 13: 1465–1474.

Fung, P. Y. H., Kirschbaum, M. U. F., Raison, R. J. and Stucley, C. The potential for bioenergy production from Australian forests, its contribution to national greenhouse targets and recent developments in conversion processes. *Biomass Bioenerg* 2002; 22: 223–236.

Galbraith, D., Smith, P., Mortimer, N., Stewart, B., Hobson, M., McPherson, G. et al. Review of greenhouse gas life cycle emissions, air pollution impacts and economics of biomass production and consumption in Scotland. SEERAD project FF/05/08 final report 2006.

Gan, J. B., and Smith, C. T. A comparative analysis of woody biomass and coal for electricity generation under various CO_2 emission reductions and taxes. *Biomass Bioenerg* 2006; 30: 296–303.

Ganesh, A., and Banerjee, R. Biomass pyrolysis for power generation a potential technology. *Renew Energ* 2001; 22: 9–14.

Goor, F., Davydchuk, V. and Ledent, J. F. Assessment of the potential of willow SRC plants for energy production in areas contaminated by radionuclide deposits: Methodology and perspectives. *Biomass Bioenerg* 2001; 21: 225–235.

Gustavsson, L. Energy efficiency and competitiveness of biomass-based energy systems. *Energy* 1997; 22: 959–967.

Gustavsson, L., and Madlener, R. CO_2 mitigation costs of large-scale bioenergy technologies in competitive electricity markets. *Energy* 2003; 28: 1405–1425.

Hamelinck, C. N., Suurs, R. A. A. and Faaij, A. P. C. International bioenergy transport costs and energy balance. *Biomass Bioenerg* 2005; 29: 114–134.

Hatje, W., and Ruhl, M. Use of biomass for power- and heat-generation: Possibilities and limits. *Ecol Eng* 2000; 16: 41–49.

Heller, M. C., Keoleian, G. A. and Volk, T. A. Life cycle assessment of a willow bioenergy cropping system. *Biomass Bioenerg* 2003; 25: 147–165.

Hoogwijk, M., Faaij, A., de Vries, B. and Turkenburg, W. Exploration of regional and global cost-supply curves of biomass energy from short-rotation crops at abandoned cropland and rest land under four IPCC SRES land-use scenarios. *Biomass Bioenerg* 2009; 33: 26–43.

IEA Bioenergy. Sustainable Production of Woody Biomass for Energy, 2002, available from http://www.ieabioenergy.com/library/157_PositionPaper-SustainableProductionofWoodyBiomassforEnergy.pdf (accessed 1/11/2009).

IEA Bioenergy. Potential Contribution of Bioenergy to the World's Future Energy Demand, 2007.

Junfeng, L., and Runqing, H. Sustainable biomass production for energy in China. *Biomass Bioenerg* 2003; 25: 483–499.

Junginger, M., Faaij, A., van den Broek, R., Koopmans, A. and Hulscher, W. Fuel supply strategies for large-scale bio-energy projects in developing countries. Electricity generation from agricultural and forest residues in Northeastern Thailand. *Biomass Bioenergy* 2001; 21: 259–275.

Kaygusuz, K. Sustainable development of hydropower and biomass energy in Turkey. *Energy Convers Manage* 2002; 43: 1099–1120.

Koh, M. P., and Hoi, W. K. Sustainable biomass production for energy in Malaysia. *Biomass Bioenerg* 2003; 25: 517–529.

Kumar, A., Cameron, J. B. and Flynn, P. C. Biomass power cost and optimum plant size in western Canada. *Biomass Bioenerg* 2003; 24: 445–464.

Kumar, A., Flynn, P. and Sokhansanj, S. Biopower generation from mountain pine infested wood in Canada: An economical opportunity for greenhouse gas mitigation. *Renew Energ* 2008; 33: 1354–1363.

la Cour Jansen, J. Toxicity of wastewater generated from gasification of woodchips 2003. Lunds Tekniska Hogskola, Lunds Universitet 2003.

Lettens, S., Muys, B., Ceulemans, R., Moons, E., Garcia, J. and Coppin, P. Energy budget and greenhouse gas balance evaluation of sustainable coppice systems for electricity production. *Biomass Bioenerg* 2003; 24: 179–197.

Mann, M. K., and Spath, P. A summary of life cycle assessment studies conducted on biomass, coal, and natural gas systems Milestone Report for the U.S. Department of Energy's Biomass Power Program Systems Analysis Task Milestone Type C (Control). Golden, Colorado, National Renewable Energy Laboratory 2000.

Matsumura, Y., Minowa, T. and Yamamoto, H. Amount, availability, and potential use of rice straw (agricultural residue) biomass as an energy resource in Japan. *Biomass Bioenerg* 2005; 29: 347–354.

Matthews, R. W. Modelling of energy and carbon budgets of wood fuel coppice systems. *Biomass Bioenerg* 2001; 21: 1–19.

Matthews, R., and Robertson, K. Answers to ten frequently asked questions about bioenergy, carbon sinks and their role in global climate change. Greenhouse Gas Balances of Biomass and Bioenergy Systems, IEA Bioenergy Task 38 2005.

McCarl, B. A., Adams, D. M., Alig, R. J. and Chmelik, J. T. Competitiveness of biomass-fueled electrical power plants. *Ann Oper Res* 2000; 94: 37–55.

McIlveen-Wright, D. R., Williams, B. C. and McMullan, J. T. A re-appraisal of wood-fired combustion. *Bioresource Technol* 2001; 76: 183–190.

McKendry, P. Energy production from biomass (part 1): Overview of biomass. *Bioresource Technol* 2002; 83: 37–46.

Miranda, M. L., and Hale, B. Protecting the forest from the trees: The social costs of energy production in Sweden. *Energy* 2001; 26: 869–889.

Møller, I. S. Criteria and indicators for sustainable production of forest biomass for energy. IEA Bioenergy EXCO58 Meeting 2006.

Norton, B. Renewable electricity—what is the true cost? *Power Eng J* 1999; 13: 6–12.

Parikka, M. Global biomass fuel resources. *Biomass Bioenerg* 2004; 27: 613–620.

Rafaschieri, A., Rapaccini, M. and Manfrida, G. Life cycle assessment of electricity production from poplar energy crops compared with conventional fossil fuels. *Energy Convers Manage* 1999; 40: 1477–1493.

Raison, R. J. Opportunities and impediments to the expansion of forest bioenergy in Australia. *Biomass Bioenerg* 2006; 30: 1021–1024.

Sáez, R. M., Linares, P. and Leal, J. Assessment of the externalities of biomass energy, and a comparison of its full costs with coal. *Biomass Bioenerg* 1998; 14: 469–478.

Siewert, A., Niemelä, K. and Vilokki, H. Initial Operating Experience of Three New High-Efficiency Biomass Plants in Germany. PowerGen Europe Conference 2004 Barcelona, Spain 2004.

Stahl, K., and Neergaard, M. IGCC power plant for biomass utilisation, Värnamo, Sweden. *Biomass Bioenerg* 1998; 15: 205–211.

St Clair, S., Hillier, J. and Smith, P. Estimating the pre-harvest greenhouse gas costs of energy crop production. *Biomass Bioenerg* 2008; 32: 442–452.

Strezov, V., Evans, T. and Hayman, C. Thermal conversion of elephant grass (pennisetum purpureum schum) to biogas, bio-oil and charcoal. *Bioresource Technol* 2008; 99: 8394–8399.

Stucley, C. R., Schuck, S. M., Sims, R. E. H., Larsen, P. L., Turvey, N. D. and Marino, B. E. Biomass energy production in Australia: Status, costs and opportunities for major technologies 2004. Rural Industries Research and Development Corporation, RIRDC 2004.

Styles, D., and Jones, M. B. Energy crops in Ireland: Quantifying the potential lifecycle greenhouse gas reductions of energy-crop electricity. *Biomass Bioenerg* 2007; 31: 759–772.

Tampier, M., Smith, D., Bibeau, E. and Beauchemin, P. A. Identifying Environmentally Preferable Uses for Biomass Resources, Stage 2 Report: Life-Cycle GHG Emission Reduction Benefits of Selected Feedstock-to-Product Threads. Envirochem Services Inc. Prepared for Natural Resources Canada and National Research Council Canada, North Vancouver, British Columbia, Canada, July 19, 2004.

Thornley, P. Increasing biomass based power generation in the UK. *Energy Policy* 2006; 34: 2087–2099.

Toonen, M. Challenges and Opportunities for Ecological and Economical Use of Biomass Crops 2005. Powerpoint presentation available from www. rrbconference.com/bestanden/downloads/120.pdf (accessed 1/11/2009).

Van Belle, J.-F. A model to estimate fossil CO_2 emissions during the harvesting of forest residues for energy—With an application on the case of chipping. *Biomass Bioenerg* 2006; 30: 1067–1075.

van den Broek, R., van den Burg, T., van Wijk, A. and Turkenburg, W. Electricity generation from eucalyptus and bagasse by sugar mills in Nicaragua: A comparison with fuel oil electricity generation on the basis of costs, macro-economic impacts and environmental emissions. *Biomass Bioenerg* 2000; 19: 311–335.

van den Broek, R., van Wijk, A. and Turkenburg, W. Electricity from energy crops in different settings—A country comparison between Nicaragua, Ireland and the Netherlands. *Biomass Bioenerg* 2002; 22: 79–98.

van den Broek, R., Vleeshouwers, L., Hoogwijk, M., van Wijk, A. and Turkenburg, W. The energy crop growth model SILVA: Description and application to eucalyptus plantations in Nicaragua. *Biomass Bioenerg* 2001; 21: 335–349.

Vande Walle, I., Van Camp, N., Van de Casteele, L., Verheyen, K. and Lemeur, R. Short-rotation forestry of birch, maple, poplar and willow in Flanders (Belgium) II. Energy production and CO_2 emission reduction potential. *Biomass Bioenerg* 2007; 31: 276–283.

Wihersaari, M. Greenhouse gas emissions from final harvest fuel chip production in Finland. *Biomass Bioenerg* 2005; 28: 435–443.

World Energy Council (WEC). 2007 Survey of Energy Resources, London, 2007.

Wu, H., Fu, Q., Giles, R. and Bartle, J. Production of mallee biomass in Western Australia: Energy balance analysis. *Energ Fuel* 2007; 22: 190–198.

Yoshida, Y., Dowaki, K., Matsumura, Y., Matsuhashi, R., Li, D., Ishitani, H. et al. Comprehensive comparison of efficiency and CO_2 emissions between biomass energy conversion technologies—Position of supercritical water gasification in biomass technologies. *Biomass Bioenerg* 2003; 25: 257–272.

Yu, Y., Bartle, J. and Wu, H. Production of mallee biomass in Western Australia: Life cycle greenhouse gas emissions. Chemeca 2008: Towards a Sustainable Australiasia. Engineers. Australia 2008: 1260–1272.

3

Combustion of Biomass

Tao Kan and Vladimir Strezov

CONTENTS

3.1 Introduction

Amongst the thermochemical conversion technologies of biomass fuels, combustion is the only proven technology for heat and power production available for installations in the range of a few kilowatts to more than 100 MW due to its high-level technical maturity, considerable heat production efficiency and essential economic feasibility (Nussbaumer 2003). For example, the energy output/input ratios for corn combustion can reach 6.5 to 7.7, which is superior to the value for making ethanol from corn (Duxbury 2006).

As a direct, mature and widely applied technology for converting biomass into energy, biomass combustion can be broadly defined as the burning of any biogenic substance (excluding fossil fuels and fossil fuel–derived products; see Fine 2002). Biomass combustion is a complex process involving a series of consecutive exothermic chemical reactions between a biomass fuel and an oxidant. During the combustion, energy is released in the form of heat as well as visible light radiation in the form of glows or flames.

Since humans first learned how to make fire a quarter of a million years ago or more, the combustion of fuels, especially the combustion of biomass, has served as a necessity for driving the modernisation of the human society (Jenkins et al. 2011). Thus far, direct combustion of biomass for large-scale applications has reached the stage of commercialisation in many European countries and the United States, and the co-firing of biomass with coal is in the process of commercial proliferation. Current research in biomass combustion science deals with further optimisation of furnace design, more accurate control of the combustion process, increase in the overall biomass-to-energy conversion efficiency, extension of raw material types and the vital minimisation of economic cost. Refractory hazardous emissions from biomass combustion is another important issue that needs to be addressed for sustainable development. The deleterious emissions include toxic gases (such as CO and NO_x), particulate materials (PM) and significant amount of persistent organic pollutants (POPs) including polycyclic aromatic hydrocarbons (PAH), volatile organic compounds (VOC) and others (Demirbas 2008).

In this chapter, the fundamentals of biomass combustion involving different stages of the combustion process and indexes for combustion evaluation are first introduced. Various types of combustion technologies, including multitudinous types of biomass combustors with different power capacities, are then classified. A description of the widespread technology of co-combustion of biomass with coal is also presented. The pollutant emissions from biomass combustion as well as the corresponding eliminating measures are discussed here. The final section elaborates the current status of biomass combustion activities.

3.2 Fundamentals of Biomass Combustion

The fundamentals of biomass combustion involve the general mechanisms of combustion, process evaluation indexes for combustion performance and factors affecting combustion.

3.2.1 Combustion Process

3.2.1.1 General Mechanism of Biomass Combustion

Taking into consideration the commonly existing major constituents C, H, O, N and S and the trace elements N, P, K, Cl, Si, Ca and others, the general reaction of biomass combustion in ambient air can be described with the following equation:

$$C_aH_bO_cN_dS_eCl_fSi_gP_hM1_iM2_jM3_k...yH_2O + air\ (O_2 + 3.76N_2)$$

$\rightarrow$ intermediates (char, tars, gases like CO, H_2, CO_2 and C_mH_n, etc.)

$\rightarrow CO_2 + CO + CH_4 + C + H_2O + O_2 + N_2 + NO_2 + NO + N_2O + NH_3 + SO_2 +$
$HCl + K_2SO_4 + KCl + PAHs +...$

where M1, M2, M3… = K, Na, Ca, Mg, Zn, Fe, Al, Ti, Cr, etc.

The overall biomass combustion process mainly involves four basic stages, that is, drying, devolatilisation, combustion of volatiles and combustion of char (Nussbaumer 2003).

3.2.1.1.1 Drying

The freshly harvested biomass may contain high moisture content, which varies from biomass to biomass (typically 50% for green wood, for example). The moisture level in the biomass can still vary at levels of 10% to 20% even after elaborate drying and torrefaction (thermal upgrading of biomass by heating to 200°C–300°C). Moisture content is a limiting factor and if it exceeds 65%, heat liberated by combustion is not sufficient to satisfy evaporation and the autothermal combustion (Jenkins et al. 1998).

During drying, the free water evaporates first, which is followed by the bound water. It is believed that the drying process is limited by the heat transfer inside the particle (Yang et al. 2008). Specifically, the length of the drying phase is greatly influenced by biomass properties such as moisture content, size and density. The evaporation of moisture from biomass takes away large amounts of energy and effectively keeps the biomass fuel at a low temperature. This cooling phenomenon disables the ignition of biomass before sufficient extraction of water. At the same time, morphological and macromolecular structures of the biomass material undergo distinct transformation (Koppmann et al. 2005).

3.2.1.1.2 Devolatilisation

After most moisture in biomass evaporates, biomass proceeds to the devolatilisation stage. At the early stage, typically, the volatile loss is approximately 75% (Jenkins et al. 1998). Dry biomass thermally decomposes into volatiles (including tars and volatile gases) and solid char, as shown with the following expression:

$$\text{Dry biomass} \rightarrow \text{tars} + \text{volatile gases} + \text{solid char}$$

When the temperature reaches 220°C, the polymer structures begins to fracture. At the temperature range of 250°C to 500°C, methane, oxygenated compounds such as aldehydes, methanol and furanes as well as aromatics (e.g. benzenes and phenols) are released (Koppmann et al. 2005) The composition of volatiles greatly depends on the fuel properties, pyrolysis temperature and its increasing rate. Product distribution of biomass pyrolysis has been a subject of intensive investigations in the past, and numerous computational models have also been proposed via the network pyrolysis programmes, FG-Biomass, CPD and FlashChain (Williams et al. 2012).

Devolatilisation is a vital process that determines the flame position and flame temperature. The flame temperature then determines the rate of char combustion as well as the formation of NO_x pollutants (Williams et al. 2013).

3.2.1.1.3 *Combustion of Volatiles*

Emitted volatiles, including tars and volatile gases, are ignited and combusted, producing flames and releasing heat and light. It may appear as either a laminar premixed flame or a laminar diffusion flame, or a mixture of the two (Stott 2000). This violent oxidation generates considerable energy, which contributes to the initial phases of drying and devolatilisation, and then the sustainability of the combustion process. Various products are formed during combustion:

$$\text{Tars} + \text{volatile gases} + \text{air} \rightarrow CO + CO_2 + H_2O + \text{soot} + \text{PAHs} + \text{other pollutants}$$

When volatiles are ignited, the particle temperature will increase to a much higher value, which in turn boosts the rates of devolatilisation and char combustion (Yang et al. 2008). The emitted volatiles, mostly oxy-compounds, react with air quickly. The oxidation reaction is highly exothermic and its rate can be expressed as a function of several parameters such as temperature, pressure and concentrations of volatiles and oxygen (Yang et al. 2008).

3.2.1.1.4 *Combustion of Char*

Upon devolatilisation, char is formed, which then reacts with oxygen in the air with the following char combustion reaction:

$$\text{Char} + \text{air} \rightarrow CO + CO_2 + \text{other pollutants}$$

Combustion of char takes place at the same time as the combustion of volatiles, appearing in the form of glowing combustion behind the flaming front

(Sullivan and Ball 2012). During the process of char oxidation, oxygen molecules pass through the flaming front and are then rapidly absorbed on the reactive sites on the char surface to proceed with char oxidation. Compared with the combustion of volatiles, the combustion of char is more exothermic, with a lower activation energy and much slower reaction speed (Branca and Di Blasi 2004). The trace element potassium plays a significant catalytic role in the process of char combustion. As the reaction proceeds, the reactivity of char decreases due to the evaporation of potassium at high temperature.

The distinct separation amongst the thermal stages of drying, devolatilisation and volatile and char combustion zones have been successfully separated with thermogravimetric studies of combustion of small biomass particles (Skreiberg 1997). Nevertheless, during the firing of large particles in practical applications, the above zones overlap to some extent as the consecutive reactions take place simultaneously at different points in the combustor (Nussbaumer 2003).

The biomass combustion process can be also divided into three principal phases of ignition, flaming and smoldering, according to the apparent changes in the combustion phenomenon. The ignition phase mainly involves drying. Sufficient heat provision is essential for releasing flammable hydrocarbon gases before the flash point or fire point is achieved to start the ignition (Stott 2000). In the flaming phase, volatiles, including tars and gases, are released from thermally decomposing biomass and subsequently mixed with air and oxidised, taking the shape of flames. Supposing that ignition has taken place and there are no exoteric interferences, biomass will burn irreversibly at extremely high reaction rates under sufficient air supply. Radical reactions take place in the flames, and polyaromatics are formed. The smoldering phase features incomplete flameless combustion of char, producing mainly carbon monoxide rather than carbon dioxide (Koppmann et al. 2005).

3.2.2 Evaluation of Biomass Combustion System

3.2.2.1 Combustion Efficiency

To simplify the evaluation of biomass combustion performance, some metrics have been proposed. The most commonly applied one is combustion efficiency (CE), which is defined as the ratio of carbon released as CO_2 to total carbon amount emitted, as shown in the following equation (Demirbas 2008; Koppmann et al. 2005; Ward and Hardy 1991):

$$CE = \frac{[C]_{CO_2}}{[C]_{CO_2} + [C]_{CO} + [C]_{CH_4} + [C]_{NMHC} + [C]_{PC}} \times 100\%$$

where $[C]_{CO_2}$ is the amount of carbon dioxide released, $[C]_{CO}$ is the amount of carbon monoxide released, $[C]_{CH_4}$ is the amount of methane released,

$[C]_{NMHC}$ is the amount of nonmethane hydrocarbons released, and $[C]_{PC}$ is the amount of the particulate carbon released.

CE is an evident indicator for assessing the completeness of the combustion process. Compared with complete combustion, an incomplete combustion results in higher emission levels of PM, polyaromatic hydrocarbons, CO and other hazardous products.

3.2.2.2 Furnace Efficiency

In some cases, the efficiency of the combustion process (also known as *furnace efficiency*) can also be calculated with the following equation in terms of the energy recovery rate (Quaak et al. 1999):

$$\eta_{comb} = \frac{\text{thermal energy available in flue gas}}{\text{chemical energy in supplied biomass}} \times 100\%$$

Calculated on the basis of lower heating value (LHV) of wet biomass fuels and flue gas, the value of η_{comb} typically ranges between 65% and 99%, depending on combustion stoichiometry and heat lost from the combustor. Furnace efficiency is determined by the extent to which the combustion system is insulated and designed (Quaak et al. 1999).

3.2.2.3 Boiler Efficiency

In most industrial applications of biomass combustion, heat exchangers are integrated into the furnaces for heating water or producing steam. The performance of these heat exchangers (also considered as boilers) plays an essential role in elevating the overall efficiency of combustion systems. Boiler efficiency is depicted by the following formula (Quaak et al. 1999):

$$\eta_{boil} = \frac{\text{thermal energy available in water or steam in the boiler}}{\text{thermal energy in flue gas from combustion}} \times 100\%$$

where the two thermal energies are simultaneously based on HHV or LHV.

3.2.2.4 Economic Cost and Pollutant Emissions

It is an essential target to achieve the product price with sufficient market competitiveness by minimising the economic cost and reducing the pollutant emissions to meet the increasingly stringent emission standards. The economic cost and pollutant emissions involve many parameters such as type of biomass fuels, type of combustors/combustion technologies, application scales, operational conditions and others. Besides, they also vary with and benefit from advancements in theoretical approach, control engineering and pollutant reduction technologies. The affecting factors, classification and reduction measures relating to pollutant emissions are discussed further in this chapter.

3.2.3 Factors Influencing Combustion Performance

The performance of biomass combustion is determined by a combination of various parameters such as fuel properties, fuel feeding control, combustion air distribution and amounts, operational conditions (temperature, pressure and fuel retention time) and furnace types and designs (Peterson and Haase 2009).

The types and characteristics of biomass fuel are key factors. Biomass can be catalogued into four main types based on the source including woody, herbaceous, agricultural residues and animal wastes. Biomass can be also classified according to the biochemical constituents, that is, lignin, cellulose and hemicellulose. For different biomass types, the flame temperature varies. For example, the maximum flame temperature for wood combustion falls in the range of 1300 to 1700 K, whereas for rice husk, it is within 1000 to 1300 K due to its lower energy value compared with wood fuels (Indian Institute of Science 2013).

An increase in particle size results in the delay of ignition of volatiles. Additional tars are cracked inside the biomass particle when increasing the particle size (Yang et al. 2008). Fuel size also has a major effect on the pollutant emissions due to the coupling between heat and mass transfers and chemical changes during the biomass conversion (Williams et al. 2012).

The detailed influences of moisture and ash contents on flame stability and flame temperature were researched by Sami et al. (2001). The increase in moisture or ash contents (or both) lowers the flame temperature. It was also found that for the combustion of sawdust, when the ash percentage is lower than 25%, the flame stability can still be ensured even when the moisture content reaches as high as 40% (Sami et al. 2001).

The elemental composition of biomass also has a significant effect on the biomass combustion behaviour. For example, K, Na and Cl elements reduce the melting temperature of ash, which thereby exacerbates the ash deposition, fouling and corrosion on the combustor's inner surface (Villeneuve et al. 2012).

Due to the complexity of biomass combustion, it is necessary to predict how and to what extent biomass properties affect the combustion process and to improve the process design and control (Jenkins et al. 1998; Sommersacher et al. 2012).

Environmental factors, such as the humidity of air and wind speed, also exert their effects on combustion. Amongst the operational parameters, excess air ratio (ER) is the principal parameter, which is defined as the ratio of air supplied to the stoichiometric amount of theoretically required air for the complete combustion of biomass into CO_2 and H_2O. An increase in the value of ER will lead to a decrease in the temperature of flue gas from combustion, which then lowers heat recovery from the gas. Practically, excessive air is introduced into the combustor to maximise combustion quality because the ideal mixing of biomass particles with air is hard to achieve. Generally, operations at low ER of less than 1.5 enable both high efficiency and high temperature, which benefits the complete burnout of the feedstock (Nussbaumer 2003). Given constant biomass fuel, combustion facility and operational conditions, an optimal ER value can be ascertained through tests. For example, the values for wood fuels typically drop in the range of 1.6 to 2.5 (Quaak et al. 1999).

3.3 Types of Combustion Technologies

The applications of biomass combustion range variously from traditional cooking to advanced combined heat and power (CHP) production. Currently, the annual consumption of biomass energy for traditional and modern applications are 33.5 and 16.6 EJ, respectively (Koppejan 2009). There are four major types of biomass materials that are utilised in large quantities and of industrial interest, that is, agricultural products (including harvesting residues, processing residues and animal wastes), forestry products (including harvesting residues, primary processing wastes and secondary processing wastes), domestic and municipal wastes (including domestic/industrial and urban green wastes) and energy crops (including wood, grasses and other crops; see Cremers 2009).

Usually, the preprocessing of biomass fuel is required before it is fed into the combustor. Physical processing methods such as drying and grinding are common first preprocessing steps of biomass preparation because water content and particle size of the material have significant effects on combustion performance. Additionally, some types of combustors have the requirement of keeping the water content and particle size of biomass fuel in respective designed ranges. Chemical preprocessing steps, such as leaching in water, diluted acid or alkaline solutions, are also extensively utilised to remove the metal constituents in biomass responsible for slagging inside the reactors and pipes. In addition, physicochemical pretreatments such as steam explosion or even thermal pyrolysis are gaining interest. Steam explosion of biomass can separate lignocellulosic materials into their three main components: lignin, cellulose and hemicellulose. This process utilises steam to process the biomass at elevated pressures for a few minutes and then suddenly decreasing the pressure (Agbor et al. 2011; Kumar et al. 2009).

A high variety of technologies and combustors are now available, amongst which the commercial scale combustors are mainly spin-offs from and analogous to the technologies utilised for coal combustion. On the basis of capacity, the biomass combustion systems can be grouped into small-scale systems (<200 KW_{th}), medium-scale systems (200 KW_{th}–20 MW_{th}), large-scale systems (>20 MW_{th}) and co-firing with coal in coal-fired power stations (some can reach hundreds of MW_{th} or even 1000 MW_{th}; see Miguez et al. 2012; Obernberger 2011; Williams et al. 2012).

3.3.1 Small-Scale Devices and Systems

Small-scale combustion devices and systems mainly refer to stoves and boilers with capacities of less than 200 kW. Small-scale combustion systems can be distinguished, thus describing wood stoves, fireplace inserts, heat-storing stoves, wood log boilers, wood pellet boilers and wood chip boilers, where wood chips, pellets and log wood are the primary fuel types (Obernberger 2011).

The most widely used small-scale stoves can be classified into several types by their structures. Some common types of stoves employed in India are summarised below (Bhaskar Dixit 2006). Sawdust stoves work with sawdust packed to approximately 250 kg/m³, and pulverised fuel (PF) stoves work on gasification mode for a part of the burn time and can obtain excellent flame quality. Gasifier stoves can accept wood pellets and chips using staged primary and secondary air. Ejector stoves with community cooking applications are at a power level of 25 kW or higher.

3.3.2 Medium-Scale and Large-Scale Industrial Systems

Medium and large-scale systems have found their applications in a variety of heat and power supplies that range from district heating to process heating and cooling as well as CHP production, applying various fuels such as wood chips, forest residues and straw.

3.3.2.1 System Structure

Commercial-scale systems are different from smaller residential systems in many aspects. For example, automated feed and control systems are incorporated to realise commercial applications. Besides, components for reduction of pollution emissions are required to guarantee that the levels of pollution emissions can meet the increasingly strict emission regulations.

A typical integrated biomass combustion system involves several distinct components. A simplified process scheme is depicted in Figure 3.1.

Biomass fuel is fed and then burned in a combustor to produce hot flue gas, which is either introduced into a heat exchanger to generate hot steam or directly used to supply heat. In the systems involving a boiler, the steam can

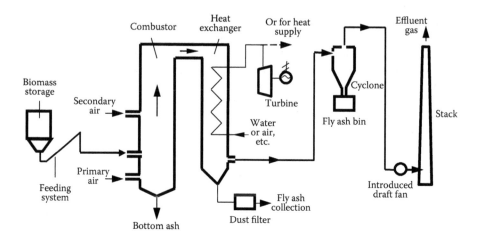

FIGURE 3.1
Basic components of an integrated boiler system for biomass combustion.

be either employed to supply heat for space heating or some industrial processes (such as food, paper and chemical industries), or used to produce electricity. In the boiler, water is evaporated into steam and superheated, which is subsequently fed into a steam turbine and expanded to a low temperature and pressure by using condensers. A generator is connected to produce electricity (Quaak et al. 1999). In power stations for pure electricity production, the heat from condensers is liberated into the environment and wasted. In CHP applications, this part of heat is recycled and applied for heating or in industrial applications (food, paper and chemical industries).

Although steam-driven turbines are utilised in most combustion systems for the purpose of power generation, hot, pressurised air or other organic mediums can be also applied to drive the turbine. In some of the cases, the organic Rankine cycle (ORC) is applied instead of conventional steam cycles, using special chemicals such as *n*-pentane or sobutane as the working fluid (Peterson and Haase 2009).

The biomass combustion process produces considerable ash in the combustor, in which the heavier ash material falls through the grate (there is no grate for some types of combustors) forming bottom ash. The bottom ash is then periodically removed manually or with the aid of special equipment. The light fly ash is entrained out of the combustor by the gas flow. Downstream devices, such as cyclone separators, packed bed filters, bag filters, electrostatic precipitators and scrubbers, are often employed to remove the particulates from the gas flow. Scrubbers or absorbents, including dolomite, can be used to control gaseous chemical pollutants such as SO_2 and H_2S.

The main energy loss from the boiler arises from the release of hot flue gas from the stack. The stack is a vertical pipe with a great height, which is the final passageway of flue gas prior to its discharge into the atmosphere. In the stack, the temperature of the flue gas is maintained at no lower than 120°C to hamper the condensation of the moisture in the flue gas (Quaak et al. 1999). Otherwise, the condensed water will absorb HCl, NO_x, SO_2, which may cause serious corrosion to the boiler and stack material.

3.3.2.2 Types of Combustors

As the core component in the combustion system, biomass combustors can be generally categorised into two main groups: direct combustors and gasifier combustors. In the less commonly used gasifier combustors, biomass fuel is first thermally decomposed in an inert atmosphere to form combustible gas, followed by the combustion of gas. Although better control of the biomass combustion and improvements in slagging and fouling can be obtained by applying this two-step process, the reactor is structurally complicated and costly (Ciolkosz 2010).

Based on the flow states inside the reactor, the commonly used biomass combustors can be divided into three basic types: stokers, fluidised beds and pulverised fuel (PF)/dust/suspension/entrained flow combustors (Nussbaumer 2003; Williams et al. 2012).

3.3.2.2.1 Stokers

Modern stoker systems are composed of four main components, including (i) biomass fuel feeding system, (ii) grate for supporting biomass fuel and its combustion, (iii) secondary air supply system and (iv) ash discharge system (EPA Combined Heat and Power Partnership 2013). In the stoker combustor, biomass fuel is fed to the grate in which biomass combusts with the primary air coming through the grate. Here, biomass drying, devolatilisation and char combustion occur simultaneously in consecutive stages, whereas the combustion of volatiles takes place in another region. Moderate secondary air is supplied to help burn out the volatiles and minimise pollutant emissions. Stokers primarily consist of two types, that is, overfeed type and underfeed type. Overfeed stokers can be further divided into horizontal feed type and gravity feed type, and overfeed stokers mainly cover mass feed type (including water-cooled vibrating grate and moving grate) and spreader type (EPA Combined Heat and Power Partnership 2013). Other specially designed stokers, such as cyclone-fired types, can be also found in the market.

For the overfeed type of stokers, biomass is introduced over the grate and air beneath the grate. Slagging can be suppressed by water-cooling the grate and walls. Biomass fuels with different biomass particle dimensions, high moisture and high ash contents can be accepted in this system. However, underfeed stokers are suitable for biomass fuels with small particles and low ash content. In underfeed stokers, the biomass fuel is fed from beneath the combustion chamber and then conveyed upward on a grate. Better control of biomass supply behaviours can be easily realised (IEA Bioenergy Task 32 2002). The schematic diagram of an underfeed stoker is shown in Figure 3.2.

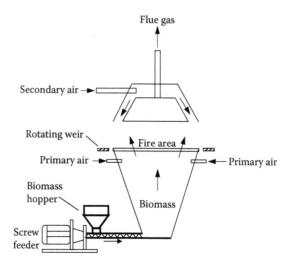

FIGURE 3.2
Schematic diagram of an underfeed stoker combustor. (From Purvis, M.R.I. et al., *Journal of the Institute of Energy* 73: 70–77, 2000.)

3.3.2.2.2 Fluidised Beds

In a fluidised bed combustor, a perforated gas distributor is installed in the lower part of the reactor and adequate bed material with good heat-conducting ability such as sand, limestone particles or other inert noncombustible materials, is filled onto the distributor. During the bed operation, the bed material is fluidised by the air that passes through the distributor. Biomass fuel is often introduced into the bed by screw feeders or other biomass transportation devices and subsequently contacts the hot bed material medium. Owing to this uniform contact between the feedstock and bed material, biomass fuel is heated instantaneously to reach its ignition point. Typically, the biomass fuel is combusted at a bed temperature of 700°C to 1000°C.

On the basis of fluidisation state inside the bed, fluidised bed combustors can be classified into two main types: bubbling fluidised beds (BFB) and circulating fluidised beds (CFB). In a BFB combustor (Figure 3.3), the bed material stays in the suspension condition in the bed. Compared with the BFB combustors, CFB combustors (Figure 3.4) are operated in a more turbulent fluidisation mode with higher air velocity. Bed material particles entrained out of the bed are then separated from the flue gas flow and circulated into the bed. Pressurised fluidised beds in which high-pressure streams can be generated may also be applied in some cases. Higher system efficiency can be achieved by pressurised fluidised beds; however, the propagation of this technology is restrained due to its high complexity and cost.

Compared with the stokers, more homogeneous temperature and concentration distributions as well as longer residence times can be obtained in fluidised bed combustors, enabling more efficient combustion of biomass with

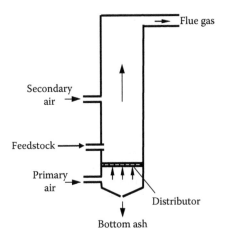

FIGURE 3.3
Schematic diagram of a BFB combustor.

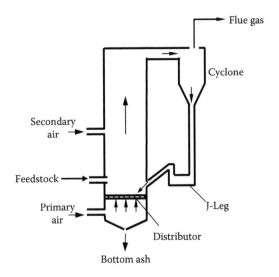

FIGURE 3.4
Schematic diagram of a CFB combustor.

lower excess air ratio and lower reaction temperature. Generally, stoker combustors will render 30% to 40% carbon in the ash as well as additional volatiles and carbon monoxide in the flue gas, whereas fluidised beds can obtain
nearly complete combustion of biomass (EPA Combined Heat and Power
Partnership 2013). Another advantage of fluidised bed combustors is that low
NO_x emissions can be obtained as a result of good mixing and low excess air
demand. Additives, such as limestone, can be added into the bed material

to capture sulphur in flue gas, enabling low SO_x emissions. Although fluidised bed systems attract great interest for large-scale applications, they are more expensive than the stokers with greater parasitic loads than stokers, which means that efficient dust precipitators and boiler cleaning systems are required (IEA Bioenergy Task 32 2002; Peterson and Haase 2009).

3.3.2.2.3 Pulverised Fuel (PF) Combustion

In PF combustion, biomass should be ground to a particle size of less than 6 mm and dried with typical moisture content of less than 15 wt% before combustion. As shown in the schematic diagram of a pulverised-fuel combustor (Figure 3.5), an auxiliary burner is necessary to start the consecutive combustion process before the temperature increases to a certain value and before feeding the fuel (IEA Bioenergy Task 32 2002). The fuel is then injected into the furnace with the primary air and is combusted in the flame whilst in a state of suspension inside the furnace. The addition of secondary air enables complete combustion of the fuel. PF combustion of biomass is

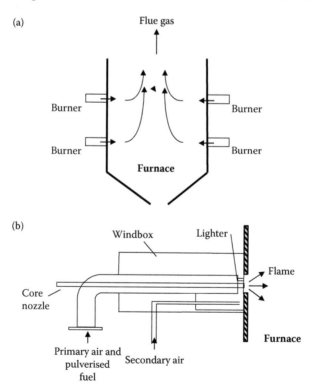

FIGURE 3.5
Schematic diagram of key parts of a typical pulverised fuel combustor: (a) overall view of the combustor and (b) auxiliary burner. (From Chaplin, R.A. Fossil fuel combustion systems. www.eolss.net/Sample-Chapters/C08/E3-10-02-03.pdf. Accessed April 2013.)

suitable for applications with capacities between 5 and 10 MW (Nussbaumer 2003), achieving boiler efficiencies of as high as 80%. However, a disadvantage is that strict drying and grinding processes are essential to ensure that the biomass meets the required standards.

3.3.3 Co-Firing of Biomass with Coal

Biomass co-firing with coal in traditional coal-fired boilers is gaining popularity for power or CHP production. A number of advantages can be obtained by biomass co-firing, including: (1) co-firing is often applied in existing coal-fired facilities, thus no or only few modifications are required; (2) lower SO_2 emissions can be achieved by biomass co-firing because biomass features lower sulphur content compared with coal; (3) compared with sole coal firing, biomass co-firing can contribute to the reduction of CO_2 emissions because biomass is considered to be a CO_2 neutral fuel; (4) compared with the dedicated biomass combustion, the utilisation efficiency of biomass can be increased when it is co-fired with coal (Mehmood 2011).

A wide range of combustor types, including pulverised coal combustors, stokers and fluidised beds, can be employed to perform co-firing. According to the biomass feeding mode, three basic co-firing technologies can be catalogued:

1. Direct co-firing, in which biomass is premixed with coal and then fed into the combustor along with coal
2. Parallel co-firing, in which biomass and coal are combusted in separate combustors and the steam streams produced from different combustors then converge
3. Indirect co-firing, in which the biomass fuel is first gasified separately and the produced gas is then combusted in the downstream coal boiler

3.3.4 Summary of Biomass Combustion Technologies/Combustors

The main biomass combustion technologies/combustors are summarised in Table 3.1. Numerous factors influence the efficiency of biomass combustion systems. Direct biomass combustion systems that generate electricity through steam turbines commonly possess a conversion efficiency ranging between 15% and 35% (usually 18%–20% for small size plants of ≤25 MW$_e$; see Peterson and Haase 2009; Valero and Biomass Group of CIRCE 2013). The efficiency of power generation in the co-firing systems (32%–36%) is generally higher than that for exclusively biomass combustion (Valero and Biomass Group of CIRCE 2013).

Some considerations should be taken into account when selecting a biomass combustor, which include available fuel types, energy capacity, compatibility

TABLE 3.1

Comparison of Various Biomass Combustion Technologies/Combustors

Biomass Combustion Technology	Combustor/Reactor Type	Capacity Range	Typical Fuel Type	Fuel Requirements Feed Size	Moisture Content
Direct combustion	Open fires, fireplaces, simple stoves, cookers for household heating and cooking	<10 KW$_{th}$	Wood logs, wood residues, straw	In large range	<20%
	Stoker: (I) Underfeed (i) horizontal feed, side-ash discharge type (ii) gravity-feed, rear-ash discharge type (II) Overfeed (i) mass feed: water-cooled vibrating grate, moving grate (including chain and travelling grates) (ii) spreader stoker	4–300 MW$_{th}$ (many in the 20–50 MW$_{th}$ range)	Sawdust, bark, chips, hog fuel, shavings, end cuts, sander dust	6–50 mm	10%–50%
	Other types: balanced draft, cyclone-fired, shaker hearth, cigar burner, and wall-fired				
	Fluidised bed: (I) BFB (II) CFB (III) Pressurised fluidised bed	Up to 500 MW$_{th}$ (many in 20–25 MW$_{th}$)	Wood residue, peat, wide variety of fuels	<50 mm	<60%
	PF combustor	5–10 MW$_{th}$	Sawdust, rice husk, bagasse	<6 mm	<15%
	Gasifier combustor	—	—	—	—
Co-firing	Pulverised coal combustor	Up to 1000 MW$_{th}$	Sawdust, bark, shavings, rice husk, bagasse	<6 mm	<20%
	Stoker and fluidised bed	Up to 300 MW$_{th}$	Sawdust, bark, shavings, hog fuel	<50 mm	10%–50%

Sources: Quaak, P. et al. Energy from biomass: A review of combustion and gasification technologies. *World Bank Technical Paper*, No. 422 Energy series, The World Bank, Washington, D.C., 1999; IEA Bioenergy Task 32. Biomass combustion and co-firing: An overview. 2002. http://www.ieabcc.nl. Accessed December 2012; Nussbaumer, T., *Energy & Fuels* 17: 1510–1521, 2003; Nussbaumer, T. Biomass combustion in Europe: Overview on technologies and regulations. New York State Energy Research and Development Authority, Albany, NY, USA, April 2008; Asthana, A.K. Biomass as Fuel in Small Boilers. Asian Productivity Organisation, Tokyo, Japan, 2009; EPA Combined Heat and Power Partnership. Biomass Conversion Technologies. http://www.epa.gov/chp/documents/biomass_chp_catalog_part5.pdf. Accessed January 2013.

with existing facilities, efficiency, parasitic loads, maintenance needs, availability of support and assistance, durability, safety and fuel compatibility (Ciolkosz 2010). For example, different fuel types and fuel requirements are required for different combustor types, as shown in Table 3.1. Except for biomass particle size and moisture content, the heating value of fuel may be another consideration. For example, BFB combustors are generally suitable for fuels with LHVs, whereas circulating fluidised bed combustors tend to be contrary (EPA Combined Heat and Power Partnership 2013).

3.4 Pollutant Emissions from Biomass Combustion

There are two main causes responsible for atmospheric pollution: (i) natural causes such as forest fires by lighting and volcanic eruptions; and (ii) human activities from stationary and mobile sources. Although pollutants caused by natural or deliberate forest fires are the major source of pollution from biomass combustion, the reduction of pollutants released from industrial installations for dedicated biomass combustion and co-firing are of great interest internationally. Emission regulations relating to biomass combustion are now becoming increasingly stricter and one of the limiting factors for the development of this technology.

3.4.1 Pollutant Types

Pollutants from biomass combustion, as a result of combustion process, can be distinguished into three main categories: (i) pollutants from incomplete combustion, including CO, NH_3, N_2O, VOCs, PAHs, PM, etc.; (ii) pollutants from complete combustion, including CO_2, NO_x (NO and NO_2) and SO_2; and (iii) other pollutants including hazardous metals (such as Cd and Hg).

Gaseous and particulate emissions from biomass combustion have different effects on the environment. CO_2, CH_4 and N_2O are the gases that contribute to the greenhouse effect. NO_x and SO_2 are partly responsible for the formation of acid precipitation. CO, CH_4 and N_2O are known as tropospheric ozone precursors through complex atmospheric reactions (Palacios-Orueta et al. 2005).

Air toxins released from biomass combustion include POPs, PAHs, dioxins (PCDDs), furans (PCDFs), VOCs, such as aliphatic hydrocarbons and benzene derivatives and aldehydes, as well as phenol and its derivatives (Demirbas 2008). PAHs can affect the respiratory system and skin. Dioxins, which can be formed in any combustion process in the presence of carbon, oxygen and chlorine are of great concern due to their carcinogenicity (Demirbas 2008). The turnover of VOCs will result in the formation of ozone and other photo-oxidants, which can cause damage to the regional environment and population health (Koppmann et al. 2005).

Emission of PM in the atmosphere is one of the most important indexes of ambient air quality. It can severely harm the respiratory system and cardiovascular system of the human body. PM emissions are generally defined as PM_{10} and $PM_{2.5}$, where PM_{10} represents inhalable coarse particulates with particle size of less than 10 μm (such as particles around motor roads and dusty plants) and $PM_{2.5}$ refers to fine particles with a diameter of smaller than 2.5 μm (such as those existing in smoke; see Villeneuve et al. 2012). In Europe, the maximum allowed values of PM_{10} (1 year mean) and $PM_{2.5}$ (1 year mean) are now 40 and 25 μg/m³, respectively. For large combustion plants that consume solid fuels with rated thermal input of 50 to 100 MW and more than 100 MW, PM emission limit values of 50 and 30 mg/Nm³, respectively, are recommended by the European parliament (Villeneuve et al. 2012). Furthermore, other heavy metal emissions such as cadmium and lead cannot be neglected.

3.4.2 Measures for Pollutant Reduction

There are a great number of factors that affect the formation rate and level of pollutant emissions such as the type and properties of fuels, combustion parameters and processes and reactor types.

Different types of fuel commonly feature diverse specific fuel properties. For example, native wood is believed to be both suitable for household heating and large facilities due to its low contents of ash and nitrogen, whereas herbaceous biomass (e.g. straw) is dedicated to larger plants owing to the high ash and nitrogen contents (Nussbaumer 2003). Fuel NO_x and SO_2 emission levels have a direct correlation to the nitrogen and sulphur contents of the biomass fuel fed into the combustor. Ash-related components, such as K, Cl, Na, Mg and P, are highly responsible for the emission of PM. In fact, K, Na and Cl can also decrease the melting point of ash, which aggravates ash fouling, slagging and corrosion on the combustor's surface (Villeneuve et al. 2012). The corresponding contents of metals in biomass fuels are the root factor for discharge of hazardous metals. High water content in fuels may lead to incomplete combustion, subsequently resulting in emissions of CO, VOCs, PAHs and other pollutants. Correspondingly, pretreatment of biomass fuels is often required to adjust the fuel's properties. For example, remarkable improvements in ash fusion temperature can be obtained by leaching the elements of alkali metals and chlorine from the fuel. Water content of the biomass feedstock can be reduced to an appropriate designed level by elaborative torrefaction.

Combustion parameters (such as air/fuel ratio, fuel feeding rate and pressure) and boiler configurations are also vital factors affecting the pollutant emissions. The concentrations of unburned pollutants, such as CO, VOCs and PAHs, can be reduced to levels close to zero by achieving high efficiency and complete combustion through good mixing of the biomass with the primary air and mixing of the produced combustible gases with the excess air. Accurate control of the staged combustion (including air staging and fuel staging) as well as optimum air/fuel ratio has been developed and often employed to get closer to the above objective. With respect to the NO_x reduction, some good primary (inside the combustor) and secondary approaches are available. Primary methods, such as air staging and fuel staging, can be based on the concept of nitrogen-related intermediates interacting in the reduction zone to form N_2 (such as $NO + NH_2 = N_2 + H_2O$) in the absence of O_2 (Nussbaumer 2003). Flue gas recirculation (FGR), an old technology used in oil and gas combustion, is another commonly used primary measure. In the FGR, flue gas from biomass combustion is recirculated to mix with the combustion air, which reduces NO_x production by lowering the temperature in the flame zone, reducing the availability of oxygen and increasing the residence time of the recirculated NO_x (Houshfar et al. 2012). Secondary measures, such as selective noncatalytic reduction (SNCR) and selective catalytic reduction (SCR), are also available for NO_x reduction on the basis of the same principles as air staging and fuel staging. Primary measures are preferable because they can be applied in existing boilers at low cost, without many modifications to the combustors, whereas the secondary measures generally cost more. Furthermore, combustor types also play a significant role in the aspect of pollutant emissions. Metal species and contents in deposit residue from different combustor types may remarkably differ (Jenkins et al. 1998). Stokers and fluidised beds commonly produce more heavy hydrocarbons than PF combustors.

3.5 Current Status of Biomass Combustion

Biomass combustion for heat and electricity production is a market-proven technology. Stoker boilers are standard facilities for heat and power production from coal as well as biomass. Biomass combustion technologies that integrate steam boilers can be traced back to one century ago. In the 1920s, stoker-fired boilers were first applied for coal combustion. The first travelling grate spreader stoker boiler for wood combustion was introduced in the late 1940s (EPA Combined Heat and Power Partnership 2013). The more recently developed fluidised bed boilers for biomass combustion are also commercially available throughout the world, especially from providers from Europe and the United States. Although fluidised bed boilers are the most recent boiler types for biomass combustion, with a short history, they have shown promising prospects in the reduction of some pollutant emissions such as NO_x and SO_2. Co-firing of biomass with coal, as a mature technology, has been extensively applied in terms of large-scale power stations for electricity or CHP production.

TABLE 3.2

Primary Energy Consumption and Turnover of Biomass Combustion Plants in EU in 2008 and Outlook for 2020

Year/Growth Rate	Approximate Primary Energy Consumption, PJ (Petajoule)/a	Approximate Turnover of Biomass Combustion Plants, Million €/a		
		Turnover of Small-Scale Plants	Turnover of Medium-Scale and Large-Scale Plants	Total Turnover
Year 2008	3800	3500	2800	6300
Year 2020	7700	9800	6700	16,500
Expected growth rate from 2008 to 2020	~100%	~180%	~140%	~160%

Source: Obernberger, I. Biomass combustion—Current status and future developments. 2011. http://www.bios-bioenergy.at/. Accessed December 2012.

The commercialisation of biomass combustion is also expected to be rapidly augmented around the world, especially in some zones or countries. Taking the European Union (EU), for example, the primary energy consumption and the turnover of biomass combustion plants are listed in Table 3.2.

An average annual growth rate of the turnover of biomass combustion plants at approximately 8% is expected from 2008 to 2020. The turnover of small-scale plants in EU for 2008 was slightly higher than for the medium-scale and large-scale plants. The gap between them may become larger in the near-term future.

Some efforts have been devoted to building and supplementing the databases relating to projects for biomass applications. The work known as 'IEA Task 32,' which was organised and performed by the International Energy Agency (IEA) with the participation of 14 country members, is a representative example. The objective of IEA Task 32 was 'to stimulate the expansion of the use of biomass combustion and co-firing for the production of heat and power to a wider scale,' which is to be achieved by 'generating and disseminating information on technical and nontechnical barriers and solutions' (IEA Bioenergy Task 32 2002).

3.5.1 Status of Direct Combustion of Biomass

In the European market, small-scale combustion facilities, including stoves and boilers, with capacities less than 200 kW are widespread. Elaborately designed combustors have been developed, amongst which fixed grate, moving grate and retort are the three main combustor types, with respective market occupancy rates of 79%, 14% and 5% (Miguez et al. 2012). Five types of fuels are mostly used, that is, wood pellets, wood logs, chips, chips blended with pellets and multifuels.

The distribution of manufacturers of small-scale biomass combustion facilities in different European countries is shown in Table 3.3. Germany, Austria, Italy, Denmark, Sweden and Switzerland are the dominant countries in the number of manufacturers. The distribution of boiler types differentiated by biomass fuel type in the European market is also listed (see Table 3.4).

In the United States, small-scale and medium-scale systems of biomass direct combustion are extensively employed and commercially available. Information about some of the system manufacturers in the United States are listed in Table 3.5, including manufacturer name and headquarter location, system type, system scale and biomass fuel type. As can be seen from Table 3.5, a wide range of system scales are available in the US market, and the fixed-bed boiler is the primary type used in small-scale and medium-scale biomass combustion systems (<20 MW$_{th}$).

Fluidised bed boilers or other boilers of special design are generally options when large-scale systems (>20 MW$_{th}$) are required. Foster Wheeler, CE-Lurgi, Gotaverken and B&W-Studsvik are the primary suppliers of CFB boilers for biomass. Fluidised bed (FB) combustion technology is becoming the increasingly dominant technology in the domain of large-scale applications in the global market. One of the reasons for this is that FB combustion technology enables the utilisation of a very broad range of biomass fuels. Additionally, compared with co-firing facilities, the typical size of dedicated direct biomass combustion plants is normally and obviously smaller. Apart from leading countries, such as Germany and the United States, other countries such as China, India, Brazil and Thailand are also developing their

TABLE 3.3

Number of Manufacturers of Small-Scale Combustion Facilities in European Countries

	Country Name						
	Germany	Austria	Italy	Denmark	Sweden	Switzerland	Rest of EU Countries
Number of manufacturers	75	41	18	15	10	6	21

Source: Miguez, J.L. et al., *Renewable & Sustainable Energy Reviews* 16: 3867–3875, 2012.

TABLE 3.4

Distribution of Boiler Types on Basis of Biomass Fuel Type in the European Market

Fuel Type	Pellet Only	Wood Log Only	Chips Only	Wood Log and Chips	Others
Percentage (%)	31	22	17	2	28

Source: Miguez, J.L. et al., *Renewable & Sustainable Energy Reviews* 16: 3867–3875, 2012.

TABLE 3.5

Information about Some of the System Manufacturers in the United States

Manufacturer Name	Headquarter Location	System Type	System Scale (MW_{th})[a]	Biomass Fuel Type
Bioheat USA (Fröling)	Lyme, NH	Fixed-bed boiler	0.02–0.06+	Pellets, wood chips
Heatmor	Warroad, MN	Small-scale furnace	0.08–2.5	Wood
Biomass Combustion Systems	Worcester, MA	Fixed-bed boiler	0.9–11.7	Wood
Hurst Boilers	South Coolidge, GA	Fixed-bed boiler	0.1–16.4	Wide range
Advanced Recycling Equipment	St. Marys, PA	Fixed-bed boiler	0.2–17.6	Wide range
McBurney	Norcross, GA	Medium to large industrial boiler of special design	5.9–23.4	Wide range
NRG Energy	Minneapolis, MN	BFB boiler	10–25	Wide range
Energy Products of Idaho	Coeur d'Alene, ID	Fluidised bed boiler	4.4–46.9	Wide range

Source: Peterson, D.; Haase, S. Market Assessment of Biomass Gasification and Combustion Technology for Small- and Medium-Scale Applications. Technical Report NREL/TP-7A2-46190, National Renewable Energy Laboratory, Cole Boulevard, Golden, CO, 2009.

[a] Calculated from the data provided by Peterson and Haase 2009.

technologies and experience in direct combustion of biomass, although their technologies now lag behind.

Development of domestic and community appliances for clean and efficient residential cooking and heating is a subject of discussion and debate, because these inefficient appliances will discharge considerable amounts of pollutants (Jenkins et al. 2011). They are being reformed with the purposes of boosting efficiency and reducing emissions of pollutants.

3.5.2 Status of Co-Firing

Co-firing was started in the 1980s in Europe and the United States (Mehmood 2011). At present, more than 245 industrial co-firing plants, which typically have capacities of more than 20 MW_{th}, are distributed around the world, mostly in Europe and in the United States. The global distribution of co-firing power plants is illustrated in Table 3.6. Finland, the United States and Germany lead the way over other countries in the number of co-firing

TABLE 3.6

Global Distribution of Co-Firing Power Plants

Region	Country	Number of Biomass Co-Firing Power Plants
Europe	Finland	78
	Germany	27
	United Kingdom	21
	Sweden	15
	Poland	10
	Denmark	9
	Italy	7
	Netherlands	6
	Austria	5
	Hungary	5
	Spain	2
	Belgium	3
	Norway	1
North America	United States	40
	Canada	7
Asia Pacific	Australia	8
	Indonesia	2
	Thailand	1

Sources: Al-Mansour, F., and Zuwala, J., *Biomass & Bioenergy* 34: 620–629, 2010; EPA Combined Heat and Power Partnership. Biomass Conversion Technologies. http://www.epa.gov/chp/documents/biomass_chp_catalog_part5.pdf. Accessed January 2013; European Biomass Industry Association (EUBIA). Experiences in Europe and List of Biomass Co-firing Plants, 2012. http://www.eubia.org/. Accessed December 2012; IEA Bioenergy Task 32, 2012. http://www.ieabcc.nl/database/co-firing.php. Accessed December 2012; Univerity of Applied Sciences (Germany). Decision support system (DSS) for the application of renewable energy (RE) from biogas and biomass combustion. *A Handbook within the Framework of the BiWaRE Project 'Biomass and Waste for Renewable Energy'*. June 2005.

power plants. All types of combustors have been employed in co-firing applications, and the major type is the PF type. The proportions of PF, CFB, BFB, stoker and others were 56%, 29%, 11%, 8% and 31%, respectively, in 2008 (Mehmood 2011).

Table 3.7 lists examples of biomass co-firing power stations in one developing countries. In 2009, approximately 20 grate and CFB boilers were commissioned or under construction in China, but only a few were operating co-firing units (Kärki 2009). In Thailand, several biomass combustion plants are under operation, some of which are listed in Table 3.7.

TABLE 3.7

Selected Biomass Co-Firing Plants in Thailand

Owner/Developer Name	Plant Location	Industry	Brief Description
Electricity Generating Public	Yala, South	Wood	21 MW co-firing plant
Chia Meng	Nakom Ratchasima, Northeast	Rice	2.5 MW co-firing plant
TRT Parawood	Surat Thani, South	Rubber wood	2.5 MW co-firing plant
The Southern Palm	Surat Thani, South	Palm oil	44 MW co-firing plant, postponed

Source: Univerity of Applied Sciences (Germany). Decision support system (DSS) for the application of renewable energy (RE) from biogas and biomass combustion. *A Handbook Within the Framework of the BiWaRE Project 'Biomass and Waste for Renewable Energy'.* June 2005.

The following gives three examples of some of the major installations of biomass co-firing power generation:

Alholmens Kraft Power Station, Finland (Kärki 2009)

The Alholmens Kraft Power Station (also known as Jakobstad Power Station), located in Pietarsaari, Finland and commissioned in 2001, is the world's largest biomass-fired power station, which produces electricity, district heating and process steam. Metso is the designer of the power station with Kværner (a Norway-based engineering and construction services company) as its boiler manufacturer. This power station uses the largest biomass-fired CFB boiler in the world with a capacity of 550 MW_{th} and employs 400 people. The boiler is operated at a temperature of 545°C and 16.5 MPa pressure. This power station normally applies 45% peat, 10% forest residues, 35% industrial wood and bark residues and 10% heavy fuel oil or coal as the mixture fuel. The boiler is designed to accept a variety of fuel types, in which blends of wood and coal ranging from 100% wood to 100% coal can be accepted.

Studstrup Power Station Unit 4, Denmark (Kärki 2009; Overgaard et al. 2004)

Based on 10 years of experience in biomass research and development, the 350 MW_e Studstrup Power Station Unit 4 was commissioned in 1985 and commenced its commercial operations in 2002. This power station is based on PF technology. Straw is used as the biomass fuel due to its high availability in Denmark. After the straw bales are milled, the pulverised straw is fed separately without premixing with coal, to ensure successful straw–coal co-firing. The straw is subsequently combusted in the boiler, which is a once-through single reheat type equipped with 24 low NO_x combustors in two levels arranged as opposed wall firing.

A maximum straw capacity of 20 tons/h can be achieved, which is calculated from a straw share of 10% on energy basis at full load.

Bay Front Station, United States (Wiltsee 2000)

Bay Front Station, located in Ashland, WI, is owned by Northern
States Power Company. This station has an output rate of 75 MW$_e$,
using coal, wood, shredded rubber and natural gas as raw feedstock.
Units 1 and 2, which generate 40 MW$_e$ of the 75 MW$_e$ nominal capacity, apply spreader stoker boilers. They were originally designed to
combust coal only. In 1979, after modification of the boilers, the fuel
for the spreader stoker boilers was transformed from coal only to
multiple blends of coal, wood and shredded rubber. Approximately
220,000 tons of wood wastes from mills, 30,000 tons of railroad ties
and 2000 tons of scrap tires were consumed annually.

3.5.3 Summary of Current Status of Technologies

Large-scale biomass combustion technologies are of great interest for industrial development due to their economic feasibility. The current status of
various biomass combustion technologies for large-scale applications is
summarised in Table 3.8. The three main technologies already available at
commercial scales include direct combustion in boilers, co-firing of coal and
biomass blends and biomass gasification, followed by co-firing of the producer gas and coal. However, the technology featured by separate biomass
combustors with an integrated steam cycle is still under demonstration.
Co-firing of bio-oils produced from biomass pyrolysis in coal boilers also
draws some attention and is currently at the stage of research and development or demonstration.

TABLE 3.8

Summary of Current Status of Biomass Combustion Technologies for Large-Scale
Applications

Technologies		Current Status
Direct combustion in boilers		Commercialisation
Direct combustion: separate biomass combustors with an integrated steam cycle	Fuels are burned in different combustors	Demonstration
	Only one steam turbine is integrated to separate biomass combustors	
Direct co-firing	Feedstock of mixture of coal and biomass	Commercialisation
	Separate biomass feeding	
Indirect co-firing	First gasify biomass and then co-fire gas	Commercialisation
	First pyrolyse biomass and then co-fire bio-oil	R&D, demonstration

Source: Kärki, J. Biomass utilisation in large scale heat and power production. VTT Technical
Research Centre of Finland, Beijing, September 2009.

Direct co-firing is gaining more attraction compared with indirect co-firing, mainly due to the relatively low investment costs of transforming existing coal power plants into co-firing plants. Despite, indirect co-firing allows very high co-firing ratios and separation of the biomass ash from the coal ash (Maciejewska et al. 2006), indirect co-firing method is currently not economically feasible.

References

Agbor, V. B.; Cicek, N.; Sparling, R.; Berlin, A.; Levin, D. B. (2011). Biomass pretreatment: Fundamentals toward application. *Biotechnology Advances* 29: 675–685.

Al-Mansour, F.; Zuwala, J. (2010). An evaluation of biomass co-firing in Europe. *Biomass & Bioenergy* 34: 620–629.

Asthana, A. K. (2009). Biomass as Fuel in Small Boilers. Asian Productivity Organisation, Tokyo, Japan.

Bhaskar Dixit, C. S. (2006). Biomass Combustion Devices. *International Training Programme*, Bangalore, India, March, 2006.

Branca, C.; Di Blasi, C. (2004). Parallel- and series-reaction mechanisms of wood and char combustion. *Thermal Science* 8: 51–63.

Chaplin, R. A. Fossil fuel combustion systems. www.eolss.net/Sample-Chapters/C08/E3-10-02-03.pdf. Accessed April 2013.

Ciolkosz, D. (2010). *Commercial-Scale Biomass Combustion Equipment*. Pennsylvania State University, Pennsylvania, USA.

Cremers, M. F. G. (2009). Technical status of biomass co-firing. *Deliverable 4 in IEA Bioenergy Task 32*, Arnhem, the Netherlands, August, 2009.

Demirbas, A. (2008). Hazardous emissions from combustion of biomass. *Energy Sources Part a-Recovery Utilisation and Environmental Effects* 30: 170–178.

Duxbury, J. M. (2006). Energy and Greenhouse Gas Budgets for Biomass Fuels. In D. W. Wolfe; V. Grubinger; B. Burtis (Ed.), *Climate Change and Agriculture: Promoting Practical and Profitable Responses*; Cornell University; NY.

EPA Combined Heat and Power Partnership. Biomass Conversion Technologies. http://www.epa.gov/chp/documents/biomass_chp_catalog_part5.pdf. Accessed January 2013.

European Biomass Industry Association (EUBIA). (2012). Experiences in Europe and List of Biomass Co-firing Plants. http://www.eubia.org/. Accessed December 2012.

Fine, P. M. (2002). The contribution of biomass combustion to ambient fine particle concentrations in the United States. PhD Thesis, California Institute of Technology, Pasadena, California.

Houshfar, E.; Khalil, R. A.; Lovas, T.; Skreiberg, O. (2012). Enhanced NO_x reduction by combined staged air and flue gas recirculation in biomass grate combustion. *Energy & Fuels* 26: 3003–3011.

IEA Bioenergy Task 32. (2002). Biomass combustion and co-firing: An overview. http://www.ieabcc.nl. Accessed December 2012.

IEA Bioenergy Task 32. (2012). http://www.ieabcc.nl/database/co-firing.php. Accessed December 2012.

Indian Institute of Science. Technologies for Biomass Utilisation. http://cgpl.iisc.ernet. in/site/Portals/0/Publications/Presentations/Gasification%20&%20Power/ Technology%20for%20Biomass%20Utilisation.pdf. Accessed January 2013.

Jenkins, B. M.; Baxter, L. L.; Miles, T. R.; Miles, T. R. (1998). Combustion properties of biomass. *Fuel Processing Technology* **54**: 17–46.

Jenkins, B. M.; Baxter, L. L.; Koppejan, J. (2011). Biomass Combustion. In R. C. Brown (Ed.), *Thermochemical Processing of Biomass: Conversion into Fuels, Chemicals and Power*; John Wiley & Sons Ltd; The Atrium, United Kingdom.

Kärki, J. (2009). *Biomass Utilisation in Large Scale Heat and Power Production*. VTT Technical Research Centre of Finland, Beijing, September 2009.

Koppejan, J. (2009). Challenges in biomass combustion and co-firing: the work of IEA Bioenergy Task 32. *IEA Bioenergy Conference*, Vancouver, British Columbia, Canada, August, 2009.

Koppmann, R.; von Czapiewski, K.; Reid, J. S. (2005). A review of biomass burning emissions, part I: Gaseous emissions of carbon monoxide, methane, volatile organic compounds, and nitrogen containing compounds. *Atmos. Chem. Phys. Discuss.* **5**: 10455–10516.

Kumar, P.; Barrett, D. M.; Delwiche, M. J.; Stroeve, P. (2009). Methods for pretreatment of lignocellulosic biomass for efficient hydrolysis and biofuel production. *Industrial & Engineering Chemistry Research* **48**: 3713–3729.

Maciejewska, A.; Veringa, H.; Sanders, J.; Peteves, S. D. (2006). Co-firing of biomass with coal: Constraints and role of biomass pre-treatment. http://edepot.wur. nl/18761. Accessed April 2013.

Mehmood, S. (2011). Energy and Exergy Analysis of Biomass Co-firing Based Pulverised Coal Power Generation. Master thesis, University of Ontario Institute of Technology, Canada.

Miguez, J. L.; Moran, J. C.; Granada, E.; Porteiro, J. (2012). Review of technology in small-scale biomass combustion systems in the European market. *Renewable & Sustainable Energy Reviews* **16**: 3867–3875.

Nussbaumer, T. (2003). Combustion and co-combustion of biomass: Fundamentals, technologies, and primary measures for emission reduction. *Energy & Fuels* **17**: 1510–1521.

Nussbaumer, T. Biomass combustion in Europe: Overview on technologies and regulations. For New York State Energy Research and Development Authority, Albany, NY, USA, April 2008.

Obernberger, I. (2011). Biomass combustion—Current status and future developments. http://www.bios-bioenergy.at/. Accessed December 2012.

Overgaard, P.; Sander, B.; Junker, H.; Friborg, K.; Larsen, O. H. (2004). Two years operational experience and further development of full-scale co-firing of straw. *Proceedings of the 2nd World Biomass Conference*, Rome, Italy, May 2004.

Palacios-Orueta, A.; Chuvieco, E.; Parra, A.; Carmona-Moreno, C. (2005). Biomass burning emissions: A review of models using remote-sensing data. *Environmental Monitoring and Assessment* **104**: 189–209.

Peterson, D.; Haase, S. (2009). Market Assessment of Biomass Gasification and Combustion Technology for Small- and Medium-Scale Applications. Technical Report NREL/TP-7A2-46190, National Renewable Energy Laboratory, Cole Boulevard, Golden, Colorado, USA.

Purvis, M. R. I.; Tadulan, E. L.; Tariq, A. S. (2000). NO_x Emissions from the underfeed combustion of coal and biomass. *Journal of the Institute of Energy* **73**: 70–77.

Quaak, P.; Knoef, H.; Stassen, H. (1999). Energy from Biomass: A Review of Combustion and Gasification Technologies. *World Bank technical paper*, No. 422 Energy series, The World Bank, Washington, D.C., USA.

Sami, M.; Annamalai, K.; Wooldridge, M. (2001). Co-firing of coal and biomass fuel blends. *Progress in Energy and Combustion Science* 27: 171–214.

Skreiberg, Ø. (1997). Theoretical and Experimental Studies on Emissions from Wood Combustion. PhD Thesis, Norwegian University, Trondheim.

Sommersacher, P.; Brunner, T.; Obernberger, I. (2012). Fuel indexes: A novel method for the evaluation of relevant combustion properties of new biomass fuels. *Energy & Fuels* 26: 380–390.

Stott, P. (2000). Combustion in tropical biomass fires: A critical review. *Progress in Physical Geography* 24: 355–377.

Sullivan, A. L.; Ball, R. (2012). Thermal decomposition and combustion chemistry of cellulosic biomass. *Atmospheric Environment* 47: 133–141.

Univerity of Applied Sciences (Germany); Technische Universitat Dresden (Germany); Cardiff University (UK); Can Tho University (Vietnam); King Mongkut's University of Technology Thonburi (Thailand). (2005). Decision Support System (DSS) for the application of RENEWABLE ENERGY (RE) from Biogas and Biomass Combustion. *A handbook within the framework of the BiWaRE Project Partners 'Biomass and Waste for Renewable Energy'*, June 2005.

Valero, A.; Biomass Group of CIRCE. Co-firing of low rank coal and biomass: A chance for biomass penetration in the renewables. http://www.icrepq.com/pdfs/PL2.%20VALERO.pdf. Accessed January 2013.

Villeneuve, J.; Palacios, J. H.; Savoie, P.; Godbout, S. (2012). A critical review of emission standards and regulations regarding biomass combustion in small scale units (<3 MW). *Bioresource Technology* 111: 1–11.

Ward, D. E.; Hardy, C. C. (1991). Smoke emissions from wildland fires. *Environ. Intern.* 17: 117–134.

Williams, A.; Jones, J.; Pourkashanian, M.; Ma, L.; Darvell, L.; Baxter, X.; Gudka, B.; Saddawi, A. Some Aspects of Modelling Biomass Combustion. http://www.supergen-bioenergy.net/Resources/user/docs/Researchers%20meeting%20-%20Solihull/18%20-%20Alan%20Williams,%20University%20of%20Leeds%20-%20Some%20Aspects%20of%20Modelling%20Biomass%20Combustion%20[Compatibility%20Mod.pdf. Accessed January 2013.

Williams, A.; Jones, J. M.; Ma, L.; Pourkashanian, M. (2012). Pollutants from the combustion of solid biomass fuels. *Progress in Energy and Combustion Science* 38: 113–137.

Wiltsee, G. (2000). Lessons Learned from Existing Biomass Power Plants. *A report for National Renewable Energy Laboratory (NREL)*, Golden, Colorado, USA, February 2000.

Yang, Y. B.; Sharifi, V. N.; Swithenbank, J.; Ma, L.; Darvell, L. I.; Jones, J. M.; Pourkashanian, M.; Williams, A. (2008). Combustion of a single particle of biomass. *Energy & Fuels* 22: 306–316.

4

Gasification of Biomass

Tao Kan and Vladimir Strezov

CONTENTS

4.1 Introduction

Biomass gasification converts various biomass fuels into combustible gases
(producer gas) in the presence of a limited supply of oxygen or suitable oxi-
dants such as carbon dioxide or steam. Biomass gasification is usually performed at high temperatures (>800°C), resulting in producer gas usually
consisting of hydrogen (H_2, 12%–20%), carbon monoxide (CO, 17%–22%),
methane (CH_4, 2%–3%), carbon dioxide (CO_2, 9%–15%), water vapour (H_2O),
nitrogen (N_2) and various impurities such as tar vapours, the composition of
which depends on the gasifier's design and operational conditions (Quaak et
al. 1999; McKendry 2002a).

   After the impurities are removed from the producer gas, the resulting
syngas is mainly composed of CO and H_2. Producer gas is typically used
to run internal combustion engines or gas turbines to provide heat in boilers for electricity and heat generation, whereas syngas can be converted
into pure hydrogen, complex liquid transportation fuels such as gasoline

and diesel or other value-added chemicals like methanol and fertilisers (Alauddin et al. 2010). The heating value of synthesis gas (or syngas) is usually about approximately 4 to 6 MJ/m^3 when using air as the gasifying agent, whereas it can reach as high as 12 to 20 MJ/m^3 using pure O_2 (McKendry 2002a).

The history of gasification can be traced back to the middle of the 19th century, when producer gas from coal was initially used for home heating. Small-scale to medium-scale biomass gasification facilities have also been utilised to make producer gas for more than half a century (Reed 2002). During World War 2, Germany was forced to synthesise transportation fuels from coal-derived syngas through the Fischer–Tropsch [n CO + $(2n + 1)$ H_2 → $C_nH_{2n+2} + n$ H_2O] and Bergius processes [n C + $(n + 1)$ H_2 → C_nH_{2n+2}]. The enthusiasm for gasification was then diminished by the availability of abundant petroleum oil. Modern developments in gasification are characterised by two major periods. The first period is from the 1970s until the mid-1980s and is characterised by coal gasification, which was dominated by the United States because of the 1973 oil embargo. The second period is characterised by developments in biomass gasification, which started in the mid-1990s with the increasing awareness of climate change (Kirkels and Verbong 2011; Babu 1995; Klass 1995; McGowin and Wiltsee 1996). Besides the United States, Canada and a number of European countries such as Germany, Austria, Sweden and Finland have become leaders in biomass gasification, and many other countries including the Netherlands, China and Japan have also contributed to the development of biomass gasification (Kirkels and Verbong 2011).

The main steps involved in the overall biomass gasification flow can be listed as upstream processing of biomass, gasification, and downstream processing (including producer gas cleaning, gas composition adjustment and gas end use). Upstream processing of biomass is generally required for meeting the standards specific for the gasifier type and the quality demand of the producer gas. Size reduction of biomass particles can be achieved by knife mills and tub grinders. Some dryers, such as perforated bin dryers, band conveyor dryers and rotary cascade dryers, are often used to dry the biomass fuels (Cummer and Brown 2002).

In this chapter, some pivotal concepts relating to biomass gasification will be preferentially presented in Section 4.2. The types of frequently used biomass gasifiers are then introduced in Section 4.3. The influences of different parameters on gasification performance are described in Section 4.4. Various technologies for the downstream producer gas cleaning, as depicted in Section 4.5, also play a key role in the improvement of gas quality, upgrading of operational efficiency, and the subsequent industrialisation of biomass gasification. The current status of biomass gasification activities is also presented in this chapter.

4.2 Biomass Gasification Concepts

4.2.1 Gasification Zones and Reactions

Gasification in a gasifier is a complex process in which producer gas is obtained through a series of chemical reactions and physical transformations (Souza-Santos 2004). Taking the variability of biomass types and properties into account, the biomass gasification process exhibits complex reactions. A typical biomass gasification process in a gasifier can be distinguished as four separate zones, in which certain predominant processes take place, respectively.

4.2.1.1 Drying Zone

After a biomass fuel with a certain moisture content is fed into the gasifier drying of the biomass takes place in the drying zone as a result of heat transfer from the partial combustion zone in the gasifier and from external heating outside the gasifier.

Typically, a biomass fuel has a moisture content ranging from 5 to 35 wt%. In this zone, both the surface and inherent moisture evaporate at a temperature of approximately 100°C to 200°C, resulting in a reduced moisture content of less than 5% (Puig-Arnavat et al. 2010). The extracted moisture is then combined with the water vapour produced in the partial combustion zone. A portion of the total water vapour reacts with the carbon-containing compounds, such as char and CH_4, to form gas species of hydrogen and carbon oxides whilst the rest will still remain in the effluent producer gas. Simultaneously, some corrosive organic acids are also released from the biomass in the drying zone.

The drying rate strongly depends on the type of gasifier used. The latent heat of moisture vaporisation requires substantial energy, which, to a great extent, influences the other gasification stages. Generally, higher energy efficiency is achieved when biomass feedstock has lower intrinsic moisture. The upstream pretreatment of biomass for moisture reduction consumes energy that will affect the overall efficiency of gasification flow.

4.2.1.2 Pyrolysis Zone

In the pyrolysis zone, the pyrolysis of biomass fuel occurs at a temperature range of approximately 200°C to 700°C in the absence of an oxidation agent. Large molecules of cellulose, hemicellulose and lignin break down into volatile medium molecules and solid char. Some medium molecules then decompose into smaller molecules (such as methane, ethane, ethylene, hydrogen, carbon dioxide and carbon monoxide) through secondary pyrolysis, whereas some of them aggregate and polymerise, resulting in the formation of bio-oil and tar.

The overall pyrolysis reaction can be depicted with the following formula:

$C_aH_bO_cN_dS_e$ + heat → solid char + tar + oil + gases ($NH_3 + N_2 + H_2S + H_2O + H_2 + CH_4 + C_2H_6 + CO + CO_2$, etc.)

4.2.1.3 Partial Combustion Zone

Heterogeneous and highly exothermic reactions of char, small gaseous molecules, tar and oil vapours with the gasifying agent (i.e. oxygen, air or steam) take place in this zone, and the temperature can be elevated to as high as 1200°C to 1500°C, even up to 1800°C. Some important chemical reactions are listed as follows (taking air or oxygen gasification, for example):

Oxidation reactions:		
	$C + 1/2\,O_2 → CO$	−123 kJ/mol
	$C + O_2 → CO_2$	−409 kJ/mol
	$CO + 1/2\,O_2 → CO_2$	−283 kJ/mol
	$H_2 + 1/2\,O_2 → H_2O$	−242 kJ/mol
	$CH_4 + 2O_2 → CO_2 + 2H_2O$	−803 kJ/mol
	$NH_3 + 3/4\,O_2 → 1/2\,N_2 + 3/2\,H_2O$	−383 kJ/mol
	$H_2S + 3/2\,O_2 → SO_2 + H_2O$	−563 kJ/mol

Besides the oxidation of biomass pyrolytic products into carbon monoxide and carbon dioxide, another significant function of the partial combustion zone is to provide heat for the other zones.

4.2.1.4 Reduction Zone

In the reduction zone (referred to as the gasification zone), carbon dioxide (CO_2) and water vapour (H_2O) are reduced by char into carbon monoxide and hydrogen, which mainly comprise the producer gas. During this process, the sensible heat of the gas species and char is transformed into the chemical energy of the producer gas.

The most dominant reactions taking place in the reduction zone are depicted below.

(a) Boudouard	$C + CO_2 ↔ 2CO$	+172 kJ/mol
(b) Water gas	$C + H_2O ↔ H_2 + CO$	+131 kJ/kmol
(c) Water–gas shift	$CO + H_2O ↔ H_2 + CO_2$	−42 kJ/kmol
(d) Steam re-forming	$CH_4 + H_2O ↔ 3H_2 + CO$	+206 kJ/kmol
	$CH_4 + 2H_2O ↔ 4H_2 + CO_2$	+165 kJ/kmol
(e) Hydrogasification	$C + 2H_2 ↔ CH_4$	−75 kJ/kmol
(f) Methane formation	$CO + 3H_2 ↔ CH_4 + H_2O$	−206 kJ/kmol
Other reactions	$NH_3 ↔ 1/2\,N_2 + 3/2\,H_2$	+46 kJ/kmol
	$SO_2 + 3H_2 ↔ H_2S + 2H_2O$	−207 kJ/kmol

The main reduction reactions (a) and (b) are endothermic gasification reactions of the char, being responsible for the decrease in gas temperature during the reduction process, and for producing H_2 and CO. The water–gas shift reaction (c) also contributes to the increase of H_2 content with the presence of solid char as a catalyst. The value of the water gas equilibrium constant at different temperatures theoretically determines the concentrations of CO, H_2, CO_2 and H_2O. However, the equilibrium composition of the gas will only be reached when the reaction rate and the reaction time are sufficient.

The remaining solid residue, including unreacted char and ash, should be periodically removed from the gasifier to avoid the blockage of the effluent pipes.

4.2.2 Evaluation Criteria of Gasification Performance

A series of criteria are required to evaluate the performance of the biomass gasification system so that it meets the requirements for downstream application of producer gas and to optimise the industrial economics. These criteria mainly include (1) producer gas properties; (2) gas product yield; (3) carbon conversion; and (4) efficiencies involving cold-gas efficiency, thermal efficiency and exergy efficiency.

4.2.2.1 Producer Gas Properties

The properties of producer gas are commonly characterised as the composition of the gas, contents of impurities (such as tar and alkali metals), lower heating value (LHV) and higher heating value (HHV). The composition of the gas obtained from a gasifier depends on numerous variables such as biomass properties, gasifying agent, operating temperature and pressure, and thus it is difficult to predict the exact composition of producer gas (Puig-Arnavat et al. 2010).

Depending on the end use applications of the producer gas, the gas-cleaning requirements can range from as-received to mild (if used for engine and turbine applications) to strict (in case of synthesis applications). This is because the catalysts used for synthesis are sensitive to impurities and can be poisoned; hence, the ideal target levels for all particulate and gaseous contaminants are very low, much lower than 1 ppm (Göransson et al. 2011). Ciferno and Marano (2002) summarised desirable syngas characteristics for different end products; for example, the desired H_2/CO molar ratio for methanol production is 2.0.

LHV, one of the most significant quality indexes for fuels, defines the energy content of a gas fuel. The LHV (kJ/m^3) of the producer gas can be calculated from the gas composition according to the following equation (Dai et al. 2000):

$$LHV_{gas} = (30.0 \times CO + 25.7 \times H_2 + 85.4 \times CH_4 + 151.3 \times C_nH_m) \times 4.2 \text{ kJ/m}^3$$

where CO, H_2, CH_4 and C_nH_m (C_2H_4 and C_2H_6) are the molar fractions of the species in the producer gas.

4.2.2.2 Gas Product Yield

The yields expressed in Nm^3/kg biomass fuel of H_2, CO, CO_2 and C_xH_y (total amount of hydrocarbons up to C_3) in the producer gas are important indicators of the gasification process. The gas yield per unit of biomass, especially H_2 and CO, is expected to be maximised during the process (Qin et al. 2012). The properties of a typical producer gas and the yield generated from an atmospheric bubbling fluidised-bed (BFB) gasifier with a steam–oxygen gasifying agent are shown in Table 4.1.

4.2.2.3 Carbon Conversion

The biomass utilisation ratio can be assessed by calculating the carbon conversion of the biomass fuel, which can be expressed as follows (Neathery 2010):

$$\text{Carbon conversation } \% = \left(1 - \frac{m_{ash} \times \%C_{ash}/100}{m_{biomass} \times \%C_{biomass}/100}\right) \times 100\%$$

where m_{ash} (kg/h) = mass rate of ash residue exiting the gasifier; $\%C_{ash}$ (%) = weight percentage of carbon in the ash residue; $m_{biomass}$ (kg/h) = mass rate of biomass feedstock; and $\%C_{biomass}$ (%) = weight percentage of carbon in the biomass feedstock.

Incomplete combustion of biomass feedstock is essential to producing combustible producer gas rich in H_2 and CO as opposed to CO_2 and H_2O. On the other hand, some problems may arise from incomplete combustion, such as a reduction in system efficiency and an increase in ash residue. Thus,

TABLE 4.1

Typical Producer Gas Properties and Yield Generated from an Atmospheric BFB Gasifier

Gas Composition (vol.%)							Tars (g/kg, daf)	Char (g/kg, daf)	Gas Yield (Nm³/kg, daf)	LHV (MJ/ Nm³)
H_2[a]	CO[a]	CO_2[a]	CH_4[a]	C_2H_n[a]	N_2[a]	Steam[b]				
13.8–31.7	42.5–52.0	14.4–36.3	6.0–7.5	2.5–3.6	0	38–61	2.2–4.6	5–20	0.86–1.14	10.3–13.5

Source: Gil, J. et al., *Energy & Fuels* 11: 1109–1118, 1997.
Note: daf, dry ash–free basis.
[a] Dry basis.
[b] Wet basis.

a balanced carbon conversion (neither 100% nor 0%) should be obtained to meet the requirements of the desired producer gas.

4.2.2.4 Efficiencies

4.2.2.4.1 Cold-Gas Efficiency

The energy efficiency of the gasification system can be expressed as a cold-gas efficiency (η), which is defined as the ratio of the total heating value output of the producer gas to the heating value input of the biomass feedstock, and is expressed with the following formula:

$$\eta = \frac{LHV_{gas} \times f_{gas}}{LHV_{biomass} \times f_{biomass}} \times 100\%$$

where LHV_{gas} (kJ/m³) is the LHV of the producer gas; f_{gas} (m³/h) is the flow rate of the producer gas; $LHV_{biomass}$ (kJ/kg) is the LHV of the biomass feed; and $f_{biomass}$ (kg/h) is the flow rate of the biomass feed.

Sometimes, cold-gas efficiency is also calculated on the basis of HHV. In general, cold-gas efficiency varies in the range of 60% to 75%, depending on the properties of biomass feedstock, gasifying agent, type and design of gasifier and its operating conditions.

4.2.2.4.2 Thermal Efficiency

Thermal efficiency is an index of the power generation from the system compared with the original energy contained in the biomass fuel, which is defined by (Damartzis et al. 2012)

$$\eta_t = \frac{P_{NET}}{M_{biomass} \times LHV_{biomass}} \times 100\%$$

where P_{NET} (MW) is the net power output from the gas engines or turbines.

4.2.2.4.3 Exergy Efficiency

Exergy analysis is an effective way of designing and analysing biomass gasification flow using mass and energy conservations with the second law of thermodynamics. The exergetic efficiency is defined as useful exergy outputs from the gasifier divided by the necessary exergy input into the gasifier (Abuadala et al. 2010). For an adiabatic gasifier using air as the gasifying agent, exergy efficiency (%) is expressed with (Puig-Arnavat et al. 2010):

$$\psi = \frac{n_{gas} \times (e_{ch,gas} + e_{ph,gas})}{e_{ch,biomass} + n_{air} \times e_{air}} \times 100\%$$

where n_{gas} (kmol) is the molar quantity of producer gas; n_{air} (kmol) is the molar quantity of air; $e_{ch,gas}$ (kJ/kmol) is the chemical exergy of producer gas; $e_{ph,gas}$ (kJ/kmol) is the physical exergy of producer gas; $e_{ch,biomass}$ (kJ/kmol) is the chemical exergy of biomass fuel; and e_{air} (kJ/kmol) is the specific molar exergy of air.

4.3 Types of Biomass Gasifiers

Gasifiers can be classified based on the type of gasifying agent (air-blown, oxygen-blown, steam-blown, air/steam-blown, etc.), temperature (slagging or nonslagging), pressure (atmospheric or pressurised), transport process (updraft, downdraft, fluidised bed or entrained flow) and the method of heat supply (indirectly or directly heated; see Zhang 2010). Direct gasification (or autothermal gasification) takes place in cases in which the gasifiying agent partially oxidises the biomass and provides the necessary heat for gasification. In indirect cases, biomass pyrolysis and gasification are performed in one reactor whilst partial combustion takes place in another reactor. Low-temperature direct gasification (<900°C) can be conducted in a fixed bed, bubbling fluidized bed (BFB) or circulating fluidised bed (CFB), whereas high-temperature direct gasification (>1300°C) is performed in an entrained-flow gasifier (Göransson et al. 2011). In this section, biomass gasifiers are catalogued into three types based on the fluid dynamics, that is, fixed bed/moving bed, fluidised bed and entrained flow. Other technologies and gasifiers in development are also introduced in this section.

4.3.1 Fixed Bed/Moving Bed Gasifiers

Fixed bed gasifiers are the traditional reactors for gasification, which are usually operated at temperatures of approximately 1000°C or lower (McKendry 2002b). In fixed bed gasifiers, the biomass fuel is fed from the top section into the reactor and the gasifying gas passes through the feedstock, which can be supported on a grate at a lower 'fixed' position. This type of gasifier is also called a moving-bed gasifier because the biomass fuel falls downward in the gasifier as a moving plug (Basu 2010). Based on the flow direction of the gasifying agent, the fixed bed gasifiers can be further classified into four types: (1) updraft (countercurrent), (2) downdraft (cocurrent), (3) sidedraft (crossflow) and (4) open core.

4.3.1.1 Updraft/Countercurrent Gasifier

The updraft gasifier is one of the oldest and structurally simplest types of all designs. The biomass fuel is fed at the top, whilst air (in Section 4.3.1, air is the default gasifying agent) is introduced at the bottom via a grate,

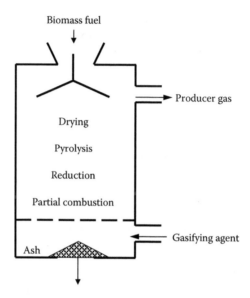

FIGURE 4.1
Schematic of an updraft gasifier. (Modified from Basu, P., *Biomass Gasification and Pyrolysis: Practical Design and Theory.* Elsevier Inc.; Kidlington, Oxford, UK, 2010.)

thus, biomass and air move in countercurrent mode (Figure 4.1). Biomass fuel drops downward and sequentially passes through drying and pyrolysis zones. The pyrolytic solid chars and volatile gases are further converted into combustible gases (mainly CO and H_2) in the reduction zone. A proportion of the char that settles down in the reactor is combusted by the air, releasing heat in the combustion zone. Heat is then transported upward by the up-flowing air to maintain the reduction, pyrolysis and drying zones.

Updraft gasifiers can accept biomass with relatively high moisture contents (up to 60%) and high ash contents (up to 25%). The overall energy efficiency is high because the producer gas leaving the gasifier at a low temperature does not take away much heat (McKendry 2002b). However, the tar content in the producer gas from this gasifier is considerable because the gas does not pass through the combustion zone. A number of updraft gasifiers have been forced to shut down due to environmental issues such as water pollution (Rezaiyan and Cheremisinoff 2005; Marsh et al. 2007). Updraft gasifiers have been commercialised for small-scale applications such as cooking stoves in rural areas and in large plants for gasoline production from coal (e.g. by South African Synthetic Oils [SASOL]; see Basu 2010).

4.3.1.2 Downdraft/Cocurrent Gasifier

The downdraft gasifier is widely used as the preferred type for small-scale power generation from biomass gasification. There are two basic types of downdraft gasifiers, that is, the throated and throatless types. For the throated type, as shown in Figure 4.2, the cross-sectional area of a throated gasifier is reduced at the throat and then expanded. A uniform distribution of high temperature is formed in this narrow partial combustion zone, in which most of the tar can be successfully cracked (Basu 2010). The design of the throat plays a crucial role in decreasing the tar content. However, throated downdraft gasifiers are not suitable for large-scale applications because they do not offer uniform flow and temperature distribution in the gasifier. As to the throatless type, there is no constriction on the gasifier vessel because the walls are vertical (Basu 2010). The absence of a throat avoids bridging or channelling.

Air is introduced into the downdraft gasifier from nozzles set around the periphery of the reactor's middle section (Figure 4.2). This design makes the biomass fuel and air move downward cocurrently, resulting in the reversed order of the reduction and combustion zones (Zhang et al. 2010). Partial combustion of chars and volatile gases from the pyrolysis zone occurs in the middle section of the reactor and provides heat for the other zones. In the downstream reduction zone, a portion of the remaining char further reacts with the CO_2 and H_2O produced from the partial combustion zone, resulting in higher concentrations of CO and H_2. The ash produced in the reduction zone drops onto the bottom of the reactor and is removed periodically. The producer gas moves downward (thus the name,

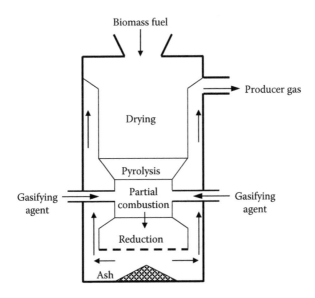

FIGURE 4.2
Schematic of a downdraft gasifier. (Modified from McKendry, P., *Bioresource Technology* 83: 55–63, 2002b.)

downdraft) and leaves the gasifier after it passes through the hot ash at the bottom (Basu 2010).

There are some disadvantages with the downdraft gasifiers. Effluent producer gas with a high temperature of approximately 900°C to 1000°C takes away substantial heat, which lowers the gasification temperature and thus the system's efficiency (McKendry 2002b). Meanwhile, there are some difficulties in handling biomass with moisture exceeding 25% and high ash content. The particulate content of producer gas is higher than that from updraft gasifiers.

However, the outstanding advantage is that the tar content of the gas is significantly reduced because the tar passes through the hot ash, and it can be destroyed via thermal cracking. Approximately 90% (or more) of tar generated during the gasification can be eliminated, and in terms of ash removal, downstream dust collection equipment can be reduced because the ash can be processed together with unreacted char in the lower end of the reactor. Moreover, the initial investment cost of downdraft gasifiers is low due to the simplicity of the reactor's structure and of the gasification process (Son et al. 2011).

4.3.1.3 Sidedraft/Cross-Flow Gasifier

In a cross-flow (also termed sidedraft) gasifier (Figure 4.3), biomass is introduced at the top of the reactor and falls downward. Air enters the reactor from one side, and the producer gas exits from the other side of the gasifier

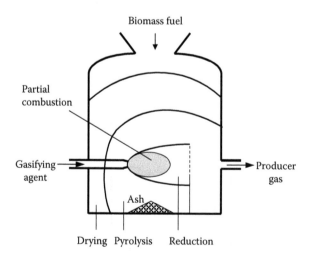

FIGURE 4.3

Schematic of a cross-flow gasifier. (Modified from Basu, P., *Biomass Gasification and Pyrolysis: Practical Design and Theory*. Elsevier Inc.; Kidlington, Oxford, UK, 2010.)

on the same horizontal level (Damartzis and Zabaniotou 2011). The partial combustion zone is formed in front of the air entrance, in which high temperatures (>1500°C) can be achieved, with the reduction, pyrolysis and drying zones surrounding the partial combustion zone (McKendry 2002b). The temperature of the gas leaving the vessel is approximately 800°C to 900°C.

A relatively small reaction zone with low thermal capacity gives a faster response time compared with all other fixed-bed types of gasifiers, which allows a cross-flow gasifier to respond well to load changes when it is used directly to run an engine (Basu 2010). The main drawbacks of the cross-draught gasifiers are the heat loss due to the high exit gas temperatures, unsuitability for high-ash or high-tar feedstock gasification and poor capabilities for CO_2 reduction and tar conversion.

4.3.1.4 Open-Core Gasifier

Figure 4.4 depicts a schematic of a typical open-core gasifier, in which air, together with the biomass fuel, is introduced into the gasifier from the top by a downstream suction force due to the vacuum formed. Gasifiers of this type are specifically designed to gasify fine biomass fuels with low bulk density and high ash content, such as rice husks. The wide-throated design is arranged to avoid biomass bridging. In addition, the water basin at the bottom of the gasifier is specifically designed to remove the ash (Quaak et al. 1999). Open-core gasifiers can also be considered as a subdesign of throatless downdraft gasifiers because the biomass and air similarly move downward in a cocurrent manner.

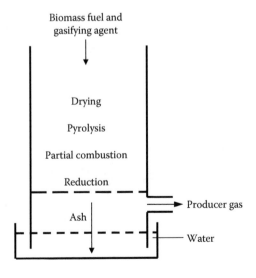

FIGURE 4.4
Schematic of an open-core gasifier.

4.3.2 Fluidised Bed Gasifiers

Fluidised-bed gasifiers are widely employed for biomass gasification. The design and gasification procedure are similar to those of coal gasification. In a fluidised bed gasifier, grainy bed materials are fluidised to offer a uniform temperature distribution, better solid–gas contact and higher heat transfer rates compared with fixed-bed gasifiers (McKendry 2002b). Additionally, fluidised-bed gasifiers can be scaled-up effectively for middle or large units. However, some problems may occur during the operation of fluidised-bed gasifiers. For example, the silica particles widely used as the bed material are likely to react with the inorganic components in the biomass, giving rise to the formation of low boiling point silicates. These silicates will melt under high temperatures and then form an adhesive layer that binds the biomass particles together, resulting in the final particle agglomerates, which stops the fluidisation state (Damartzis and Zabaniotou 2011). Fluidised-bed gasifiers can be further classified into three main types, that is, bubbling fluid bed (BFB), circulating fluid bed (CFB), and twin bed/dual fluidised bed (DFB).

4.3.2.1 Bubbling Fluidised-Bed Gasifier

In a BFB gasifier (Figure 4.5), the gasifying agent is evenly introduced from the bottom of the reactor through a distributor consisting of a perforated plate or several nozzles. Bubbles form at the distributor and then grow larger as they move upward. The biomass fuel is generally fed into the reactor by screw feeders and then blown upward by the gasifying gas. During the conversion process of biomass into producer gas, the gasifying agent in the

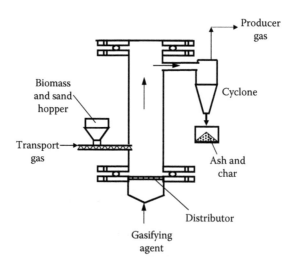

FIGURE 4.5
Schematic of a BFB gasifier.

bubbles exchanges with the gases and vapours produced from the pyrolysis and partial combustion of the biomass. The biomass rapidly and simultaneously undergoes drying, pyrolysis, partial combustion and reduction. The residence time is short, and the temperatures are in the range of 700°C to 900°C.

Cyclones are usually positioned after the fluidised-bed reactor to recycle the entrained inert bed material particles as well as the ash and char. The low tar content of the producer gas is obtained owing to the direct contact of tar with the high-temperature bed material (McKendry 2002b).

4.3.2.2 Circulating Fluidised-Bed Gasifier

A CFB gasifier, shown schematically in Figure 4.6, is an extension of the BFB gasifiers. CFBs have become the preferential choice for nearly all medium-scale to large-scale gasification projects for power production from biomass due to their high throughput, easy scale-up and adaptability for various biomass fuels (Morris et al. 2005). In a CFB gasifier, hot bed material and solid char are circulated in the reactor and cyclone (Damartzis and Zabaniotou 2011) whilst the ash is separated and removed from the circulating stream. The CFB gasifiers are operated in a more turbulent fluidisation mode with higher fluidisation velocity compared with BFBs. The gasifying bed in the CFBs can be operated at a temperature of 800°C to 1000°C, depending on the biomass feedstock and the downstream application of the producer gas. The temperature of the exiting gas is similar to the bed temperature producing low tar content.

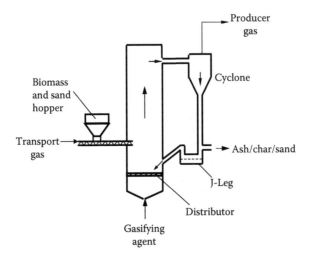

FIGURE 4.6
Schematic of a CFB gasifier.

4.3.2.3 Twin-Bed/Dual Fluidised-Bed Gasifier

Air is often used as a gasifying agent because of its low cost and convenient availability. The main issue in using air as a gasifiying agent is that the nitrogen in the air will inevitably dilute the producer gas resulting in its low heating value. Oxygen gasification can avoid this issue, but its application is limited by the high cost of oxygen. Twin-bed gasifiers (also called DFB gasifiers) have been developed to address the 'nitrogen dilution' problem. The DFB gasifier system consists of a CFB combustor (i.e. the riser shown in Figure 4.7) in which residue char is combusted to supply heat, and a BFB gasifier in which biomass pyrolysis and char gasification take place. Inert bed material, used as a heat carrier, is circulated between the CFB and BFB reactors. Preheated steam is commonly used as the gasifying agent in the BFB gasifier at a temperature of 700°C to 900°C to generate producer gas (Göransson et al. 2011). The residue char and the tar generated from the BFB move into the riser combustor where they are oxidised by the fed air. Sequentially, the flue gas that has nitrogen is discharged after the contained particles are recovered by the cyclone. Thus, a producer gas with negligible contents of nitrogen and tar is achieved. Other advantages of a DFB gasifier involve no or simple pretreatment requirements of the biomass fuel, convenient biomass feeding and no need for oxygen (Zhang 2010). However, there are still some remaining issues, such as high dust content in the producer gas, which is close to that from fixed beds, and higher investment and operating costs compared with fixed-bed gasifiers.

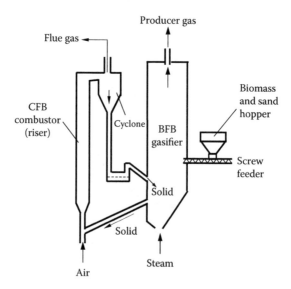

FIGURE 4.7
Schematic of a twin bed/DFB gasifier.

4.3.3 Entrained Flow

Entrained-flow gasifiers, schematically presented in Figure 4.8, with capacities of several hundred MW_{th} have been the most successful and widely commercialised types of gasifiers for integrated gasification combined-cycle (IGCC) coal power plants. The entrained-flow gasifiers are usually operated using pure oxygen under high pressures of 2 to 8 MPa and high temperatures of 1200°C to 1600°C (Göransson et al. 2011; Collot 2006). Additionally, uniform fine particle distribution (<0.1–0.4 mm) is also required. Producer gas with very little or no methane and other hydrocarbons can be obtained (Zhang 2010). Very low or no tar content in the final producer gas is another advantage (Qin et al. 2012).

Entrained-flow gasifiers have been applied for coal gasification; however, they are not recommended for biomass gasification, especially for the gasification of fibrous woody materials, because of the difficulty in particle preparation of the fibrous biomass into the fine granules required to meet the short residence time (Huber et al. 2006). Another serious problem is that the ash in biomass fuels tends to melt and aggregate into corrosive slag at high temperatures in the entrained-flow gasifiers (Damartzis and Zabaniotou 2011).

4.3.4 Other Biomass Gasifier Types/Gasification Technologies

Besides the abovementioned types of biomass gasifiers, there are additional gasifier types or gasification technologies that are widely investigated and reported in the literature.

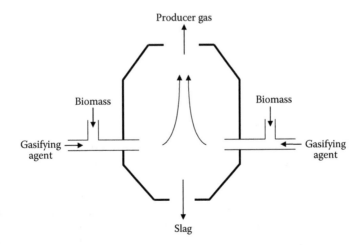

FIGURE 4.8
Schematic of an entrained-flow gasifier. (Modified from Marsh, R. et al., Advanced thermal treatment for solid waste—A wastemanager's guide. *Proceedings of the 22nd International Conference on Solid Waste Management and Technology*. Philadelphia, PA, 2007.)

4.3.4.1 Hydrothermal Gasification

Supercritical water with temperature and pressure higher than its critical point (647 K and 22.1 MPa) exhibit special characteristics. For instance, the ion product of water increases dramatically, and water behaves as a weakly polar solvent that is able to hydrolyse many compounds. Meanwhile, it can dissolve organic substances and provide a homogeneous phase for reactions. Because the reaction medium is water, wet biomass can be directly used as a feedstock. Moreover, due to the short reaction times, much less char formation, low cost of water and high energy efficiency, the *in situ* process of water gas shift reaction, as well as the absence of additional pollution, the subcritical and supercritical water gasification of biomass is considered to be an effective route for biomass conversion.

The relevant research was started in 1971 by the U.S. Bureau of Mines with the conversion of carbohydrates in hot compressed water in the presence of CO and Na_2CO_3 for the production of hydrogen. Since then, a number of investigations have been conducted on the hydrothermal gasification (HTG) of biomass under wide temperature conditions of 250°C to 800°C, pressures of around 5 to 50 MPa and residence times from minutes to hours. Experiments are usually performed in laboratory batch, fixed bed, continuous stirred-tank reactors, quartz capillary and fluidised bed reactors (Azadi and Farnood 2011). During the HTG process, products in three phases, that is, solid char, liquid tar/bio-oil and gas fuel are generated. The gas product is mainly composed of carbon monoxide, hydrogen, carbon dioxide and methane. Two groups of catalysts, that is, the platinum group metal catalysts and alkali salts, are commonly applied to improve gas yield during HTG of biomass.

For the process of biomass HTG, some obstacles still exist on its way to commercialisation, such as (1) it requires a great deal of heat input for endothermic reactions and for the maintenance of its high reaction temperature and (2) the gasification efficiency and gas yield decrease with an increase in dry solids in the feed (Basu 2010).

4.3.4.2 Plasma Gasifiers

Plasma gasification (also known as plasma pyrolysis) is a special gasification process in which biomass is converted into the basic components of gas (such as hydrogen and carbon monoxide) at an extremely high temperature of 3000°C or even higher in an oxygen-starved atmosphere (Zhang et al. 2010). Molten metals and vitrified inorganic slag are also produced. The plasma torch is the key device in which an electric arc is generated between two electrodes. Under these extremely high temperatures, the biomass fuel can be successfully processed in just a few milliseconds, and the effluent producer gas has a high temperature of 1000°C to 1200°C.

Plasma gasification of biomass is regarded as a clean and promising technology with extremely low tar generation and little environmental impact

(Zhang et al. 2010). One of the remaining problems is the reduced life span of the reactor liner due to the high operating temperature and the presence of chlorine in the feedstock (Basu 2010).

4.3.5 Comparison of Biomass Gasification Technologies

A great number of fixed-bed biomass gasifiers have been set up around the world because of their small scale, simple structure designs, high energy efficiency and low cost. However, fixed-bed gasifiers generally offer producer gas with low heating value. Detailed comparisons between fluidised-bed and fixed-bed gasifiers have been reviewed extensively by Warnecke 2000. Table 4.2 summarises the advantages and disadvantages of the main types of biomass gasifiers.

In the application of biomass gasification, the selection of the types of biomass gasifiers is one of the key steps. The selection depends on various conditions such as the properties of the biomass feedstock and the downstream applications. For example, the downdraft gasifier is the preferred option for transportation applications when combined with an internal combustion engine. Fixed-bed gasifiers are recommended for smaller plants of 10 kW_{th} to 10 MW_{th} capacity, and fluidised-bed gasifiers are generally used for medium-sized units of 5 MW_{th} to 100 MW_{th}, whereas the entrained-flow type gasifiers are more appropriate for large-scale facilities of more than 50 MW_{th} (Basu 2010). In case of biomass gasification, small-scale to medium-scale facilities close to abundant biomass resources are preferable because the biomass is sparsely distributed with low density and low heating value. Other key factors that should be considered when selecting a biomass gasifier include the capital cost of the gasifier, investment of the downstream gas cleaning, operational and maintenance costs and energy consumption of feedstock pretreatment (McKendry 2002b).

4.4 Effects of Operating Conditions on Gasification Performance

Biomass gasification performance is highly dependent on the operating conditions such as biomass feeding rate, type of gasifying agent, air equivalence ratio, steam to biomass ratio, temperature, pressure and heating rate.

4.4.1 Type, Properties and Feeding Rate of Biomass

It is well-known that biomass covers a wide range of carbon-containing materials, such as wood waste, agricultural residues (e.g. rice husk and

TABLE 4.2

Advantages and Disadvantages of the Main Types of Biomass Gasifiers

Gasifier/Type	Characterisation	Advantages	Disadvantages
Fixed bed	Biomass gasified using a gasifying agent, generally air at low velocity	Can process large and coarse particles; Producer gas of lower temperature	Producer gas with high dust content; High gasifying agent consumption
(I) Updraft		Simple, inexpensive process; Accepts biomass of high moisture and ash content; High carbon conversion and thermal efficiency; Low dust content in gas	High tar production; Small feed size; Potential bridging; Potential clinkering
(II) Downdraft		Simple process; Only traces of tar in gas	Limited ash and moisture contents for feedstock; Limit to scale-up capacity
Fluidised bed	Inert bed materials and/or catalysts are filled and then fluidised in bed by a gasifying agent that flows through the bed at a high enough velocity	Better gas–solid contact; Uniform temperature distribution; Low particulate content in gas; Accepts biomass of high ash; Flexible biomass feed rate	High producer gas temperature; Complex design and operation; Possibility of high carbon content in fly ash
I) CFB		Flexible process	Corrosion and attrition problems; High demand for operational control
II) DFB		Negligible nitrogen and tar content in gas; No or simple biomass pretreatment; No demand for pure oxygen	High dust content in gas; High investment and operating costs
Entrained flow	Very fine particles of feedstock are 'entrained' in a flow of gasifying agent (generally oxygen or steam)	Very low contents of tar and CO_2; High exit gas temperature	Requirement for very fine (<0.1–0.4 mm) biomass particle; Not suitable for high ash content feedstock; High oxygen demand; Ash slagging

Source: Rampling, T. Fundamental research on the thermal treatment of wastes and biomass: Literature review of part research on thermal treatment of biomass and waste. ETSU B/T1/00208/Rep/1, 1993; Damartzis, T., and Zabaniotou, A., *Renewable and Sustainable Energy Reviews* 15: 366–378, 2011; Kirkels, A. F., and Verbong, G. P. J., *Renewable & Sustainable Energy Reviews* 15: 471–481, 2011.

coconut shells), peat, charcoal and animal wastes, which differ greatly in properties (i.e. chemical composition, volatile matter, ash content, moisture content, bulk density, heating value and morphological characteristics). For a specific biomass fuel, it is highly important to clarify which type of gasifier is suitable to operate and the preferred end applications of the product gas.

For different woody biomass fuels, the three basic constituents (i.e. cellulose, hemicellulose and lignin) differ in their contents. It was found that lignin produces approximately three times more H_2 than hemicellulose, whereas cellulose produces the lowest amount of H_2 (Yang et al. 2007). An increase in cellulose content elevated the gasification peak temperature and prolonged the gasification time (Lv et al. 2010). Other indexes of biomass, such as ash and moisture contents, also influence (to some extent) gasification performance.

An optimum feeding rate of biomass fuel is required to maximise the energy efficiency of gasification process, because overfeeding will lead to plugging and consequently a decrease in biomass conversion efficiency, whereas starve-feeding also reduces the gas yield (Kumar et al. 2009a).

4.4.2 Type and Flow Rate of Gasifying Agent

4.4.2.1 Type of Gasifying Agent

Air, oxygen and steam are the most common biomass gasifying agents, with carbon dioxide as an alternative option. The heating value of the producer gas depends on the applied gasifying agents. Table 4.3 lists the advantages and disadvantages of the different gasifying agents. A mixture of air/steam with a variable ratio is a favourable option as a gasifying agent that maximises the benefits of each fluidising gas (Damartzis and Zabaniotou 2011).

4.4.2.2 Equivalence Ratio

Equivalence ratio (ER) indicates the flow rate of air (or oxygen) supply as well as the quantitative relationship between air (or oxygen) and biomass. ER is defined as the amount of air (or oxygen) introduced into the gasifier to the stoichiometrically demanded air (or oxygen) for complete biomass oxidation, as expressed by the following equation (Cao et al. 2006):

$$ER = \frac{\text{air used (kg)/biomass used (kg)}}{\text{stoichiometrically demanded air (kg)/biomass used (kg)}}$$

ER is an important parameter affecting the gasification performance, such as the product gas composition, heating value and the cold-gas efficiency. A high ER (>1) approaches the combustion process, giving a product of mainly CO_2, whereas a low ER (<0.25) favours the pyrolysis process, producing

TABLE 4.3

Advantages and Disadvantages for Different Gasifying Agents

Gasifying Agent	Advantages	Disadvantages
Air	1. Most widely used due to its low cost and availability 2. High temperature of 900°C–1100°C can be achieved 3. Produces moderate char and tar content	1. Low heating value of the gas product: 4–7 MJ/Nm^3 2. Not suitable for synthesis of bioautomotive fuels 3. Large amount of N_2 in syngas (e.g. >50 vol.%) 4. Difficult determination of ER (usually 0.2–0.4)
Steam	1. Additional hydrogen is produced by the methane steam re-forming 2. High heating value of the gas product: 10–18 MJ/Nm^3 3. H_2-rich syngas (e.g. >50 vol.%)	1. High cost due to the indirect or external heat supply for water vaporisation 2. High tar content in syngas 3. Requires catalytic tar reforming
Pure oxygen	1. High temperature of 1000°C–1400°C can be achieved 2. High heating value of the gas product: 12–28 MJ/Nm^3 3. No N_2 in syngas	High cost and safety implications
Carbon dioxide	1. Produces highly reactive char to boost thermochemical conversion 2. High H_2 and CO and low CO_2 in syngas	1. Requires indirect or external heat supply 2. Requires catalytic tar re-forming

Source: Saxena, R.C. et al., *Renewable and Sustainable Energy Reviews* 12: 1909–1927, 2008; Reprinted from *Biomass Gasification and Pyrolysis: Practical Design and Theory*, Basu, P. Copyright 2010, with permission from Elsevier; Wang, L. et al., *Biomass & Bioenergy* 32: 573–581, 2008.

mainly syngas (CO + H_2; Damartzis et al. 2012). Therefore, there is an optimum ER value for the desired gas composition. Wood gasification studies in a downdraft reactor reported an increase in the low heating value when the ER is increased to 0.35, followed by a decline in the low heating value with a further increase in the ER due to further consumption of the combustible gas and nitrogen dilution. The cold-gas efficiency also follows a similar trend, resulting in a cold-gas efficiency of 69% to 72% at ER = 0.35 (Son et al. 2011). Kumar et al. (2009b) presented an increase in gas yields, carbon conversion and energy efficiencies when ER was increased from 0.07 to 0.25. Additionally, the tar content of the producer gas is suppressed by higher ER values.

4.4.2.3 Steam to Biomass Ratio

Steam to biomass ratio (S/B) is a basic operating parameter involved in steam gasification, which is calculated from the flow rate of steam divided by the flow rate of the biomass feed. At higher S/B ratio, the obtained steam partial pressure in the reactor is higher, which promotes the water gas, water–gas shift and methane steam re-forming reactions to generate additional hydrogen. Gas yields, gas heating value and carbon conversion efficiencies are improved as the S/B ratio is increased (Lv et al. 2004), whereas the tar content in the producer gas decreases with higher S/B ratio (Ruoppolo et al. 2012). However, an additional heat supply is required to maintain the high gasification temperature if the steam feeding is increased, which may become economically unfeasible. Meanwhile, the increase in the producer gas H_2 content is accompanied by an increase in CO_2 concentration due to the water–gas shift and methane steam re-forming reactions. Thus, some technologies for the simultaneous capture of CO_2, such as CaO absorbent, were then developed.

4.4.2.4 Superficial Velocity or Residence Time

Superficial velocity (SV; m/s) is defined as the gas flow rate divided by the internal cross-section of the gasifier (Yamazaki et al. 2005). The residence time can be calculated from the SV and the bed height (or length). SV is one of the most important measures of gasifier performance because it determines the time available for reactions to occur and hence controls biomass consumption, gas, char and tar production.

Yamazaki et al. (2005) investigated the effect of SV in the downdraft gasification of wood chips on gas composition, tar yield and particle yield. With variation of SV in the range of 0.3 to 0.7 m/s, H_2 and CO concentrations increased, whereas CO_2 showed the opposite tendency due to the short residence time and channelling phenomenon in the gasifier. The tar yield decreased, with the SV reaching a minimum of 1.4% in the range of 0.3 to 0.4 m/s followed by higher tar yields for SV of greater than 0.4 m/s. The particle yield increased nearly linearly with SV due to the char entrainment by gas flow from char bed and greater soot formation. Reed et al. (1999), on the other hand, reported a decrease in both the tar and particulate contents in producer gas, with increased SV in the range of 0.05 to 0.44 m/s.

4.4.3 Temperature

A high gasification temperature of typically more than 800°C is preferred to obtain high carbon conversion of the biomass fuel as well as clean producer gas with lower tar content. The effect of temperature on producer gas composition depends on the thermodynamic behaviour of the endothermic and exothermic reactions that take place in the gasifier (Alauddin et al. 2010). Bed temperatures ranging from 700°C to 900°C promote carbon-conversion efficiencies ranging from 80% to 90% with gas yields ranging from 1.5 to 2.5 m^3/kg. Air gasification at temperatures from 700°C to 900°C promotes H_2 and CO production, whereas CH_4 and CO_2 contents decrease (Gonzalez et al. 2008). Similar results were obtained in an entrained flow gasification of wood at the temperature range of 1000°C to 1350°C (Qin et al. 2012). However, Alauddin et al. (2010) states that an increase in the gasification temperature reduces the gas heating value, because high temperature promotes biomass combustion, which consequently results in higher CO_2 production rates. Steam gasification of pine wastes in an atmospheric fluidised bed in the temperature range of 700°C to 850°C increased the H_2 and CO_2 concentrations, whereas the CO concentration and the heating value of the producer gas decreased with temperature (Franco et al. 2003). The air–steam gasification of pine sawdust in a fluidised bed was reported to first increase the gas LHV for temperatures of up to 800°C, and then decreased with further increases in temperature due changes in the H_2/CO ratio (Lv et al. 2004).

Higher temperatures reduce the char and tar content. From the viewpoint of achieving low tar content, the temperature should be as high as possible. However, there are several factors that restrict the operating temperature, such as cost and practicality in case of steam gasification. Also, some alkali components in biomass vaporise at very high temperatures, which subsequently causes agglomeration problems.

4.4.4 Pressure

Pressurised gas at high temperature and with few impurities is often required for the production of synthetic liquid fuels or some chemicals, and for combined heat and power (CHP) applications (Kitzler et al. 2011). The reaction rate, as well as the concentration of the components in the produced gas, is influenced by pressure. For example, elevated pressure promotes the production of methane (Kitzler et al. 2011) and reduces tar formation. Knight (2000) reported a decrease in the total tar amount, and the phenols in the tar were almost eliminated when the pressure was increased from 0.8 to 2.1 MPa. The main disadvantage of pressurised biomass gasification is the higher cost and complexity of the gasifier.

4.5 Producer Gas Cleaning

The downstream processing generally includes producer gas cleaning, reforming to alter the gas composition and final utilisation of the gas, which can be for heating, power generation or liquid fuel synthesis.

The generation of unwanted impurities in the gasifier, such as particulates, tar, alkali metals, nitrogen compounds and sulphur compounds, poses serious problems for its end use applications. Particulates may damage the equipment by clogging the internal combustion engine. The tar may also be responsible for operating failures, equipment blocking and fouling. Sulphur compounds must also be removed before the gas is used for Fischer–Tropsch

TABLE 4.4

Gas Quality Requirements for Power Generation and Fuel Synthesis

Impurities	Power Generation		Fuel Synthesis
	Internal Combustion Engine	Gas Turbine	
Particles, mg/Nm³	<50	<2–30	<0.02
Particle size, μm	<10	<5	
Tar, mg/Nm³	<100		<0.1
Alkali metals, mg/Nm³		<0.2	
Sulphur, mg/Nm³			<0.1

Source: Milne, T.A. et al., Biomass Gasifier 'Tar': Their Nature, Formation and Conversion. Biomass Energy Foundation Press; Golden, CO, 1998; Graham, R.G., and Bain, R. Biomass gasification: Hot gas clean-up. Report for the IEA Biomass Gasification Working Group from Ensyn Technologies and the National Renewable Energy Laboratory, Golden, CO. 1993; Stevens, D.J. Hot gas conditioning: Recent progress with larger-scale biomass gasification systems. NREL/SR-510-29952, National Renewable Energy Laboratory, Golden, CO, 2001.

synthesis in the process of liquid fuel production to avoid catalyst poisoning (Damartzis and Zabaniotou 2011). Thus, cleaning the producer gas is necessary and the quality restrictions of the gas are determined by its downstream end use. For example, the gas quality requirements for power generation and fuel synthesis are listed in Table 4.4.

There are generally two categories of technologies for producer gas treatment: the conventional wet cold-gas cleaning and the dry hot-gas cleaning (McKendry 2002b). Wet cold-gas cleaning is a conventional technology with the drawbacks of higher energy losses and wastewater production, which then needs further management. This process involves particle, alkali and HCl removal by cyclones, filters, scrubbers and packed beds with sorbents, whereas hot-gas cleaning is more attractive due to its higher energy efficiency and environmentally friendly characteristics, in which the solid contaminants are removed by ceramic candle filters or metallic filters, and fluid contaminants are controlled by sorbents (Göransson et al. 2011).

4.5.1 Particulate Removal

The particulates in the producer gas are mainly composed of unconverted char, biomass ash and entrained fine bed material particles. Table 4.5 shows the particulate content of the raw producer gas from different atmospheric air-blown gasifiers.

Routine mechanic capture devices, such as cyclones, are widely used for initial separation of large particulates with a diameter size of more than 50 μm. The separation efficiency can be greatly improved by applying

TABLE 4.5

Particulate Level in Raw Producer Gas from Atmospheric
Air-Blown Biomass Gasifiers

	Fixed Bed Downdraft Gasifier	Fixed Bed Updraft Gasifier	CFB Gasifier
Particles, g/Nm^3	0.1–8	0.1–3	8–100

Source: Pathak, B.S. et al., *International Energy Journal* 8, 15–20, 2007.

cyclones in a series. The cyclones should be positioned inside the gasifier or thermally well-insulated to avoid tar deposition on their inner walls. Smaller particulates of less than 50 μm are then removed by scrubbers and filters. In a wet scrubber, liquid (usually water) is sprayed to wash the hot gas. Approximately 60% to more than 90% of particulates measuring more than 2 μm in diameter can be controlled using the wet scrubbing system. The wastewater with certain amounts of ash and char as well as tars and bio-oils is collected by a bottom wastewater basin. This process results in considerable loss of sensible heat of the producer gas as a result of the quench spray.

Filters can capture particulates larger than 0.5 μm when the producer gasses pass through various porous media. The types of filters mainly consist of metals or ceramic porous candle filters, bag filters and packed bed filters (Kumar 2009). Candle filters, especially ceramic filters, are applicable for hot-gas cleaning. Fabric bag filters can operate at temperatures as high as 350°C, with a high filtration efficiency of more than 99.95%. In packed bed filters, particulates are captured by the bed material as the gas passes through the bed. The drawback of the filters is the serious clogging by the tar after a certain working period.

Electrostatic precipitators (ESPs) are widely used in coal-fired power plants, metallurgical industries and cement industries due to their high collection efficiency of more than 90% over the entire range of particle sizes, down to approximately 0.5 μm, and their very low pressure drop (Basu 2010; Han and Kim 2008). When the gas passes through the ESP, solid and liquid particles are charged by high electrical voltages and then collected. The ESP is suitable for large-scale applications due to its high cost.

4.5.2 Tar Removal

The presence of tar in the producer gas is regarded as the most cumbersome issue for biomass gasification. Tar is sometimes responsible for plant operating failures as it tends to condense and deposit in downstream equipment, such as fuel lines, particulate filters and injectors in internal combustion engines, fuel cells and others, resulting in several technical problems including pipe blockage and filter clogging as well as an increase in operational costs. Thus, tar elimination from the producer gas is an essential step for downstream gas applications. Meanwhile, the gasification energy efficiency

TABLE 4.6

Tar Content in Raw Producer Gas from Various Biomass
Gasifiers

	Fixed Bed Downdraft Gasifier	Fixed Bed Updraft Gasifier	CFB Gasifier
Range of tar content, g/Nm^3	0.01–6	10–150	2–30
Mean tar content, g/Nm^3	0.5	50	8

Source: Pathak, B.S. et al., *International Energy Journal* 8, 15–20, 2007;
Morf, P. Secondary Reactions of Tar during Thermochemical
Biomass Conversion Dissertation. PhD, Eidgenoessische
Technische Hochschule Zurich, Switzerland, 2001.

is also improved due to the potential production of combustible gases from
tar, such as H_2, CO and CH_4.

Tar is mainly formed in the pyrolysis zone of the gasifiers. It consists of a
complex mixture of condensable hydrocarbons, including single-ring to five-
ring aromatic compounds, oxygen-containing hydrocarbons, such as phenolic compounds, and complex polycyclic aromatic hydrocarbons (PAHs).
Based on its molecular weight, the components in tar can be classified into
five groups, that is, light aromatic (one ring), light PAH compounds (two to
three rings), heavy PAH compounds (four to seven rings), heterocyclic aromatic hydrocarbons and heavy tars undetectable by gas chromatography
(Li and Suzuki 2009). The amount and nature of tar largely depends on the
feedstock properties, type of gasifier, gasifying agent and operating conditions (McKendry 2002b). For instance, Table 4.6 shows the tar content in raw
producer gas from different gasifiers.

The tar maturation scheme from primary products to larger aromatic
hydrocarbons as a function of process temperature was proposed by Elliott
(1988) and then summarised by Milne et al. (1998), as presented in Table 4.7.

Considerable efforts have been devoted to tar removal from raw producer gas. Tar removal technologies are generally classified as primary and

TABLE 4.7

Tar Maturation Scheme

Organics in Tar	Mixed Oxygenates	Phenolic Ethers	Alkyl Phenolics	Heterocyclic Ethers	PAH	Larger PAH
Temperature, °C (for transformation into next organic)	400	500	600	700	800	900

Source: Elliott, D.C. Relation of reaction time and temperature to chemical composition of
pyrolysis oils. In E.J. Soltes and T.A. Milne (ed.), *Pyrolysis Oils from Biomass*; ACS
Symposium Series 376; Denver, CO, 1988; Milne, T.A. et al., Biomass Gasifier 'Tar':
Their Nature, Formation and Conversion. Biomass Energy Foundation Press; Golden,
CO, 1998.

secondary removal technologies. Although the secondary removal technologies have been proven to be effective, the primary technologies are receiving more attention due to their *in situ* tar formation control.

4.5.2.1 Primary Removal Technologies

The primary removal technologies aim to suppress or eliminate the tars inside the gasifiers, which can be further categorised into direct and indirect methods. The direct approaches include modifications of the gasifier design and optimisation of operational parameters (such as feeding rate of feedstock, gasification temperature, pressure, steam-to-biomass ratio, ER, gas residence time, etc.) to avoid tar generation. The indirect approaches refer to the addition of in-bed catalysts into the gasifier, which promoted cracking of the tar into lighter hydrocarbons and other combustible gases such as H_2 and CO.

4.5.2.1.1 Modifications of Gasifier Design

The type of gasifier used influences the amount of tar formation. Downdraft-fixed bed gasifiers tend to be the preferred type of reactor design compared with the other types due to their superiority in minimum tar generation. In a throated downdraft gasifier, the design of the throat is very critical for tar formation. High temperature and its uniform distribution are obtained in the narrow combustion zone so that the tar produced can be cracked as much as possible in the throat zone.

Secondary air injection into the gasifier is efficient in reducing the tar content. A part of tar is combusted by the additional air supply, and the remaining tar is thermally cracked by secondary air injection. The optimal secondary-to-primary air ratio of approximately 20% was reported for forest residue gasification under laboratory-scale fluidised-bed conditions during which approximately 90 wt.% of the tars were reduced at the temperature range of 840°C to 880°C, resulting in a tar content of 0.4 g/m^3 in the producer gas (Pan et al. 1999). Sun et al. (2009) reported a decrease in the tar content in an air cyclone gasification of rice husk from 4.4 to 1.6 g/m^3 when secondary air was injected into the oxidation zone.

High efficiency of tar removal is achieved in a two-stage gasifier design, the basic concept of which is to separate the pyrolysis zone from the reduction zone (Devi et al. 2003). A tar content of 50 mg/Nm^3 in the producer gas was reported for wood gasification in two-stage gasifiers (Bui et al. 1994). Cao et al. (2006) claimed efficient tar formation control of less than 10 mg/Nm^3 in a fluidised-bed gasifier through elevated temperatures in the freeboard region maintained through a partial fuel gas and secondary air supply.

4.5.2.1.2 Optimisation of Operational Parameters

Higher gasification temperature, greater ER and longer gas residence time are beneficial to the reduction of tar formation. Pan et al. (1999) reported a decrease in the tar content of the producer gas from 6.7 to 2.5 g/m^3 when the temperature was increased from 800°C to 1000°C during fluidised-bed gasification of forest residues. A proportion of tar can be further combusted and cracked under greater ER and longer gas residence times, resulting in a reduction of the tar content.

4.5.2.1.3 Addition of In-Bed Catalysts

In-bed catalysts are extensively applied to help increase the gasification rate and convert tar into valuable combustible gases via steam reforming, dry reforming, thermal cracking, hydroreforming and hydrocracking or water–gas reactions in the gasifier, thereby reducing the tar yield and increasing overall carbon conversion efficiency (Abu El-Rub et al. 2004). The thermal cracking of tar takes place at a temperature range of 900°C to 1200°C, with catalytic cracking at 750°C to 900°C, whereas steam reforming can occur at 650°C.

During the catalytic gasification of biomass, the most significant reactions relating to tar conversion can be expressed as follows:

steam reforming	$C_nH_m \text{ (tar)} + H_2O \rightarrow n\,CO + (n + m/2)\,H_2$
water–gas shift reaction	$CO + H_2O \leftrightarrow H_2 + CO_2$
dry reforming	$C_nH_m \text{ (tar)} + n\,CO_2 \rightarrow 2n\,CO + m/2\,H_2$
cracking	$C_nH_m \text{ (tar)} \rightarrow n\,C + m/2\,H_2$

Catalysts can be utilised directly as bed materials or as additives to the biomass fuels. The criteria for selection of the catalysts were proposed as follows (Sutton et al. 2001):

1. Must be effective in tar removal
2. Should provide a suitable gas composition for the intended end uses
3. Should be resistant to deactivation caused by carbon deposition and poisoning by impurities
4. Should be easily regenerated and strong enough to resist attrition
5. Should be inexpensive

The catalysts can be divided into two major groups: minerals and synthetic catalysts. Minerals are formed naturally and thus are cost-effective. They include dolomite, limestone, olivine, clay minerals and iron ore. The synthetic catalysts are produced by chemical methods at a relatively high cost such as alkali metal-based catalysts (e.g. Li, Na, K, Rb, Cs and Fr), transitional metal-based catalysts (e.g. Ni, Pt, Ru and Rh), char and others (Abu El-Rub et al. 2004). Tar conversion in excess of 99% can be obtained using dolomite, nickel-based catalysts and other catalysts under a defined biomass-to-oxidant ratio and at elevated temperatures of typically 800°C to 900°C (Sutton et al. 2001; Balat et al. 2009). Dolomite, with the general chemical formula $CaMg(CO_3)_2$, is known for its high tar-cracking capability. Although dolomite is efficient in tar reduction, it still has some limitations: (1) it is difficult to convert heavy tars using dolomite; (2) dolomite is easily broken during biomass gasification; (3) dolomite loses catalytic activity as a result of its melting and due to its low melting point (Zhang 2003). Olivine was reported to possess the same efficiency in tar removal as dolomite but with much greater attrition resistance (Rapagna et al. 2000).

Alkali metal-based catalysts are often utilised to effectively improve hydrogen yield by direct addition into biomass feedstock (i.e. dry mixing or wet impregnation). However, the disadvantage of this method is the difficulty of recovering added alkali metal catalysts during the process and, consequently, an increase in the ash content in the producer gas.

Ni-based catalysts are very active in promoting the tar conversion and the water–gas shift reaction as well as decreasing the amount of nitrogenous compounds. The major shortcoming of Ni-based catalysts is the fast deactivation caused by carbon deposition and poisoning by sulphur, chlorine and alkali metals.

4.5.2.2 Secondary Removal Technologies

Secondary tar removal technologies involve the conditioning of the hot exit producer gas after the gasifier in downstream vessels.

4.5.2.2.1 Physical Approaches

A great deal of tar is also eliminated along with the particulate removal through physical approaches such as cyclone separation, gas scrubbing, filtration via filters and electrostatic precipitation.

4.5.2.2.2 Chemical Approaches

Chemical approaches, including thermal cracking and catalytic steam reforming, are also applied to control tar and simultaneously produce hydrogen. Thermal cracking or catalytic steam reforming is preferably conducted inside the gasifier (i.e. the primary removal) compared with the secondary tar removal.

4.5.3 Nitrogen, Sulphur and Chlorine Removal

Nitrogen in the biomass is mainly converted into ammonia and molecular nitrogen during the gasification process. NO_x contaminants are further produced from the combustion of ammonia, if it is not removed in advance. Ammonia can be removed by wet scrubbing, if cold product gas is desired, or by hot-gas cleaning technologies such as catalytic conversion using dolomites and nickel-based and iron-based catalysts (Kumar et al. 2009a). Sulphur content in the biomass results in low concentrations of SO_2 and H_2S, which can be removed by wet scrubbing or using absorbents like dolomite or CaO. Similarly, the elimination of HCl is typically performed by wet scrubbing or absorption on active materials such as CaO/MgO (McKendry 2002b).

4.5.4 Alkali Compounds Removal

The alkali compounds (such as CaO, K_2O, P_2O_5, MgO, SiO_2, Na_2O, etc.) can volatilise during gasification, which will then sinter, agglomerate and condense, causing the corrosion of the gasifier, downstream ceramic filters and turbine blades. They are also sometimes responsible for the operation failure of fluidisation in the fluidised bed. Removal of the alkali compounds is performed by cooling the producer gas to approximately 500°C followed by gas filtration (McKendry 2002b).

4.6 Current Status of Biomass Gasification Activities

Biomass gasification applications are used to convert biomass to producer gas and then into various products, including co-firing, heat and power generation, Fischer–Tropsch synthesis to gasoline and diesel, hydrogen production, catalytic synthesis of methanol and dimethyl ether (DME), ethanol production through syngas fermentation and production of other petrochemical substitutes. Figure 4.9 depicts the development in accumulated capacity of the main applications of biomass gasification. Obviously, heat and power generation in domestic or industrial heating, CHP and co-firing are the dominant options.

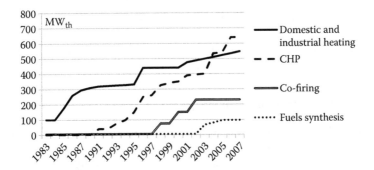

FIGURE 4.9
Accumulated capacity of main applications of biomass gasification. (From Hellsmark, H. The Formative Phase of Biomass Gasification, 2007. Chalmers University of Technology, Göteborg, Sweden.)

By 2011, 87 gasification facilities in pilot, demonstration and commercial stages of development were active, according to the International Energy Agency (IEA 2011), amongst which nearly half of all gasification facilities (47%) are commercial, 27% are pilot plants and 26% are demonstration plants. Of these facilities, 59% are currently in operation, 14% are in construction and 3% are being commissioned, whereas 16% are planned and 8% are on hold (IEA 2011).

4.6.1 Heat and Power Generation

A number of large-scale commercial plants and demonstrations have been successfully implemented around the world for heat and power generation through biomass gasification.

4.6.1.1 Heating Applications

The simplest application of producer gas from biomass gasification is to supply heat through combustion in boilers or kilns used in the cement, pulp and paper industries. In the 1980s, when fuel oil prices were high, several commercial heating or boiler plants were set up in Europe. Most of them are still in operation to provide circulating hot water. In some developing counties, efforts have been devoted to heat applications of biomass gasification. For example, in China by 2004, approximately 160 and 370 sets (not all of which may have been recorded in the IEA database) of gasification systems have been operated for domestic cooking and wood-drying processes, respectively (Salam et al. 2010).

4.6.1.2 Co-Firing with Coal

After the producer gas from biomass gasification is cleaned, it can be co-fired with coal in the coal-firing boiler to produce heat or electricity. The co-firing application with coal has the advantages of, first, having low technical risk because the hot producer gas is directly used in the coal-firing boiler and hence, the tar problem is avoided. Second, the overall cost of co-firing the producer gas with coal is relatively low.

4.6.1.3 Combined Heat and Power with Gas Engine

As shown in Figure 4.9, the CHP application has gained increasing attraction and became the primary biomass gasification application after 2003. Several demonstration and commercial CHP projects were completed in the 1990s and 2000s. However, only limited facilities of CHP with gas engines have been installed due to the uncompetitive price of electricity obtained from this technology.

4.6.1.4 Biomass Integrated Gasification Combined Cycle

As an advanced CHP application, biomass IGCC (BIGCC) became the centre of attention in the 1990s in response to the successful demonstrations of coal IGCC (Kirkels and Verbong 2011). However, only a few BIGCC plants were successfully implemented due to the high installation costs and technical risks.

4.6.1.4.1 SYDKRAFT Plant at Varnamo, Sweden

The most successful and attractive BIGCC demonstration based on Foster Wheeler technology was installed at Varnamo, Sweden with outputs of 6 MW of electricity and 9 MW of heat using wood chips as feedstock. This plant was operated between 1993 and 1999 for a total of 8500 hours; however, it was shut down due to unfavourable economic costs. In this project, the producer gas was produced from a high-pressure circulating bed gasifier, which was sequentially conditioned using a hot-cleaning technique and then combusted in a gas turbine.

4.6.1.4.2 Arbre Plant

The Arbre plant, using Termiska Processor AB (TPS) CFB as the biomass gasifier, is located at North Yorkshire, United Kingdom. This project was initiated in July 1998 with a net electrical output of 8 MW_e and an efficiency of 30.6% using coppice chips as the raw material (Maniatis 2001).

4.6.1.5 Integrated Gasification Fuel Cell

Biomass gasification can also be combined with downstream high-temperature efficient fuel cells for CHP applications, which is known as integrated gasification fuel cell (IGFC). In high-temperature fuel cells, such as molten carbonate fuel cells (MCFCs) and solid oxide fuel cells (SOFCs), hydrogen and oxygen are used to produce electricity and heat by-products in the presence of electrically conductive electrolyte materials (Wang et al. 2008).

4.6.1.6 Heat and Power Generation Plants

Table 4.8 shows the typical data of some power generation technologies from biomass, whereas Table 4.9 summarises the main plants installed for various heat and power generation applications.

4.6.2 Catalytic Synthesis of Methanol, DME and Alcohols

Methanol and DME are regarded as clean liquid fuels and alternatives to conventional gasoline and diesel. Methanol is also widely used for the production of various chemicals and fuels, such as formaldehyde, methyl tert-butyl ether (MTBE), biodiesel (via reacting with triacylglycerols) and others.

114 *Biomass Processing Technologies*

TABLE 4.8

Typical Data for Some Power Generation Technologies from Biomass in 2006

			Typical Costs	
Technologies	Efficiency % (LHV)	Typical Size (MW$_e$)	Capital ($/kW)	Electricity ($/kWh)
Co-firing	35–40	10–50	1100–1300	0.05
IGCC	30–40	10–30	2500–5500	0.11–0.13
Gasification + Engine CHP	25–30	0.2–1	3000–4000	0.11

Source: International Energy Agency. Biomass for Power Generation and CHP. Available at http://www.iea.org/publications/freepublications/publication/essentials3.pdf, 2007. Accessed May 2012.

TABLE 4.9

Main Plants for Various Heat and Power Generation Applications

Application	Company Name	Location	Start-Up	Scale (MW$_{th}$)
Kiln	Ahlstrom/FW	Pietarsaari, Finland	1983	34
	Ahlstrom/FW	Jakobstad, Finland	1983	35
	Ahlstrom/FW	Norrsundet, Sweden	1985	25
	Lurgi	Pöls, Austria	1985	27
	Ahlstrom/FW	Iberian Peninsula, Portugal	1986	17
	Ahlstrom/FW	Karlsborg, Sweden	1986	27
	Götaverken/Metso	Värö, Sweden	1987	30
	Lurgi	Rüdersdorf, Germany	1996	100
Boiler	TPS	Greve, Chinati, Italy	1992/1998	30
	Foster Wheeler	Varkaus, Finland	2000	40
Co-firing with coal	Foster Wheeler	Lahti, Finland	1998	60
	Lurgi	Geertruidenberg, Netherlands	2000	85
	Foster Wheeler	Ruien, Belgium	2002	50
CHP with gas engine	Repotec	Güssing, Austria	2002	8
	Carbona	Skive, Denmark	2008	28
	Ortner	Oberwart, Austria	2009	10
BIGCC	IGT/Carbona	Tampere, Finland	1991	20
	Foster Wheeler	Värnamo, Sweden	1993	18
	Renugas	Hawaii, US	1994	20
	TPS	Arbre, Yorkshire, UK	2003	30

Source: Maniatis, K. Progress in biomass gasification: An overview. Available at http://ec.europa.eu/energy/renewables/bioenergy/doc/2001_biomass_gasification_km_tyrol_tony.pdf, 2001. Accessed May 2012; Hellsmark, H.R.A. Unfolding the Formative Phase of Gasified Biomass in the European Union. The Role of System Builders in Realizing the Potential of Second-Generation Transportation Fuels from Biomass. PhD Thesis, 2010. Chalmers University of Technology, Göteborg, Sweden.

A mixture of gases composed of CO, H_2, CO_2 and H_2O is used to produce methanol at temperatures of 220°C to 300°C, and at pressures of 5 to 10 MPa over commercial $Cu/ZnO/Al_2O_3$ catalysts, as expressed with the following reactions (Huber et al. 2006):

$$CO + H_2O \leftrightarrow H_2 + CO_2$$

$$CO_2 + 3H_2 \rightarrow CH_3OH + H_2O$$

DME is then synthesised through the reaction $2CH_3OH \rightarrow CH_3OCH_3 + H_2O$. Ethanol can be produced through homologation of methanol with additional syngas in the presence of $Co(OAc)_2$ catalyst, the overall reaction of which is described as $CH_3OH + CO + H_2 \rightarrow C_2H_5OH + H_2O$.

The selective production of mixed alcohols from syngas is realised by applying metal catalysts. These catalysts are molybdenum, tungsten or rhenium and the promoters can be cobalt, nickel or iron. Mixed alcohols can be used as a gasoline replacement fuel in flexible fuel engines or blended with gasoline.

Many efforts have been dedicated to the commercialisation of methanol, DME and alcohols productions from biomass. The relevant projects at different stages (i.e. pilot, demonstration and commercial) are listed in Table 4.10.

4.6.3 Hydrogen Production

Hydrogen is recognised as a clean fuel and energy carrier especially in the fuel cell application, which is also an important chemical for ammonia production and in oil refineries. Commercial hydrogen is mainly generated from catalytic steam reforming of natural gas and oil-derived naphtha, partial oxidation of heavy oils or gasification of coal as well as electrolysis of water (Kan et al. 2010). Biomass gasification coupled with downstream treatments of producer gas provides a feasible alternative to producing hydrogen. The downstream treatments may consist of steam reforming of CH_4, water–gas shift reaction of CO to H_2 and CO_2 as well as absorption of CO_2 by various absorbents such as CaO. Pure hydrogen can be also obtained using a hydrogen-selective membrane. Hydrogen membrane separation is now mainly at the research phase, and some technical challenges, such as limited durability due to material or catalyst failure in the presence of contaminants, should be resolved (Hannula 2009).

The Gas Technology Institute (GTI; Des Plaines, IL), in collaboration with the Natural Resources Research Institute (NRRI; University of Minnesota, Duluth, MN), demonstrated the feasibility of the hydrogen-production process from biomass gasification using a hydrogen-selective palladium–copper membrane (GTI 2007).

TABLE 4.10

Projects for Methanol, DME and Alcohol Production from Thermochemical Conversion of Biomass

Company/ Organisation	Location	Product	Facility Type	Start-Up	Output
Enerkem Alberta Biofuels LP	Edmonton, Alberta, Canada	Ethanol; methanol, syngas	Commercial	2013, Under construction	30,000 t/a; 10 mmgy
Enerkem Mississippi Biofuels LLC	Pontotoc, Mississippi, US	Ethanol, methanol, syngas	Commercial	Planned	30,000 t/a; 10 mmgy
Enerkem– Varennes Cellulosic Ethanol L.P.	Varennes, Quebec, Canada	Ethanol, methanol, syngas	Commercial	Planned	30,000 t/a; 10 mmgy
Enerkem	Westbury, Quebec, Canada	Ethanol, methanol	Demonstration	2009	3900 t/a; 1.3 mmgy
Tembec Chemical Group	Temiscaming, Quebec, Canada	Ethanol	Demonstration	Operational	13,000 t/a
Chemrec AB	Örnsköldsvik, Sweden	Methanol, DME	Demonstration	2015, Planned	147,000 t/a; 100,000 t/a
Enerkem	Sherbrooke, Quebec, Canada	Methanol, ethanol, etc.	Pilot	2003	/
Range Fuels, Inc.	Denver, Colorado, US	Mixed alcohols	Pilot	2008	/
Chemrec AB	Pitea, Sweden	DME	Pilot	2011	1800 t/a

Source: IEA Bioenergy Task 39. Available at http://www.task39.org, see also http://demoplants. bioenergy2020.eu/, 2013. Accessed January 2013.
Note: mmgy, million gallons per year.

4.6.4 Ethanol Production through Syngas Fermentation

Syngas can also be converted to chemical products, including organic acids, alcohols and polyesters, using biological fermentation. During the process, the existence of certain bacteria is required to generate the desired chemicals, for example, *Butyribacterium methylotrophicum* for butanol and ethanol, Clostridial bacteria for ethanol, photosynthetic bacteria for poly-3-hydroxybutyrate and *Rhodospirillus rubrum* for H_2 and polyesters (Wang et al. 2008). Attractive ethanol production can be simply presented as the following reactions (Kumar et al. 2009a):

$$6CO + 3H_2O \rightarrow C_2H_5OH + 4CO_2$$

$$6H_2 + 2CO_2 \rightarrow C_2H_5OH + 3H_2O$$

The main advantages of the fermentation route over the catalytic technology for ethanol production from syngas include (1) no requirement for high temperature and pressure, and (2) no requirement for expensive sulphur removal from the producer gas and complex adjustment of the H_2/CO ratio (Wang et al. 2008). On its way from current R&D stage to commercialisation, the major barrier is how to increase the ethanol-producing rate and yield to acceptable levels.

References

Abu El-Rub, Z.; Bramer, E. A.; Brem, G. (2004). Review of catalysts for tar elimination in biomass gasification processes. *Industrial & Engineering Chemistry Research* **43**: 6911–6919.

Abuadala, A.; Dincer, I.; Naterer, G. F. (2010). Exergy analysis of hydrogen production from biomass gasification. *International Journal of Hydrogen Energy* **35**: 4981–4990.

Alauddin, Z. A. B. Z.; Lahijani, P.; Mohammadi, M.; Mohamed, A. R. (2010). Gasification of lignocellulosic biomass in fluidized beds for renewable energy development: A review. *Renewable and Sustainable Energy Reviews* **14**: 2852–2862.

Azadi, P.; Farnood, R. (2011). Review of heterogeneous catalysts for sub- and super-critical water gasification of biomass and wastes. *International Journal of Hydrogen Energy* **36**: 9529–9541.

Babu, S. P. (1995). Thermal gasification of biomass technology developments: End of task report for 1992 to 1994. *Biomass & Bioenergy* **9**: 271–285.

Balat, M.; Balat, M.; Kirtay, E.; Balat, H. (2009). Main routes for the thermo-conversion of biomass into fuels and chemicals. Part 2: Gasification systems. *Energy Conversion and Management* **50**: 3158–3168.

Basu, P. (2010). *Biomass Gasification and Pyrolysis: Practical Design and Theory*. Elsevier Inc.; Kidlington, Oxford, UK.

Bui, T.; Loof, R.; Bhattacharya, S. C. (1994). Multi-stage reactor for thermal gasification of wood. *Energy* **19**: 397–404.

Cao, Y.; Wang, Y.; Riley, J. T.; Pan, W. P. (2006). A novel biomass air gasification process for producing tar-free higher heating value fuel gas. *Fuel Processing Technology* **87**: 343–353.

Ciferno, J. P.; Marano J. J. (2002). Benchmarking biomass gasification technologies for fuels, chemicals and hydrogen production. Prepared for: U.S. Department of Energy National Energy Technology Laboratory; Pittsburgh, PA, USA.

Collot, A. G. (2006). Matching gasification technologies to coal properties. *International Journal of Coal Geology* **65**: 191–212.

Cummer, K. R.; Brown, R. C. (2002). Ancillary equipment for biomass gasification. *Biomass & Bioenergy* **23**: 113–128.

Dai, X. W.; Wu, C. Z.; Li, H. B.; Chen, Y. (2000). The fast pyrolysis of biomass in CFB reactor. *Energy & Fuels* **14**: 552–557.

Damartzis, T.; Zabaniotou, A. (2011). Thermochemical conversion of biomass to second generation biofuels through integrated process design—A review. *Renewable and Sustainable Energy Reviews* **15**: 366–378.

Damartzis, T.; Michailos, S.; Zabaniotou, A. (2012). Energetic assessment of a combined heat and power integrated biomass gasification-internal combustion engine system by using Aspen Plus (R). *Fuel Processing Technology* **95**: 37–44.
Devi, L.; Ptasinski, K. J.; Janssen, F. J. J. G. (2003). A review of the primary measures for tar elimination in biomass gasification processes. *Biomass & Bioenergy* **24**: 125–140.
Elliott, D. C. (1988). Relation of reaction time and temperature to chemical composition of pyrolysis oils. In E.J. Soltes and T.A. Milne (eds.), *Pyrolysis Oils from Biomass*; ACS Symposium Series 376; Denver, CO.
Franco, C.; Pinto, F.; Gulyurtlu, I.; Cabrita, I. (2003). The study of reactions influencing the biomass steam gasification process. *Fuel* **82**: 835–842.
Gas Technology Institute (GTI). (2007). Direct Hydrogen Production from Biomass Gasifier Using Hydrogen-Selective Membrane. Report prepared by GTI in collaboration with NRRI for Xcel Energy. http://www.xcelenergy.com/staticfiles/xe/Corporate/RDF-DirectHydrogenProduction-Report[1].pdf. Accessed May 2012.
Gil, J.; Aznar, M. P.; Caballero, M. A.; Frances, E.; Corella, J. (1997). Biomass gasification in fluidized bed at pilot scale with steam–oxygen mixtures. Product distribution for very different operating conditions. *Energy & Fuels* **11**: 1109–1118.
Gonzalez, J. F.; Roman, S.; Bragado, D.; Calderon, M. (2008). Investigation on the reactions influencing biomass air and air/steam gasification for hydrogen production. *Fuel Processing Technology* **89**: 764–772.
Göransson, K.; Söderlind, U.; He, J.; Zhang, W. (2011). Review of syngas production via biomass DFBGs. *Renewable and Sustainable Energy Reviews* **15**: 482–492.
Graham, R. G.; Bain, R. (1993). Biomass Gasification: Hot Gas Clean-up. Report for IEA Biomass Gasification Working Group from Ensyn Technologies and National Renewable Energy Laboratory, Golden, CO.
Han, J.; Kim, H. (2008). The reduction and control technology of tar during biomass gasification/pyrolysis: An overview. *Renewable & Sustainable Energy Reviews* **12**: 397–416.
Hannula, I. (2009). Hydrogen production via thermal gasification of biomass in near-to-medium term. VTT Technical Research Centre of Finland. http://www.vtt.fi/inf/pdf/workingpapers/2009/W131.pdf. Accessed May 2012.
Hellsmark, H. (2007). The formative phase of biomass gasification. Chalmers University of Technology, Göteborg, Sweden.
Hellsmark, H. R. A. (2010). Unfolding the formative phase of gasified biomass in the European Union. The role of system builders in realizing the potential of second-generation transportation fuels from biomass. PhD Thesis, Chalmers University of Technology, Göteborg, Sweden.
Huber, G. W.; Iborra, S.; Corma, A. (2006). Synthesis of transportation fuels from biomass: Chemistry, catalysts, and engineering. *Chemical Reviews* **106**: 4044–4098.
International Energy Agency (IEA) Bioenergy Task 39. (2013). http://www.task39.org/ See also: http://demoplants.bioenergy2020.eu/. Accessed January 2013.
IEA (2007). Biomass for Power Generation and CHP. http://www.iea.org/publications/freepublications/publication/essentials3.pdf. Accessed May 2012.
IEA (2011). Thermal Gasification of Biomass. http://www.iea.org/impagr/cip/pdf/Task33_Newsletter_Vol1.pdf. Accessed May 2012.
Kan, T.; Xiong, J. X.; Li, X. L.; Ye, T. Q.; Yuan, L. X.; Torimoto, Y.; Yamamoto, M.; Li, Q. X. (2010). High efficient production of hydrogen from crude bio-oil via an integrative process between gasification and current-enhanced catalytic steam reforming. *International Journal of Hydrogen Energy* **35**: 518–532.

Kirkels, A. F.; Verbong, G. P. J. (2011). Biomass gasification: Still promising? A 30-year global overview. *Renewable & Sustainable Energy Reviews* **15**: 471–481.

Kitzler, H.; Pfeifer, C.; Hofbauer, H. (2011). Pressurized gasification of woody biomass—Variation of parameter. *Fuel Processing Technology* **92**: 908–914.

Klass, D. L. (1995). Biomass energy in North American policies. *Energy Policy* **23**: 1035–1048.

Knight, R. A. (2000). Experience with raw gas analysis from pressurized gasification of biomass. *Biomass & Bioenergy* **18**: 67–77.

Kumar, A. (2009). Biomass Thermochemical Gasification: Experimental Studies and Modeling. PhD Thesis, University of Nebraska-Lincoln, Lincoln, NE.

Kumar, A.; Eskridge, K.; Jones, D. D.; Hanna, M. A. (2009a). Steam–air fluidized bed gasification of distillers grains: Effects of steam to biomass ratio, equivalence ratio and gasification temperature. *Bioresource Technology* **100**: 2062–2068.

Kumar, A.; Jones, D.; Hanna, M. (2009b). Thermochemical biomass gasification: A review of the current status of the technology. *Energies* **2**: 556–581.

Li, C.; Suzuki, K. (2009). Tar property, analysis, reforming mechanism and model for biomass gasification—An overview. *Renewable and Sustainable Energy Reviews* **13**: 594–604.

Lv, D. Z.; Xu, M. H.; Liu, X. W.; Zhan, Z. H.; Li, Z. Y.; Yao, H. (2010). Effect of cellulose, lignin, alkali and alkaline earth metallic species on biomass pyrolysis and gasification. *Fuel Processing Technology* **91**: 903–909.

Lv, P. M.; Xiong, Z. H.; Chang, J.; Wu, C. Z.; Chen, Y.; Zhu, J. X. (2004). An experimental study on biomass air–steam gasification in a fluidized bed. *Bioresource Technology* **95**: 95–101.

Maniatis, K. (2001). Progress in biomass gasification: An overview. http://ec.europa.eu/energy/renewables/bioenergy/doc/2001_biomass_gasification_km_tyrol_tony.pdf. Accessed May 2012.

Marsh, R.; Hewlett, S.; Griffiths, A.; Williams, K. (2007). Advanced thermal treatment for solid waste—A wastemanager's guide. *Proceedings of the 22nd International Conference on Solid Waste Management and Technology*: Philadelphia (USA), 2007.

McGowin, C. R.; Wiltsee, G. A. (1996). Strategic analysis of biomass and waste fuels for electric power generation. *Biomass & Bioenergy* **10**: 167–175.

McKendry, P. (2002a). Energy production from biomass (part 2): Conversion technologies. *Bioresource Technology* **83**: 47–54.

McKendry, P. (2002b). Energy production from biomass (part 3): Gasification technologies. *Bioresource Technology* **83**: 55–63.

Milne, T. A.; Abatzoglou, N.; Evans, R. J. (1998). Biomass Gasifier 'Tar': Their Nature, Formation and Conversion. Biomass Energy Foundation Press; Golden, CO.

Morf, P. (2001). Secondary Reactions of Tar During Thermochemical Biomass Conversion Dissertation. Ph.D., Eidgenoessische Technische Hochschule Zurich, Switzerland.

Morris, M.; Waldheim, L.; Faaij, A.; Stahl, K. (2005). Status of large-scale biomass gasification and prospect. In H. Knoef (Ed.), *Handbook of Biomass Gasification*; BTG Biomass Technology Group; Netherlands.

Neathery, J. K. (2010). Biomass Gasification. In M. Crocker (Ed.), Thermochemical Conversion of Biomass to Liquid Fuels and Chemicals. Royal Society of Chemistry; Cambridge, UK.

Pan, Y. G.; Roca, X.; Velo, E.; Puigjaner, L. (1999). Removal of tar by secondary air in fluidized-bed gasification of residual biomass and coal. *Fuel* **78**: 1703–1709.

Pathak, B. S.; Kapatel, D. V.; Bhoi, P. R.; Sharma, A. M.; Vyas, D. K. (2007). Design and development of sand bed filter for upgrading producer gas to IC engine quality fuel. *International Energy Journal* **8**: 15–20.

Puig-Arnavat, M.; Bruno, J. C.; Coronas, A. (2010). Review and analysis of biomass gasification models. *Renewable and Sustainable Energy Reviews* **14**: 2841–2851.

Qin, K.; Lin, W. G.; Jensen, P. A.; Jensen, A. D. (2012). High-temperature entrained flow gasification of biomass. *Fuel* **93**: 589–600.

Quaak, P.; Knoef, H.; Stassen, H. E. (1999). Energy from biomass, a review of combustion and gasification technologies. Washington, D.C., World Bank.

Rampling, T. (1993). Fundamental research on the thermal treatment of wastes and biomass: Literature review of part research on thermal treatment of biomass and waste. ETSU B/T1/00208/Rep/1.

Rapagna, S.; Jand, N.; Kiennemann, A.; Foscolo, P. U. (2000). Steam-gasification of biomass in a fluidised-bed of olivine particles. *Biomass & Bioenergy* **19**: 187–197.

Reed, T. B.; Walt, R.; Ellis, S.; Das, A.; Deutch, S. (1999). In *Proceedings of the 4th Biomass Conference of the Americas, Oakland, California*, 1999; Elsevier Science, Ltd.; Oxford, 1999; Vol. 2, pp. 1001–1007.

Reed, T. (2002). Encyclopedia of Biomass Thermal Conversion: The Principles and Technology of Pyrolysis, Gasification & Combustion. Biomass Energy Foundation Press; Golden, CO.

Rezaiyan, J.; Cheremisinoff, N. P. (2005). *Gasification Technologies—A Primer for Engineers and Scientists*. CRC Press, Taylor & Francis Groups; Boca Raton, FL.

Ruoppolo, G.; Ammendola, P.; Chirone, R.; Miccio, F. (2012). H2-rich syngas production by fluidized bed gasification of biomass and plastic fuel. *Waste Management* **32**: 724–732.

Salam, P. A.; Kumar, S.; Siriwardhana, M. (2010). *Report on the status of biomass gasification in Thailand and Cambodia*. Prepared for: Energy Environment Partnership (EEP), Mekong Region, Asian Inst Technol; Bangkok, Thailand.

Saxena, R. C.; Seal, D.; Kumar, S.; Goyal, H. B. (2008). Thermo-chemical routes for hydrogen rich gas from biomass: A review. *Renewable and Sustainable Energy Reviews* **12**: 1909–1927.

Son, Y. I.; Yoon, S. J.; Kim, Y. K.; Lee, J. G. (2011). Gasification and power generation characteristics of woody biomass utilizing a downdraft gasifier. *Biomass & Bioenergy* **35**: 4215–4220.

Souza-Santos, M. L. (2004). *Solid Fuels Combustion and Gasification—Modeling, Simulation, and Equipment Operation*. Marcel Dekker Inc.; New York.

Stevens, D. J. (2001). Hot gas conditioning: Recent progress with larger-scale biomass gasification systems. NREL/SR-510-29952, National Renewable Energy Laboratory, Golden, CO.

Sun, S. Z.; Zhao, Y. J.; Ling, F.; Su, F. M. (2009). Experimental research on air staged cyclone gasification of rice husk. *Fuel Processing Technology* **90**: 465–471.

Sutton, D.; Kelleher, B.; Ross, J. R. H. (2001). Review of literature on catalysts for biomass gasification. *Fuel Processing Technology* **73**: 155–173.

Wang, L.; Weller, C. L.; Jones, D. D.; Hanna, M. A. (2008). Contemporary issues in thermal gasification of biomass and its application to electricity and fuel production. *Biomass & Bioenergy* **32**: 573–581.

Warnecke, R. (2000). Gasification of biomass: Comparison of fixed bed and fluidized bed gasifier. *Biomass & Bioenergy* **18**: 489–497.

Yamazaki, T.; Kozu, H.; Yamagata, S.; Murao, N.; Ohta, S.; Shiya, S.; Ohba, T. (2005). Effect of superficial velocity on tar from downdraft gasification of biomass. *Energy & Fuels* **19**: 1186–1191.

Yang, H. P.; Yan, R.; Chen, H. P.; Lee, D. H.; Zheng, C. G. (2007). Characteristics of hemicellulose, cellulose and lignin pyrolysis. *Fuel* **86**: 1781–1788.

Zhang, L. H.; Xu, C.; Champagne, P. (2010). Overview of recent advances in thermochemical conversion of biomass. *Energy Conversion and Management* **51**: 969–982.

Zhang, W. N. (2010). Automotive fuels from biomass via gasification. *Fuel Processing Technology* **91**: 866–876.

Zhang, X. (2003). The mechanism of tar cracking by catalyst and the gasification of biomass. PhD thesis, Zhejiang University, Hangzhou, Zhejiang, China.

5

Pyrolysis of Biomass

Cara J. Mulligan, Les Strezov and Vladimir Strezov

CONTENTS

5.1 Introduction

The pyrolysis process is the decomposition of carbonaceous material by thermal means, in the absence of oxygen. Typical products obtained from biomass pyrolysis are oil, gas and charcoal in varying proportions, depending on the type and conditions of the pyrolysis process. Biomass feed material is lignocellulosic, referring to the chemical composition of the material, which is composed of the lignin and cellulose that form the hard structure of the plant matter and the hemicellulose that binds the lignin and cellulose. The major categories of lignocellulosic biomass appropriate for pyrolysis are forestry residues, crop residues, paper/cardboard/organic municipal waste and sewage sludge.

Traditional biomass pyrolysis to produce charcoal has been practised throughout the world for centuries (Schenkel et al. 1998). The most basic technique involves placing biomass in a pit or mound, igniting the material and covering the pit or mound with earth to allow the hot biomass to decompose. The pyrolysis occurs over several days in limited oxygen, and heat is maintained by combustion of the evolved gases (Schenkel et al. 1998). Basic handmade earthen kilns have also been used in a similar manner. Currently, the earth kiln techniques are still widely used in developing countries for charcoal production and are well suited to the local conditions (Schenkel et al. 1998). The disadvantage is that this process is fairly inefficient and difficult to control, with most kiln operators gaining knowledge of the process through years of experience (Mangue 2000). Modern-day pyrolysis has progressed, with specialised reactor designs developed to enable improved process control and a designated product output.

Biomass pyrolysis processes can operate under fast or slow pyrolysis conditions, depending on the residence time and heating rate of the material in the reactor. Slow pyrolysis or 'conventional' pyrolysis produces a moderate proportion of charcoal with moderate to low levels of liquid. On the other hand, fast pyrolysis, sometimes referred to as flash pyrolysis, is characterised by high yields of liquid (Meier and Faix 1997). Fast and slow pyrolysis are broad terms to represent each end of the pyrolysis spectrum, so processes may operate somewhere in between and are not strictly either fast or slow pyrolysis.

Fast pyrolysis reactor designs are typically based around the principle of providing a very short and intensive heat flux to small biomass particles, often with very short solid and vapour residence times. Fast pyrolysis temperatures can range between 450°C and 550°C (Scott et al. 1999), although to obtain maximum liquid yield, the temperature is usually held around 500°C and 520°C (Bridgwater et al. 1999). A typical fast pyrolysis process has a heating rate within the range of 1000°C/s to 10,000°C/s with a residence time between 30 ms and 1.5 s (Maggi and Delmon 1994). The fast pyrolysis process generates vapours and gases that are rapidly quenched or cooled to condense the oil and avoid further decomposition reactions that favour gas formation. The final breakdown of products from the fast pyrolysis of lignocellulosic biomass sources is typically 50% to 80% liquid, with gas and charcoal accounting for the remainder in approximately equal proportions (Maggi and Delmon 1994; Scott et al. 1999; Bridgwater 2004). Fast pyrolysis processes, which are aimed at producing the maximum oil fraction, heat the biomass material at the more rapid rates of up to tens of thousands of degrees per second (Graham and Bergougnou 1984; Scott et al. 1988). A number of reactor types have been designed in an attempt to produce consistent quality products, feed handling and cost-effectiveness for successful commercialisation.

Unlike fast pyrolysis reactors, slow pyrolysis reactors are generally designed to slowly roast or bake the biomass to obtain a substantial generation of the solid charcoal product. The remainder of the products include either liquid and gas yields or gas yield alone. It is possible to achieve an equal product distribution amongst the solid, liquid and gas phases, although most processes seem to continue the reaction to drive the oil into an incondensable gas phase. The slow pyrolysis process is generally classified as having residence times in the order of minutes (Maggi and Delmon 1994; Scott et al. 1999), with heating rates reaching as low as several degrees per minute. The pyrolysis temperature will usually be at or less than 500°C (Williams and Besler 1996).

The extreme ends of slow pyrolysis are carbonisation and torrefaction. Carbonisation occurs when pyrolysis conditions are such that the biomass feed is very slowly heated to favour maximum charcoal production. Charcoal is essentially pure carbon and may be sequestered as a beneficial additive to soil to improve soil structure and water and nutrient retention (Okimori et al. 2006; Lehmann et al. 2006), where the carbon can be stored permanently in the lithosphere (Lehmann et al. 2006). The charcoal is also suitable for combustion for its energy content or use as metallurgical carbon and other specialty carbon products. The carbonisation temperature is typically 500°C, in which most volatiles are released from the biomass to form a combustible gas (Alves and Figueiredo 1986).

Torrefaction is the process of heating carbonaceous material to remove moisture and some light volatiles. The torrefaction temperature of approximately 200°C to 300°C (Bourgois and Guyonnet 1988; Prins et al. 2006), is lower compared with standard pyrolysis to avoid the reactions that break down the lignin structure of the biomass. The breakdown of hemicellulose and the removal of moisture is the goal of torrefaction, to produce a higher quality fuel for further applications such as pyrolysis, gasification or combustion (Bourgois and Guyonnet 1988).

5.2 Existing Reactor Designs for Biomass Pyrolysis

5.2.1 Fast Pyrolysis Reactors

Fast pyrolysis reactors must be designed to achieve two principles; these are rapid biomass heating rate and short product residence time. Most fast pyrolysis reactors have been developed as slight variants of one of the major generic forms described in the following sections.

5.2.1.1 Bubbling Fluidised Bed Pyrolysis

Rapid particle heating can be achieved using a bubbling fluidised bed (Figure 5.1), in which hot gas is pumped upward through the biomass particles. When the gas velocity reaches the minimum fluidisation velocity, the particle bed will suspend and behave similar to a fluid, and this characteristic creates an ideal situation for pyrolysis reactions due to the excellent mixing and heat transfer properties. Heat is usually supplied by a hot carrier gas, although approximately 90% of the heat transfer in a bubbling fluidised bed occurs directly between the biomass solids (Bridgwater 1999). Rapid quenching of

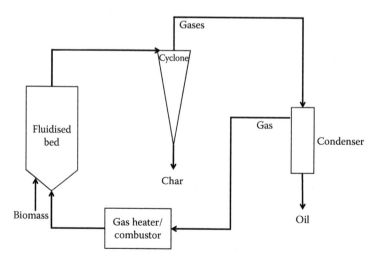

FIGURE 5.1
Bubbling fluidised bed pyrolysis process.

the vapours using a condenser is required to maximise oil production from bubbling fluidised bed pyrolysis, with reasonably high liquid product yields of up to 70% (Scott et al. 1999).

A disadvantage of bubbling fluidised bed reactors is that the products contain high levels of particulates and moderate levels of tar (Bridgwater 2003). Like most fast pyrolysis technologies, the process also requires finely ground feed material to allow a great enough surface area for heat transfer and reaction, which must be no larger than 2 mm for bubbling fluidised bed pyrolysis (Bridgwater 1999).

5.2.1.2 Circulating Fluidised Bed Pyrolysis

Similar to the bubbling fluidised bed reactor configuration, the circulating fluidised bed is able to achieve rapid particle heating using a solid heat transfer medium with particle transport through a hot gas stream. There are several different configurations of circulating fluidised beds; however, the design will generally include a reactor, where pyrolysis occurs, a separation unit such as a cyclone to separate the product vapours from the solids and charcoal, and a regenerator, to reheat the solid particles by combusting the char. The reheated solid particles are recycled back to the fluidised bed. Figure 5.2 shows a typical circulating fluidised bed schematic. Yields of oil from circulating fluidised bed reactors have been found to be approximately 65% to 70%, which is higher compared with bubbling fluidised beds because of the shorter residence times in the reactor (Lappas et al. 2002).

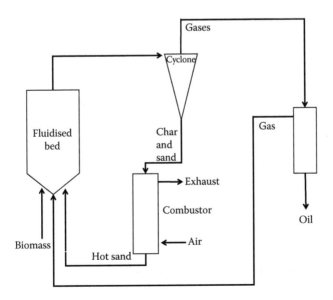

FIGURE 5.2
Circulating fluidised bed pyrolysis process.

The technology has the same disadvantages as bubbling fluidised beds, with the requirement for finely ground feed at a maximum size of 6 mm for circulating fluidised beds, and contamination of charcoal particles in the products (Bridgwater 1999). The process requires careful control to maintain the correct temperature in the pyrolysis reactor.

5.2.1.3 Rotating Cone Reactor

The rotating cone design differs from fluidised bed technology in that it uses centrifugal force to transport the biomass particles and products in a spiral through the reactor in either the upward or downward direction. The heat is transferred by hot carrier solids mixed with the biomass, which are separated from the products after pyrolysis and recycled (Wagenaar et al. 1994). One particular rotating cone reactor design employs a fluidised bed at the base of the cone, where the reheated solid carrier particles are directed back into the cone to be transported upward and eventually overflow and fall back into the fluidised bed (Janse et al. 2000a). A diagram of a general rotating cone pyrolysis process is shown in Figure 5.3.

A disadvantage of rotating cone reactors when compared with bubbling and circulating fluidised bed designs is the less effective heat transfer between the solid heat carrier particles and the biomass feed due to the lower density of solids in the reactor (Bridgwater 1999). The reactor also operates most efficiently with feed material that is less than 1 mm in size to enable

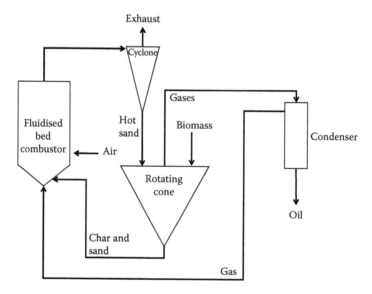

FIGURE 5.3
Rotating cone pyrolysis process.

effective heat transfer without causing a significant heat gradient to occur inside the biomass particle (Janse et al. 2000b).

5.2.1.4 Ablative Pyrolysis

The ablative pyrolysis reactor is fundamentally unique and does not rely on small particle sizes and mixing to achieve heat transfer. The process involves pressing the biomass against a hot moving surface to 'melt' the biomass (Peacocke and Bridgwater 1994), commonly achieved by forcing the biomass against a hot rotating disk. Another configuration is the ablative vortex reactor, in which a stream of gas carries the biomass particles and forces them tangentially across a hot surface (Bridgwater and Peacocke 2000). A typical ablative pyrolysis process is shown in the schematic diagram in Figure 5.4. To produce a high liquid yield, it was determined that there must be both high available heat flux and efficient removal of products (Lédé et al. 1985). Liquid yields of up to 80% have been obtained despite the comparatively long gas residence times (Peacocke and Bridgwater 1994), with evidence of liquid cracking during volatilisation to produce a generally lighter oil product than other fast pyrolysis techniques (Peacocke et al. 1994; Lédé 2003). The design has the advantage of avoiding the need for a carrier gas, and accepts large feed sizes because the material is continuously eroded away at the heat transfer front (Di Blasi 1996). The high level of contact between the heated disk and the biomass causes the charcoal to be eroded from the biomass as it is formed and allows the unreacted biomass to be heated directly (Bridgwater 1999).

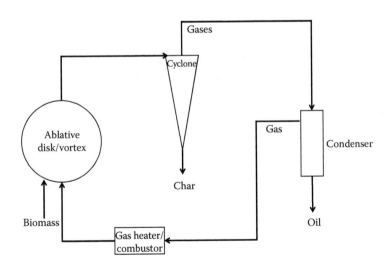

FIGURE 5.4
Ablative pyrolysis process.

Disadvantages of ablative pyrolysis designs include difficulties with effectively heating the rotating disk itself (Bridgwater 1999) and limitations with measuring the pyrolysis temperature. Temperature measurement is difficult because it is not possible to place a device such as a thermocouple at the reaction front (Lédé 2003). The reactor internals may experience excessive wear due to the high particle to surface relative velocity.

5.2.1.5 Twin Screw Reactor

The twin screw pyrolysis design uses two offset screws encased in the reactor to fluidise and transport the biomass particles through the reactor. The screws rotate in the same direction and have intertwining flights to dislodge particles caught in the thread (Raffelt et al. 2006). A heat carrier, such as sand, is mixed with the feed at the reactor entry to provide the heat for pyrolysis, with the product gas or charcoal optionally being combusted to reheat the heat carrier material. A twin screw pyrolysis process is shown in the schematic diagram in Figure 5.5. Experimental analysis has shown that the reactor is able to produce 53% to 78% liquid, 12% to 34% charcoal and 8% to 20% gas (Raffelt et al. 2006). The design avoids the use of a carrier gas and is benefitted by high shear mixing of the biomass and charcoal particles (Raffelt et al. 2006).

Similar to fluidised beds, the disadvantages of the twin screw design include the requirement for small particle sizes. The particles must have a characteristic length, or ratio of volume to surface area of less than 0.5 mm (Henrich and Weirich 2004), which is equivalent to less than 2 mm for a spherical particle but may allow larger cross-sectional areas if one dimension of the particle is smaller. The liquid product may also contain high levels of particulates and tars.

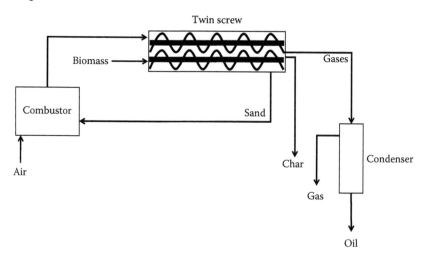

FIGURE 5.5
Twin screw pyrolysis process.

5.2.2 Slow Pyrolysis Reactors

Slow pyrolysis reactors are designed to provide slower heating rates and much more lengthy residence times than fast pyrolysis. The most commonly utilised slow pyrolysis reactor designs are described and discussed below.

5.2.2.1 Fluidised Bed Slow Pyrolysis

Fluidised bed slow pyrolysis is similar to the same technique used for fast pyrolysis but with longer residence times that allow a greater proportion of charcoal production. Experiments have shown that fluidised bed slow pyrolysis generates product ratios of around 35% to 45% liquid, 20% to 25% charcoal and 30% to 35% gas (Zabanitou and Karabelas 1999).

Pyrolysis oil is the most commercially lucrative product and thus a disadvantage of fluidised bed slow pyrolysis is that lower oil yields are produced compared with the fast pyrolysis fluidised bed process (unless charcoal rather than oil is the desired output for the specific application). It also shares the same feed size restrictions and product quality issues of fluidised bed fast pyrolysis.

5.2.2.2 Vacuum Pyrolysis

Vacuum pyrolysis employs low absolute pressures inside the reactor. The biomass is transported into the reactor on a conveyor where it is mechanically stirred during the process before being expelled as charcoal through a pressure seal. Figure 5.6 shows a diagram of a particular vacuum pyrolysis process that uses molten salt as a heat transfer medium. Vacuum pyrolysis is considered to be a slow pyrolysis technique because the heating rates are

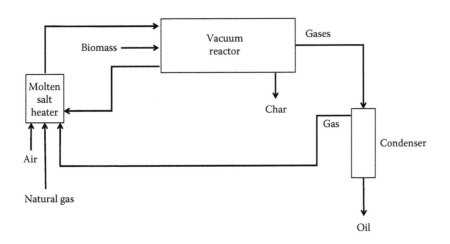

FIGURE 5.6
Vacuum pyrolysis process.

slow and the residence time is approximately 40 s. Vacuum pyrolysis produces a greater proportion of liquid due to the low pressure conditions that reduce reaction rates as well as condensation reactions in the vapour phase (Effendi et al. 2008). An advantage of the technique over high oil-producing fast pyrolysis processes is that vacuum pyrolysis achieves typical liquid yields of 30% to 65% without the requirement for small particle sizes (Bridgwater et al. 1999; Garcìa-Pèrez et al. 2002).

A disadvantage of the vacuum pyrolysis process is the higher costs associated with the requirement for large, complicated equipment (Bridgwater et al. 1999) because the pressure in the reactor must be maintained in the vicinity of 8 to 40 kPa absolute (Garcìa-Pèrez et al. 2002; Ba et al. 2004; Effendi et al. 2008). The process also has a tendency to produce greater quantities of water in the product oil (Ringer et al. 2006).

5.2.2.3 Heated Kiln Reactor

The heated kiln is characterised by much longer residence times than both fluidised bed slow pyrolysis and vacuum pyrolysis reactors. Heated kilns are the most common designs for slow pyrolysis reactors and are similar to the traditional earth-covered kiln pyrolysers for charcoal production (Zaror and Pyle 1982; Honnery et al. 2007). The reactor may be heated internally, such as from combustion of product gas (Honnery et al. 2007), or externally, which often involves a heating jacket surrounding the kiln. Figure 5.7 shows a schematic diagram of an externally heated kiln pyrolysis process. Some kilns are operated in batch mode and may not require any agitation; others are operated continuously and usually involve some type of mechanical transport. There are several different methods of mixing and transport

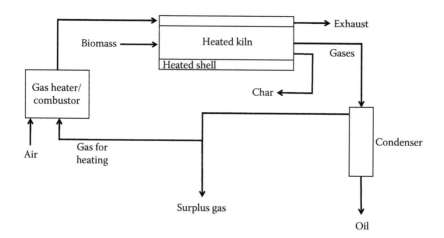

FIGURE 5.7
Heated kiln pyrolysis process.

in heated kilns, including rotating or inclining the kiln, or using internal conveyors or sweepers. All types offer a simple low-capital design, in particular, the stationary heated kiln, which has few moving parts. The product output ratio will vary depending on factors including residence times and temperature.

The major shortfall of heated kiln pyrolysis is the inefficiency of the process, which will produce very little oil and charcoal if the process conditions, such as the kiln temperature, biomass feed rate and product residence times, are not set correctly (Zaror and Pyle 1982). The process tends to have poor heat transfer characteristics if an external heating mechanism is used.

5.2.2.4 Screw Feeder/Auger Reactors

Screw feeder reactors, also known as augers are, in principle, similar to heated kilns and essentially consist of a rotating helical screw encased in a tube, in which the biomass is mixed and transported through the tube by the rotational motion of the screw. A typical auger pyrolysis process is shown in Figure 5.8. The advantage of the screw reactor is the effective mixing and transport of biomass material through the reactor. As is the case with heated kilns, the product output ratios of the screw feeder reactor will vary depending on the process conditions, including the reactor temperature and residence times of the products. Liquid yields ranging from 18% to 25% and charcoal yields between 50% and 60% have been reported (Bridgwater and Peacocke 2000).

The particle size should ideally be less than 1 mm to ensure uniform feed rates through the reactor (Day et al. 1999), which generally means that costly

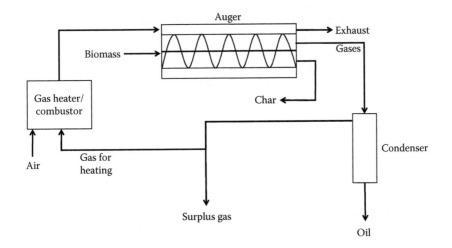

FIGURE 5.8
Auger pyrolysis process.

feed grinding is required. Blockage of the internals due to biomass compaction has also been found to be a problem. Difficulties arise with internal material temperature measurements as there is usually no clearance between the reactor wall and the flight of the screw, thus wall temperatures must be used as a sufficient estimate (Day et al. 1999).

5.3 Current State of Biomass Pyrolysis Activities

Most of the generic biomass pyrolysis reactor designs have reached the pilot or demonstration phases. Pyrolysis facilities in operation have been generally classified according to the descriptions and claims of the status made by the owning company. For example, a 50 t/day facility has been described as a commercial operation whereas another 50 t/day facility operated by a different company has been described as a demonstration plant. At this stage, there are no 'commercially proven' operations in which the plant has been functioning successfully for several years with proliferation of the design around the world. The following sections describe the significant activities in each of the development stages from pilot/demonstration to commercially operating biomass pyrolysis plants.

5.3.1 Industrial Pyrolysis Plants

Commercial biomass pyrolysis operations have been emerging in only the last decade, with Ensyn's Renfrew plant as the first industrial scale facility commissioned in 2002 (Ensyn 2013). The largest industrial-scale biomass pyrolysis facility is the Kior plant, which has a capacity of up to 500 t/day. Most commercialised plants use fast pyrolysis, most likely due to the commercial value of the oil product in preference to the char. The large-scale facilities currently in full operation are listed in Table 5.1, with a description of each plant following the table. The feed capacity can be based on wet or dry biomass and has been indicated if the information was available.

5.3.1.1 Kior

In 2012, Kior began operating a 500 t/day facility in Columbus, OH, processing woody wastes, in particular pine waste. The company utilises a proprietary process that is based on catalytic pyrolysis; however, the design of the pyrolysis reactor itself has not yet been revealed. The catalytic pyrolysis process combines biomass pyrolysis and oil upgrading into a single step, which, in the Kior process, is followed by hydrotreating to produce gasoline, diesel and fuel-oil blends. The gas product is combusted in a cogenerator, which produces steam and electricity to operate the process (Kior Inc. 2013).

TABLE 5.1

Industrial-Scale Pyrolysis Facilities

Company	Process	Description	Location	Capacity	Feed	Primary Product	References
Kior	Fast pyrolysis	Catalytic pyrolysis (reactor type unknown)	Columbus, OH	500 t/day (dry)	Pine woody biomass	Oil	Kior Inc. 2013
Mitsubishi Heavy Industries/ Mie Chuo Kaihatsu	Slow pyrolysis	Indirect heating rotary kiln	Mie Prefecture, Japan	100 t/day	Woodchips	Gas	Koga et al. 2007; JSIM 2001; Machida et al. 2004
Ensyn	Fast pyrolysis	Circulating fluidised bed	Rhinelander, Wisconsin	40 t/day (dry)	Hardwood wastes	Oil	Ringer et al. 2006; Ensyn 2013; Bridgwater 2012
			Renfrew, Canada	100 t/day (dry)	Wood residues		

5.3.1.2 *Mitsubishi Heavy Industries/Mie Chuo Kaihatsu*

Operating in Japan since 2005, the indirectly heated rotary kiln technology of Mitsubishi Heavy Industries (MHI) processes 100 t/day and is currently the only commercial form of slow pyrolysis. Built for Mie Chuo Kaihatsu, the plant is different from other pyrolysis facilities in that it has a major focus on producing gas rather than bio-oil (Machida et al. 2004). The woodchip feed is heated to between 400°C and 500°C in the kiln, thus limiting the formation of dioxins (Koga et al. 2007). The plant dimensions are 2.4 × 20.5 m and it consists of two concentric cylinders with the internal tube containing the biomass and the external tube providing the heating jacket. The gaseous and solid products are separated using a cyclone before combustion of the gas to provide the heat for the kiln and a boiler that powers a 1400 kW steam turbine. The main applications of the produced charcoal are as a fuel, reductant, adsorbent and soil improver. The oil is not recovered from the plant (Japan Society of Industrial Machinery Manufacturers [JSIM] 2001; Koga et al. 2007). MHI is also in the process of constructing a 30 t/day sewage sludge pyrolysis facility for Bio Fuel Co., Inc. using the same rotary kiln design (Koga et al. 2007).

5.3.1.3 *Ensyn*

A 36 t/day plant owned by Ensyn commenced operations in 1996 (Bridgwater 1999) and was the first large-scale biomass pyrolysis facility constructed. The company currently has six operational pyrolysis facilities; however, only the Rhinelander and Renfrew plants are commercial scale, processing 40 t/day and 100 t/day, respectively (Ringer et al. 2006; Ensyn 2013). The Rhinelander plant has been in operation since 2002 and the Renfrew plant since 2006, with larger plants in Italy and Malaysia currently in the planning phase. The technology applied by Ensyn is essentially fast pyrolysis in a circulating fluidised bed configuration with the plant being composed of compact modular units. Sand is cycled between the fluidised bed and the heater, in which the charcoal produced from the pyrolysis is left dispersed amongst the sand and combusted in the heater. The reheated sand is then fed into the pyrolyser again to maintain a temperature of 500°C. A wood feedstock will create a 75% bio-oil product, which is sold for use in combustion applications and used to produce various specialty products including natural resin and V-additive (in concrete and food additives). Approximately 13% charcoal and 12% gas is produced (Ensyn 2013).

5.3.2 Pyrolysis Plants at Pilot and Demonstration Stage

The modern biomass pyrolysis plants have been operating at demonstration scales since the early 1990s with the successful designs generally reaching commercial levels after a few years of demonstration operations. Many plants currently at pilot and demonstration scale are utilising techniques that are fundamentally very different from the existing commercial designs. Table 5.2 outlines a selection of plants at pilot and demonstration stages, with a description of each following the table.

5.3.2.1 Pytec

Ablative pyrolysis has reached demonstration scale with Pytec's 6 t/day plant in North Germany (Bridgwater 2006). The facility has been in operation since 2006 and is currently the largest scale fast pyrolyser using the ablative pyrolysis technique. The Pytec design has the flexibility to accept variable feed particle sizes, which is an advantage when woody biomass feeds are processed. The woodchip feed is hydraulically pressed against an upright heated (700°C) rotating disk, which pyrolyses the wood upon contact (Pytec 2013). The plant produces approximately 70% bio-oil with the remainder being 15% to 20% gas and 10% to 15% char. The char and noncondensable gases are combusted to, respectively, heat the reactor and dry the feedstock (Pytec 2013).

5.3.2.2 University of Science and Technology of China

The University of Science and Technology of China has designed a fast pyrolysis pilot plant (3 t/day) and demonstration plant (15 t/day) in Hefei, China to process crop residues. The system is a bubbling fluidised bed operated at 470°C to 550°C, where cold bio-oil product is used to condense the hot gases inside the reactor. Approximately 50% to 60% of the feed is converted to oil in the process. The noncondensable gas and charcoal products are combusted to provide process heat for pyrolysis and feed drying, with excess gas planned to be used as fuel for heat and power (Zhu 2006; Wu et al. 2010).

5.3.2.3 Kansai Corporation

Kansai have developed a carbonisation plant to produce charcoal (marketed as 'Biotan') from waste rice husks and pruned branches. The biomass is carbonised in a type of heated kiln described as a 'fire chamber', with the process being thermally self-sustaining. The design includes a dust separator to avoid producing smoke and soot whilst achieving complete carbonisation. Rice husk charcoal contains up to 57% silica and is primarily used as a soil conditioner (Kansai Corporation 2013).

5.3.2.4 Lurgi/Forschungszentrum Karlsruhe

Lurgi and Forschungszentrum Karlsruhe have partnered to develop a twin screw mixer pyrolysis reactor for yields of bio-oil. Based on the

TABLE 5.2

Selection of Pilot/Demonstration-Scale Pyrolysis Plants in Operation

Company	Process	Description	Location	Capacity	Feed	Primary Product	References
Pytec	Fast pyrolysis	Ablative pyrolysis	North Germany	6 t/day (demo)	Wood	Oil	Butler et al. 2011; Bridgwater 2012; Pytec 2013
University of Science and Technology of China	Fast pyrolysis	Fluidised bed	Hefei, China	120 kg/h (pilot), 15 t/day (demo)	Wood and agricultural waste	Oil	Zhu 2006; Wu et al. 2010
Kansai Corporation	Carbonisation	Heated kiln	Kyoto, Japan	12 t/day (demo)	Rice husk, greenwaste (pruned branches)	Char	Kansai Corporation 2013
Lurgi/Forschungszentrum Karlsruhe	Fast pyrolysis (followed by gasification of liquid and charcoal product)	Twin screw fluidised bed	Karlsruhe, Germany	20 kg/h (pilot), 12 t/day (demo)	Straw, agricultural waste	Oil	Henrich 2007; Butler et al. 2011; Meier et al. 2013
BTG	Fast pyrolysis	Rotating cone	Netherlands	250 kg/h (dry)	Wood	Oil	Butler et al. 2011; Bridgwater 2012; BTG 2013
Pacific Pyrolysis	Slow pyrolysis	Heated kiln	New South Wales, Australia	300 kg/h (pilot)	Various	Char	Pacific Pyrolysis 2013
Chaotech	Slow/carbonisation	Heated kiln	Queensland, Australia	100 kg/h (pilot)	Sawdust	Char	Chaotech Pty Ltd. 2013
Agri-therm	Fast pyrolysis	Fluidised bed	Mobile plants	5 t/day mobile plant	Agricultural wastes	Oil	Agri-therm 2013
ABRI-Tech	Fast pyrolysis	Auger	Ottawa, Canada	500 kg/h mobile plant	Wood waste	Oil	Meier et al. 2013

Lurgi Ruhrgas design for coal pyrolysis, the pilot plant has been adapted to accept agricultural and forestry residue. The fast pyrolysis of the biomass is followed by mixing of the product liquid and charcoal to form a slurry. The slurry is then gasified with the resulting syngas suitable for liquid fuel synthesis. Heat is provided to the pyrolysis reactor by fluidised hot sand heated by combusting a proportion of the pyrolysis gas (Henrich 2007).

5.3.2.5 Biomass Technology Group

The largest scale rotating cone transported bed reactor is the Biomass Technology Group's (BTG) 250 kg/h plant (Bridgwater 2012). The company also operated a 50 t/day plant in Malaysia that was fed with waste biomass from palm oil production (Bridgwater 2006); however, the plant is no longer running (Butler et al. 2011). In the BTG design, the biomass is fed into a rotating heated reactor that uses centrifugal force to transport the particles. Heat is supplied to the reaction vessel by hot sand mixed with the feed material, where the charcoal formed in the process is combusted to reheat the sand before it is recycled back to the reactor. The company states that in theory the process requires no external utilities, with the excess heat from the pyrolyser being recovered for feed drying and product gas used to generate electricity (BTG 2013). Bio-Oil Holding N.V., formerly associated with BTG, is also planning a 5 t/h facility to convert wood to oil in the Netherlands based on the same reactor design (Butler et al. 2011).

5.3.2.6 Pacific Pyrolysis

Pacific Pyrolysis (formerly Best Energies) has been operating a slow pyrolysis pilot plant that processes 300 kg/h of biomass and produces gas and char. The reactor has been described as a 'swept drum' (Joseph 2008). The charcoal is of interest for use as a carbon sequestering soil additive, and the gas is combusted to provide process heat with the excess being investigated as a fuel. Between 25% and 70% of the feed may be converted into charcoal, depending on process conditions (Best Energies 2008; Pacific Pyrolysis 2013).

5.3.2.7 Chaotech

Chaotech are developing a pyrolysis plant with the aim of producing char. The current small pilot plant produces up to 40 kg of charcoal per hour. The charcoal has a carbon content of approximately 80% and is being marketed as a soil improver (Chaotech Pty., Ltd. 2013).

5.3.2.8 Agri-Therm

The mobile pilot plant built by Agri-therm processes 5 t/day of agricultural waste to produce bio-oil. The plant uses a fluidised bed to fast-pyrolyse the biomass and generates electricity to sustain the process through combustion of the gas product. The plant produces 3 t/day of bio-oil and 1.5 t/day of bio-char (Agri-therm 2013).

5.3.2.9 ABRI-Tech

ABRI-Tech has developed small mobile pyrolysis plants that are currently undergoing trials. The plants incorporate a feed predryer and use a 'hot steel shot' heat transfer medium to process wood waste into bio-oil. A 50 t/day system has been developed, which produces 44% to 62% liquids. A number of these units have been sold and are currently in use (Meier et al. 2013).

5.3.3 Abandoned Pyrolysis Operations

There are a number of pyrolysis plants that have ceased operating or where no recent documentation of operations can be found. Most of these were only at pilot or demonstration scale, although at least two were considered to be industrial-scale operations. Several of the more significant plants are listed below.

- Dynamotive built two woodchip-fed flash pyrolysis facilities in Canada, which ceased operations in 2010 (Meier et al. 2013). The plant at West Lorne, Ontario began operations in 2005 and processed up to 130 t/day of dry woodchips and sawdust. The Guelph plant, also located in Ontario, began operating in 2007 and accepted 200 t/day of wood waste. Both plants used bubbling fluidised beds to carry out pyrolysis (Briens et al. 2008; Dynamotive 2008).
- Choren was operating a slow pyrolysis and gasification facility in Germany using a stirred heated kiln design. The plant processed up to 180 t/day of woody biomass and agricultural residue to produce syngas before it filed for insolvency in 2011. The technology was sold to Linde Engineering, who intends to continue the development of the pyrolysis process (Choren 2008; Balan et al. 2013).
- The largest slow pyrolysis facility with the purpose of oil production was the Evritania demonstration plant in Greece. The plant used a fluidised bed and processed up to 35 t/day of biomass (Zabaniotou and Karabelas 1999).

- The largest vacuum pyrolysis reactor was Pyrodev's 70 t/day facility in Jonquière, Québec, Canada (Garcìa-Pèrez et al. 2002; Gupta et al. 2002). It was recently reported that the facility will be moved to Oregon, United States, where it will recommence operations as a char production facility (Meier et al. 2013).
- Planning for commercial screw feeder pyrolysis units processing 50 t/day have been documented; however, there has been no further evidence in the literature of the completion of these facilities (Bridgwater and Peacocke 2000).

5.3.4 Summary of Activities

In summary, the largest commercial-scale pyrolysis facility is the Kior plant, which uses a catalytic pyrolysis process (of unknown pyrolysis reactor type), with a capacity of up to 500 t/day of biomass. This is followed by the circulating fluidised bed of Ensyn's Renfrew plant, which processes 100 t/day. Other fast pyrolysis reactor configurations that have been implemented at demonstration or pilot scale include the Lurgi twin screw reactor, the rotating cone design implemented by BTG and the ablative pyrolysis design constructed by Pytec.

Heated kilns are the most common designs for slow pyrolysis reactors, although this technology has only been developed to commercial scale for Mitsubishi Heavy Industries/Mie Chuo Kaihatsu's 100 t/day plant in Japan, which primarily produces gas. Slow pyrolysis has not yet reached large-scale commercial processing quantities for oil production. The Evritania demonstration plant in Greece, now decommissioned, was the largest plant and processed up to only 35 t/day of biomass. Table 5.3 summarises the current status of each major reactor category.

TABLE 5.3

Current Status of the Major Reactor Types

Reactor Type	Status	Maximum Size (t/day)
Circulating fluidised bed	Commercial	100
Heated kiln	Commercial	100
Twin screw	Demonstration	12
Ablative pyrolysis	Demonstration	6
Bubbling fluidised bed	Commercial (abandoned)	200
Vacuum pyrolysis	Commercial (abandoned)	70
Rotating cone	Commercial (abandoned)	50
Screw feeder/auger	Planned commercial (abandoned)	50

5.4 Comparison of Existing Biomass Pyrolysis Reactor Designs

As outlined in Section 5.3, several different design configurations have been scaled to industrial or demonstration stage. However, all designs still have several technological constraints that must be overcome before widespread adoption of biomass pyrolysis technologies can occur. The major factors restricting the rate of progress and expansion of both fast and slow pyrolysis plants include the reliance on feed material preparation, such as drying and grinding, process efficiency ceilings, scalability limitations, capital expense and product quality. Each reactor design has strengths and weaknesses in these respects. Table 5.4 summarises the general characteristics and challenges of the major reactor styles. These are generic characteristics associated with the reactor design so individual commercial projects may have developed innovations that ameliorate some of these issues.

The major factors restricting further development and expansion of pyrolysis plants include low energy efficiency due to the reactor configuration and requirement for feed pretreatment, difficulty with scaling, high capital costs due to complex designs and poor product quality. Currently, there is no single reactor design described in the literature that is able to overcome these limitations.

5.4.1 Particle Size

Fast pyrolysis reactor designs, with the exception of ablative pyrolysis, are constrained to accept feed biomass particle sizes somewhere between at least 0.5 and 6 mm in diameter depending on the process. Ablative pyrolysis is able to process particle sizes of up to 20 mm due to the constant shear on the particle. A smaller particle size will give a greater surface area to volume ratio, enabling effective heat transfer for an isothermal pyrolysis reaction and allowing complete decomposition of the biomass matter without forming an insulating charcoal layer on the particle surface. Slow pyrolysis designs are generally able to tolerate particles up to 50 mm because there is no requirement for rapid heating or minimising charcoal formation. Attaching a feed grinder to the plant to achieve small particle sizes will serve to increase both capital and operating costs, with greater energy expenditure for smaller particle sizes.

5.4.2 Feed Moisture

Existing pyrolysis reactor designs ideally operate with a feed moisture content of less than 10% (Bridgwater 2003). The higher the moisture content of the feed, the less efficient the pyrolysis process becomes. Any water present in the feed will require energy to be heated to the pyrolysis temperature, and will additionally require the heat of vapourisation at the transition from

TABLE 5.4

Characteristics and Challenges of Each Major Reactor Type

Design	Feed Size	Feed Moisture	Energy Efficiency Considerations	Scalability Limitations	Capital Intensity	Product Quality	Other Challenges	Strengths
Bubbling fluidised bed	<2 mm	<10%	Reduced by feed grinding and feed drying. Small heat energy losses from reactor and piping	Increased residence time with deeper bed, restricted to shallow beds. Bed must maintain proportion so area cannot be scaled without depth increase	Costs increased by requirements for fine grinder, dryer, cyclone/filter, condenser and burner	Oil contains water and high level of ash and charcoal particles	Clogging and fouling of gas handling system due to tars. Aerosols formed are difficult to collect and condense	High yields of oil, good mixing properties and even heat distribution
Circulating fluidised bed	<6 mm	<10%	Reduced by feed grinding and feed drying. Small heat energy losses from reactor and solids transport	Increased residence time with deeper bed, restricted to shallow beds. Bed must maintain proportion so area cannot be scaled without depth increase	Costs increased by equipment including fine grinder, dryer, cyclone/filter, condenser and combustor. Fluidised bed combustor more costly than kiln combustor	Oil contains water and high level of ash and charcoal particles	Clogging and fouling of gas-handling system due to tars. Aerosols formed are difficult to collect and condense. Process must be tightly controlled to achieve correct level of charcoal combustion to maintain steady temperature	High yields of oil, good mixing properties and even heat distribution

(continued)

TABLE 5.4 (Continued)

Characteristics and Challenges of Each Major Reactor Type

Design	Feed Size	Feed Moisture	Energy Efficiency Considerations	Scalability Limitations	Capital Intensity	Product Quality	Other Challenges	Strengths
Rotating cone	<0.2–6 mm	<10%	Reduced by feed grinding and feed drying. Some heat loss from reactor wall	Heated surface area (reactor wall) to volume (biomass) ratio restricts scalability. Limit of cone angle and height	Costs increased by requirement for fine grinder, dryer, cyclone, condenser and combustor. Fluidised bed combustor more costly than kiln combustor	Oil contains water, ash and charcoal particles	Clogging and fouling of gas-handling system due to tars. Process must be tightly controlled to achieve correct level of charcoal combustion to maintain steady temperature	High oil yields, no carrier gas required so fewer aerosols formed
Ablative pyrolysis	<20 mm	<10%	Reduced by feed drying. Some energy losses from heat escaping from heated moving surface. Inefficient reactor heating if using electricity	Heated surface area can be increased although problems may occur with maintaining uniform temperature and short vapour and charcoal residence times. Increased resistance to heated surface movement must be counteracted	Costs increased by requirement for dryer, cyclone, condenser and electrical heating element/burner	Oil contains water and some ash and charcoal particles	Clogging and fouling of gas-handling system due to tars	Greater flexibility of particle size. High oil yields, no carrier gas required

Twin screw	<2 mm	<10%	Reduced by feed grinding and feed drying. Small heat energy losses from reactor and hot gas or heat carrier solids transport	Poorer mixing with increased size. Increased residence time with deeper beds must be avoided by faster screw rotation	Costs increased by requirement for fine grinder, dryer, condenser and combustor	Oil contains water and some ash and charcoal particles	Clogging and fouling of gas-handling system due to tars. Process must be tightly controlled to achieve correct level of gas/charcoal combustion to maintain steady temperature	Able to produce high yields of oil. Good mixing properties, no requirement for carrier gas
Vacuum pyrolysis	20–50 mm	<10%	Reduced by feed drying. Some heat loss from reactor walls. Additional losses if heating walls use heat transfer medium rather than direct heating	Scalability restricted by need to maintain above the critical ratio of heated surface area of reactor walls to volume of biomass	Mechanically complex. Costs increased by requirement for dryer, condenser, vacuum pumps, airtight seals and feed and discharge devices. Expenses from heating system if using liquid heat transfer medium to supply heat to walls	Clean, minimal charcoal particles in liquid. Generates more water than other pyrolysis processes	Clogging and fouling of gas-handling system due to tars	Clean oil produced with relatively high yields despite long residence time. No carrier gas required

(continued)

TABLE 5.4 (Continued)

Characteristics and Challenges of Each Major Reactor Type

Design	Feed Size	Feed Moisture	Energy Efficiency Considerations	Scalability Limitations	Capital Intensity	Product Quality	Other Challenges	Strengths
Heated kiln	5–50 mm	<10%	Reduced by feed drying. Some heat loss from reactor wall	Scalable lengthways, limited by kiln diameter if externally heated. Not practical to increase beyond certain length	Kiln cost low due to simplicity. Costs increased by requirement for dryer, condenser and burner	Gas can contain particulates and tar, may be very acidic. High moisture content in gas and/or oil if feed is not dried before pyrolysis	Clogging and fouling of gas-handling system due to tars	Simple reactor design with a range of options for mixing. Able to produce high char yields
Auger/screw feeder	5–50 mm	<10%	Reduced by feed drying. Some heat loss from reactor wall	Scalable lengthways, limited by diameter if externally heated. Not practical to increase beyond certain length	Costs increased by requirement for dryer, condenser and burner	Gas can contain particulates and tar, may be very acidic. High moisture content in gas and/or oil if feed is not dried before pyrolysis	Clogging and fouling of gas handling system due to tars	Easy mixing and transport through reactor. Able to produce high char yields

liquid to gas. Moreover, all pyrolysis reactors designed to produce oil accomplish oil retrieval by condensing the vapours produced, including water vapour, which is mixed with the oil product. Similarly for processes producing gas, the water content of the feed will be present in the product gas. High water content in the oil or gas reduces the calorific value of the product. The moisture content of appropriate and accessible biomass typically ranges from 18% for harvested straw (Kadam et al. 2000) to 55% for wood chips (Bain et al. 1998), meaning that feed drying must be incorporated into the system in most cases. Drying will increase the capital costs and reduce the process efficiency as the energy requirement of the latent heat of vapourisation of water is not easily recovered.

5.4.3 Energy Efficiency

The energy requirement of each process depends on a number of factors. The incoming feed qualities, such as particle size and moisture content, will influence the extent of drying and grinding energy needed. The selection of biomass species determines the moisture content, product composition and chemistry and hence the energy contained in the products. The choice of auxiliary equipment, such as separators, condensers and combustors, will affect the energy expended on the process.

For most reactor designs, the process efficiency is significantly reduced by the feed drying stage due to the energy requirement of the latent heat of evaporation of the water. Drying is one of the most energy-intensive steps of pyrolysis, with moisture evaporation requiring more than 10% of the energy value of raw biomass when woody feedstocks are used. Feed grinding also represents a reasonable proportion of energy input to the process, with greater energy required for smaller particle sizes. Although the influence is not major in comparison to the energy lost from feed drying, the mechanism of heat transfer to the reactor will also slightly alter the overall efficiency of the process. Depending on the particulars of the design, some systems will have greater heat loss than others. For reactors using gas-to-solid or solid-to-solid heat transfer, the losses are from transferring the heat twice because the heat must first be transferred to the gas or carrier particles by combustion before they are introduced to the pyrolysis reactor. Additional heat loss may occur during the transport of the gas or heat carrier particles back to the reactor. Heat provided by a hot gas stream, such as in a fluidised bed, will allow both convective and conductive gas-to-solid and solid-to-solid heat transfer, and is thus a fairly rapid means of achieving uniform heating. The major mechanism of heat transfer for reactors using heat carrier particles is conduction between the solids, which will also allow a reasonable rate of transfer if there is sufficient particle mixing.

Reactors with indirect or external heating may experience heat losses through the outside surface of the heating jacket or housing around the reactor, with insulation reducing the heat loss effect. Most other designs will also experience some heat loss through the outside surfaces of the reactor. External heating has a slow rate of heat transfer because the heat must be conducted through the reactor walls before being transferred to the biomass where there is only a limited surface area available for heat transfer. Good mixing is essential as particle contact with the hot wall is much more effective than conduction through the biomass alone. Without mixing, the heat transfer will be poor and will result in a nonuniform temperature profile along the cross-section of the reactor.

In ablative pyrolysers, the biomass is indirectly heated, where the heat transfer occurs through a moving surface heated by combustion gases or electricity. Electrically heating the disk is very inefficient due to the associated inefficiencies of electricity generation so direct heating is the likely preferable option to minimise energy losses. Ablative heat transfer is very rapid, although it only occurs to one surface of the particle. Placing pressure on the biomass against the moving surface will enhance heat transfer; however, this will also increase the resistance of the moving surface and require more energy.

The consumption of gas and oil to create energy for the feed preparation steps and inefficient heating reduces the net product output, and therefore places a restrictive ceiling on the maximum efficiency of current fast and slow pyrolysis processes.

5.4.4 Scalability

Further expansion of the biomass pyrolysers is inhibited by the inability to scale-up some of the current designs, particularly those with a geometry that have a critical heating surface area to volume ratio, which are unable to provide sufficient heat contact area for an increased volume of feed material. Rotating cone reactors provide heat to the biomass through contact with the cone walls. The available heated surface area of the reactor per unit volume of biomass will decrease with either an increased volume of material or a larger reactor size. Similarly, vacuum pyrolysers with heated walls or heated tubes will be restricted by the ability to provide sufficient heat as reactor volume is increased. Ablative pyrolysers can increase the throughput volume by increasing the contact area available for ablation, although this may slightly increase the vapour and charcoal residence times, and it may be more difficult to achieve evenly distributed heating over the ablative surface.

Externally heated kilns and augers also have a limited maximum diameter to allow the biomass volume sufficient contact with the wall. These reactors can be enlarged by increasing the length of the reactor; however, the biomass must be moved faster through the kiln to maintain the same residence time. It is usually impractical to increase the length of the reactor beyond a certain point.

The fluidised bed reactors are restricted by the need to maintain correct fluidisation properties and mixing. Fluidised bed reactors are limited to a reasonably shallow bed depth if very short residence times are to be achieved. The shallow bed depth restricts the size of the bed area as the dimensions must remain within a set ratio to achieve the correct fluidisation dynamics and avoid channelling of the gas. Twin screw reactors experience longer biomass residence times and less effective mixing as size increases, although this can be countered to a certain extent by increasing the rotational velocity of the two screws.

Some facilities with scalability limitations have increased their capacity by resorting to building modular plants. Modularisation can be an expensive solution if the design is capital intensive, as is the case with most of the fast and slow pyrolysis reactors.

5.4.5 Capital Cost

Capital costs are generally higher when building a plant with a design that is more complex or has a requirement for numerous pieces of auxiliary equipment. The overall capital cost of existing systems is heightened by the cost for dryers and grinders needed to suitably prepare the feed biomass. Most reactors receive the necessary process heat from the combustion of either or both gas and charcoal products and therefore combustion equipment must be installed. The combustors may be as simple as burners for gas combustion, where heat transfer to the reactor is achieved by direct combustion heat, in the case of heated kilns and augers, or hot gas, in the case of bubbling fluidised beds. Where the heat is being transferred to the reactor via heat carrier particles such as in circulating fluidised beds, rotating cones and twin screw reactors, then the heat carrier particles are usually heated by gas or charcoal combustion. The combustion may occur using a kiln or chamber, although some processes employ more effective but more complicated and costly fluidised beds.

Most existing pyrolysis methods involve extracting the mixture of vapours and noncondensables from the reactor and then separating and condensing the products. These facilities require costly gas-handling systems that usually include a separation procedure using cyclones or hot vapour filtration, a quenching step using condensers or electrostatic precipitation and equipment for gas storage, recycling or immediate use. The gas-handling system is prone to blockage and fouling, and additional equipment may be required to manage aerosols that are formed in high gas flow rate processes.

The vacuum pyrolysis reactor design is generally mechanically complex and faces additional expenses from the purchase of vacuum pumps, seals and airtight feed entry and product discharge devices. The ablative pyrolyser may also have an increased capital expense because it is composed of several complex parts including a device for feeding and pushing biomass against the heated surface, a heating mechanism using electricity or combustion of products, housing to collect the vapour and charcoal and, in most cases, a rapidly moving surface such as a disk or blade. On the other hand, heated kiln pyrolysers offer a less expensive reactor due to the simplicity of the design, although there is still the requirement for associated feed preparation, gas handling and combustion auxiliary equipment.

5.4.6 Product Quality

Most lignocellulosic biomass pyrolysis processes are disadvantaged by the product quality, particularly of the oil, which has high oxygen content and low pH, making it unsuitable as a feedstock for refinery separation. Further upgrading of the pyrolytic oils is recommended to be able to convert them into transport fuels. The upgrading generally consists of hydrothermal processing or oil gasification and reforming.

The pyrolytic oil also contains particulates from ineffective charcoal separation and fine dust entrained in the vapours prior to condensation. In particular, the reactors that use a high-velocity gas flow, such as fluidised beds, experience problems with high levels of charcoal fines being carried through to the oil. Vacuum pyrolysis is the only technology that is able to consistently produce clean oil.

For most existing pyrolysis reactors, the water content of the oil reflects the moisture levels of the feed material. In addition to the reaction water produced, any water contained in the feed biomass will be present in the oil due to the mixture of water vapour and oil vapours being quenched together. The gas product of pyrolysis also contains particulate charcoal and moisture. The importance of clean product oil and gas depends on the expected application of the products. For example, if the products are to be used as a feed for gasification then the presence of particulates is of little relevance.

The charcoal product from most pyrolysis processes is of a quality suitable for the intended purpose, although there are no official standards for charcoal grading. A lack of industry standards and quality grading system means that the composition and properties of pyrolysis products can be variable. The lack of reliability may be causing potential consumers to be wary of the consistency and performance of the product.

References

Agri-therm. http://www.agri-therm.com/. Accessed October 2013.

Alves, S.S.; Figueiredo, J.L. (1986). "Fuel Gas from a Wood Waste Carbonization Reactor." *Fuel* **65**: 1709–1713.

Ba, T.; Chaala, A.; Garcia-Perez, M.; Rodrigue, D.; Roy, C. (2004). "Colloidal Properties of Bio-oils Obtained by Vacuum Pyrolysis of Softwood Bark. Characterization of Water-Soluble and Water-Insoluble Fractions." *Energy and Fuels* **18**: 704–712.

Bain, R.L.; Overend, R.P.; Craig, K.R. (1998). "Biomass-fired Power Generation." *Fuel Processing Technology* **54**: 1–16.

Balan, V.; Chiaramonti, D.; Kumar, S. (2013). "Review of US and EU Initiatives toward Development, Demonstration, and Commercialization of Lignocellulosic Biofuels." *Biofuels, Bioproducts and Biorefining* 7(6): 732–759.

Best Energies. http://www.bestenergies.com/. Accessed September 2008.

Bourgois, J.; Guyonnet, R. (1988). "Characterization and Analysis of Torrefied Wood." *Wood Science Technology* 22: 143–155.

Bridgwater, A.V. (1999). "Principles and Practice of Biomass Fast Pyrolysis Processes for Liquids." *Journal of Analytical and Applied Pyrolysis* 51: 3–22.

Bridgwater, A.V. (2003). "Renewable Fuels and Chemicals by Thermal Processing of Biomass." *Chemical Engineering Journal* 91: 87–102.

Bridgwater, A.V. (2004). "Biomass Fast Pyrolysis." *Thermal Science* 8: 21–49.

Bridgwater, A.V. (2006). "Biomass for Energy." *Journal of the Science of Food and Agriculture* 86: 1755–1768.

Bridgwater, A. (2012). "Review of Fast Pyrolysis of Biomass and Product Upgrading." *Biomass and Bioenergy* 38: 68–94.

Bridgwater, A.V.; Peacocke, G.V.C. (2000). "Fast Pyrolysis Processes for Biomass." *Renewable and Sustainable Energy Reviews* 4: 1–73.

Bridgwater, A.V.; Meier, D.; Radlein, D. (1999). "An Overview of Fast Pyrolysis of Biomass." *Organic Geochemistry* 30: 1479–1493.

Briens, C.; Piskorz, J.; Berruti, F. (2008). "Biomass Valorization for Fuel and Chemicals Production—A Review." *International Journal of Chemical Reactor Engineering* 6: R2.

BTG –Biomass Technology Group. http://www.btgworld.com/. Accessed October 2013.

Butler, E.; Devlin, G.; Meier, D.; McDonnell, K. (2011). "A Review of Recent Laboratory Research and Commercial Developments in Fast Pyrolysis and Upgrading." *Renewable and Sustainable Energy Reviews* 15(8): 4171–4186.

Chaotech Pty Ltd. http://www.chaotech.com.au/biomass.php. Accessed October 2013.

Choren. http://www.choren.com/. Accessed September 2008.

Day, M.; Shen, Z.; Cooney, J.D. (1999). "Pyrolysis of Auto Shredder Residue: Experiments with a Laboratory Screw Kiln Reactor." *Journal of Analytical and Applied Pyrolysis* 51: 181–200.

Di Blasi, C. (1996). "Heat Transfer Mechanisms and Multi-Step Kinetics in the Ablative Pyrolysis of Cellulose." *Chemical Engineering Science* 51: 2211–2220.

Dynamotive. http://www.dynamotive.com/. Accessed September 2008 and October 2013.

Effendi, A.; Gerhauser, H.; Bridgwater, A.V. (2008). "Production of Renewable Phenolic Resins by Thermochemical Conversion of Biomass: A Review." *Renewable and Sustainable Energy Reviews* 12: 2092–2116.

Ensyn. http://www.ensyn.com/. Accessed October 2013.

Garcìa-Pèrez, M.; Chaala, A.; Roy, C. (2002). "Vacuum Pyrolysis of Sugarcane Bagasse." *Journal of Analytical and Applied Pyrolysis* 65: 111–136.

Graham, R.G.; Bergougnou, M.A. (1984). "Fast Pyrolysis of Biomass." *Journal of Analytical and Applied Pyrolysis* 6: 95–135.

Gupta, M.; Yang, J.; Roy, C. (2002). "Predicting the Effective Thermal Conductivity of Polydispersed Beds of Softwood Bark and Softwood Char." *Fuel* 82: 395–404.

Henrich, E.; Weirich, F. (2004). "Pressurized Entrained Flow Gasifiers for Biomass." *Environmental Engineering Science* 21: 53–64.

Henrich, E. (2007). "The Status of the FZK Concept of Biomass Gasification." *2nd European Summer School on Renewable Motor Fuels*, Warsaw, Poland, August 29–31.

Honnery, D.; Ghojel, J.; Stamatov, V. (2007). "Performance of a DI Diesel Engine Fuelled by Blends of Diesel and Kiln-Produced Pyroligneous Tar." *Biomass and Bioenergy* **32**: 358–365.

Janse, A.M.C.; Biesheuvel, P.M.; Prins, W.; van Swaaij, W.P.M. (2000a). "A Novel Interconnected Fluidized Bed for the Combined Flash Pyrolysis of Biomass and Combustion of Char." *Chemical Engineering Journal* **76**: 77–86.

Janse, A.M.C.; de Jong, X.A.; Prins, W.; van Swaaij, W.P.M. (2000b). "Heat Transfer Coefficients in the Rotating Cone Reactor." *Powder Technology* **106**: 168–175.

Joseph, S. (2008). "Bring Biochar to the Market; Materials, Process and Plant Considerations." http://www.bioeconomyconference.org/images/Joseph,Stephen.pdf. Accessed November 2008.

JSIM -Japan Society of Industrial Machinery Manufacturers. (2001). "Introduction of Japanese Advanced Environmental Equipment." http://www.gec.jp/JSIM_DATA/WASTE/WASTE_3/html/Doc_433.html. Accessed October 2013.

Kadam, K.L.; Forrest, L.H.; Jacobson, W.A. (2000). "Rice Straw as a Lignocellulosic Resource: Collection, Processing, Transportation, and Environmental Aspects." *Biomass and Bioenergy* **18**: 369–389.

Kansai Corporation. http://www.kansai-sangyo.co.jp/e-index.html. Accessed October 2013.

Kior Inc. http://www.kior.com/. Accessed October 2013.

Koga, Y.; Tsuneizumi, S.; Tabata, M.; Mizutani, H.; Yamamoto, H.; Amari, T. (2007). "New Biomass Utilization Technologies such as Methane Fermentation and Pyrolysis." *Mitsubishi Heavy Industries Ltd. Technical Review* **44**: 1–5.

Lappas, A.A.; Samolada, M.C.; Iatridis, D.K.; Voutetakis, S.S.; Vasalos, I.A. (2002). "Biomass Pyrolysis in a Circulating Fluid bed Reactor for the Production of Fuels and Chemicals." *Fuel* **81**: 2087–2095.

Lédé, J.; Panagopoulos, J.; Li, H.Z.; Villermaux, J. (1985). "Fast Pyrolysis of Wood: Direct Measurement and Study of Ablation Rate." *Fuel* **64**: 1514–1520.

Lédé, J. (2003). "Comparison of Contact and Radiant Ablative Pyrolysis of Biomass." *Journal of Analytical and Applied Pyrolysis* **70**: 601–618.

Lehmann, J.; Gaunt, J. and Rondon, M. (2006). "Bio-char Sequestration in Terrestrial Ecosystems—A Review." *Mitigation and Adaptation Strategies for Global Change* **11**(2): 395–419.

Machida, K.; Cyaya, K.; Okuno, S.; Yamamoto, H.; Amari, T.; Kitta, T. (2004). "Development of Woody Biomass Gasification and Fuel Production System." *Symposium on Environmental Engineering: The Japan Society of Mechanical Engineers* **14**: 208–211.

Maggi, R.; Delmon, B. (1994). "Comparison Between 'Slow' and 'Flash' Pyrolysis Oils from Biomass." *Fuel* **73**(5): 671–677.

Mangue, P.D. (2000). "Review of the Existing Studies Related to Fuelwood and/or Charcoal in Mozambique." *Forestry Statistics and Data Collection*, FAO Corporate Document Repository.

Meier, D.; Faix, O. (1997). "State of the Art of Applied Fast Pyrolysis of Lignocellulosic Materials—A Review." *Bioresource Technology* **68**: 71–77.

Meier, D.; van de Beld, B.; Bridgwater, A.V.; Elliott, D.C.; Oasmaa, A.; Preto, F. (2013). "State-of-the-Art of Fast Pyrolysis in IEA Bioenergy Member Countries." *Renewable and Sustainable Energy Reviews* **20**: 619–641.

Okimori, Y.; Ogawa, M.; Takahashi, F. (2006). "Potential of Co$_2$ Emission Reductions by Carbonizing Biomass Waste from Industrial Tree Plantation in South Sumatra, Indonesia." *Mitigation and Adaption Strategies for Global Change* **8**: 261–280.

Pacific Pyrolysis. http://www.pacpyro.com/index.html. Accessed October 2013.

Peacocke, G.V.C.; Bridgwater, A.V. (1994). "Ablative Plate Pyrolysis of Biomass for Liquids." *Biomass and Bioenergy* **7**: 147–154.

Peacocke, G.V.C.; Madrall, E.S.; Li, C.Z.; Güell, A.J.; Wu, F.; Kandiyoti, R.; Bridgwater, A.V. (1994). "Effect of Reactor Configuration on the Yields and Structures of Pine-Wood Derived Pyrolysis Liquids: A Comparison between Ablative and Wire-Mesh Pyrolysis." *Biomass and Bioenergy* **7**: 155–167.

Prins, M.J.; Ptasinski, K.J.; Janssen, F.J.J.G. (2006). "Torrefaction of Wood Part 1. Weight Loss Kinetics." *Journal of Analytical and Applied Pyrolysis* **77**: 28–34.

Pytec. http://www.pytecsite.de/. Accessed October 2013.

Raffelt, C.; Henrich, E.; Koegel, A.; Stahl, R.; Steinhardt, J.; Weirich, F. (2006). "The BTL2 Process of Biomass Utilization Entrained-Flow Gasification of Pyrolyzed Biomass Slurries." *Applied Biochemistry and Biotechnology* **129**: 153–164.

Ringer, M.; Putsche, V.; Scahill, J. (2006). "Large-Scale Pyrolysis Oil Production: A Technology Assessment and Economic Analysis." *National Renewable Energy Laboratory Technical Report*, NREL/TP-510-37779, November.

Schenkel, Y.; Bertaux, P.; Vanwijnbserghe, S.; Carre, J. (1998). "An Evaluation of the Mound Kiln Carbonization Technique." *Biomass and Bioenergy* **14**: 505–516.

Scott, D.S.; Piskorz, J.; Bergougnou, M.A.; Graham, R.; Overend, R.P. (1988). "The Role of Temperature in the Fast Pyrolysis of Cellulose and Wood." *Industrial and Engineering Chemistry Research* **27**: 8–15.

Scott, D.S.; Majerski, P.; Piskorz, J.; Radlein, D. (1999). "A Second Look at Fast Pyrolysis of Biomass—The RTI Process." *Journal of Analytical and Applied Pyrolysis* **51**: 23–37.

Wagenaar, B.M.; Prins, W.; van Swaaij, W.P.M. (1994). "Pyrolysis of Biomass in the Rotating Cone Reactor: Modelling and Experimental Justification." *Chemical Engineering Science* **49**: 5109–5126.

Williams, P.T.; Besler, S. (1996). "The Influence of Temperature and Heating Rate on the Slow Pyrolysis of Biomass." *Renewable Energy* **7**(3): 233–250.

Wu, C.Z.; Yin, X.L.; Yuan, Z.H.; Zhou, Z.Q.; Zhuang, X.S. (2010) "The Development of Bioenergy Technology in China." *Energy* **35**(11): 4445–4450.

Zabaniotou, A.A.; Karabelas, A.J. (1999). "The Evritania (Greece) Demonstration Plant of Biomass Pyrolysis." *Biomass and Bioenergy* **16**: 431–445.

Zaror, C.A.; Pyle, D.L. (1982). "The Pyrolysis of Biomass: A General Review." *Sadhana* **5**: 269–285.

Zhu, X. (2006). "Biomass Fast Pyrolysis to Liquid Fuel in China." http://www.science.org.au/events/australiachina/xifeng.pdf. Accessed September 2008.

6

Hydrothermal Processing of Biomass

Tao Kan and Vladimir Strezov

CONTENTS

6.1 Introduction

The most advanced thermochemical technologies that convert biomass into value-added products, combustion (including co-firing with coal), gasification and pyrolysis, generally utilise dry biomass (usually with a moisture content of <20 wt%) as the feedstock. The need to process high-moisture content biomass fuels has led to the development of hydrothermal processing technologies. The term 'hydrothermal' originates from the geological domain (Jin and Enomoto 2009). Hydrothermal processing can be broadly defined as a technology that utilises subcritical or supercritical water medium at elevated temperature (typically 200°C–800°C) and pressure (typically 5–30 MPa) (Peterson et al. 2008; Pavlovic et al. 2013).

Hydrothermal processing of biomass possesses a number of advantages over other biomass processing technologies for biofuel production:

i. Acceptance of wet biomass and mixed feedstock. Moisture content is one of the main limitations for the high energy efficiency of the biomass-based systems. Wet biomass with moisture content higher than 50% (such as animal manure, algae and wastewater) is generally undesirable for further utilisation as feedstock for various technical and nontechnical reasons. For example, the biomass transportation expense will be increased, and considerable additional heat will be consumed in the drying and torrefaction of wet biomass to be able to meet the feeding requirements, both of which will result in increased operating costs. Additionally, environment-related problems such as unpleasant smell, bacteria and parasites also need to be taken into consideration (Pavlovic et al. 2013). In the case of hydrothermal technology (HTT), water in biomass is not a problem because the water is used as a reaction medium and reactant. For these reasons, HTT provides a promising alternative for processing the wet biomass, such as agricultural wastes, municipal sludge, wastes from food processing and aquatic biomass such as algae. HTT also allows a flexible mixture of different feedstock such as lignocellulose materials and wastes (Peterson et al. 2008).

ii. Selectivity of products. The target products (including a variety of liquid, solid and gaseous biofuels and chemicals) for hydrothermal processing of biomass can be highly flexible. They depend on the physical and chemical properties of water, which are extremely sensitive to the operating temperature and pressure. The HTT can achieve high selectivity of desirable products by tuning the temperature and pressure. Other adjustable operating parameters that affect the selectivity of products include the feedstock concentrations and the presence and types of heterogeneous or homogeneous catalysts.

iii. Product separation. Another outstanding advantage of hydrothermal processing over other conventional biomass conversion technologies is the separation of products from the entire reaction stream.
Through tuning the solvation properties of water near its critical
point, different matter in the stream, including products, can be
partitioned into separate phases according to the difference in their
solubilities (Peterson et al. 2008). Thus, the separation and purification of desired products can be technically achieved.

iv. Energy efficiency. The system energy efficiency is highly dependent
on the heating value of the biomass feedstock, the loading of biomass feeding and the energy recovery. In hydrothermal processing,
the integration of energy recovery into the system can be realised as
the heat in the hot effluent can be recycled to preheat the feed stream
to a high temperature (Demirbas 2009).

v. Other benefits include high biomass throughputs, no biologically
active matter (e.g. bacteria and viruses) in the products owing to
processing at high temperature (Peterson et al. 2008).

Currently, the hydrothermal processing of biomass still generally stays at
the stage of laboratory research and development and pilot/demonstration.
There are still some technical challenges to be overcome before the extensive
commercialisation of hydrothermal processing of biomass is realised.

In this chapter, the fundamental principles of subcritical and supercritical
water medium characteristics for hydrothermal processing are summarised.
Subsequently, four main types of hydrothermal technologies are described,
in particular, the liquefaction and gasification of biomass. Finally, the current
status of biomass hydrothermal processing as well as the remaining issues
to be addressed is reviewed.

6.2 Fundamentals of Hydrothermal Processing

Water can act as a solvent, reactant and catalyst during the hydrothermal
processing of biomass (Pavlovic et al. 2013). It is very important to know how
the properties of the water change with operating temperature and pressure
conditions as well as how they affect biomass reactions. The most relevant
properties involve miscibility, density, dielectric constant, ionic product,
hydrogen bonds, viscosity and diffusion coefficients (Kruse and Dinjus
2007a,b).

Subcritical water (SubCW) refers to the liquid water with a temperature
between 100°C and 374°C and a pressure higher than the corresponding saturation pressure. It is also known as 'pressurised hot water' or 'superheated

water'. In other cases, water below its saturation pressure and 374°C, and water below the critical pressure (i.e. 22.1 MPa) but above 374°C are termed as 'subcritical steam' (Basu and Mettanant 2009).

Supercritical water (SCW) refers to the water above the critical point ($T = 374$°C and $P = 22.1$ MPa), and it behaves as a phase between liquid and gas. No phase transition occurs when varying the temperature and pressure.

In the vicinity of the critical point, the water properties are very sensitive to the changes of temperature and pressure. At a pressure of 24 MPa, the effects of temperature on water density, dielectric constant and ionic product are shown in Figure 6.1.

Density plays an important role in the reaction performance. In the subcritical range, water density is high, which is beneficial to ionic reaction mechanisms. However, as shown in Figure 6.1, in the supercritical range, the water density is much lower, which favours radical reactions (such as the breakdown of C–C bonds in biomass gasification; Pavlovic et al. 2013).

The dielectric constant describes the liquid polarity. Compared with ambient water, the subcritical water possesses a much lower dielectric constant, which makes the subcritical water a good solvent for hydrophobic organic compounds (Carr et al. 2011). For example, the dielectric constant of water at 300°C and 24 MPa is similar to acetone (Kritzer and Dinjus 2001). The not too low dielectric constant also enhances the ionic reactions, making subcritical water a suitable reaction medium for synthesis reactions as well as degradation reactions (e.g. biomass liquefaction; Kruse and Dinjus 2007a).

In the supercritical range, especially by increasing the temperature to more than 500°C, the dielectric constant of the supercritical water decreases to a very low level, becoming a nonpolar solvent favouring free radical reactions.

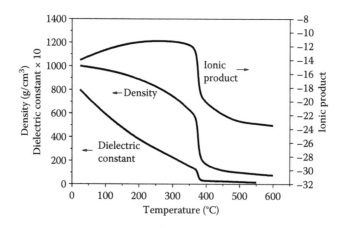

FIGURE 6.1
Water density, dielectric constant and ionic product versus temperature at 24 MPa. (From Kritzer, P. and E. Dinjus, *Chemical Engineering Journal* 83(3): 207–214, 2001.)

The ionic product (K_w, in units of $[mol/L]^2$) of water is defined as the product of the two concentrations of acid H_3O^+ and basic OH^- ions dissociated from water. The ionic product of the subcritical water can reach three orders of magnitude above that of ambient water, enabling the subcritical water to act as an acid/base catalyst (Kruse and Dinjus 2007a). In addition, for the subcritical water and the supercritical water, enhanced mass and heat transfers indicated by high diffusion coefficients and low viscosity increase the reaction rates in the water.

It is generally accepted that one of the main aims of converting biomass to biofuels is the removal of oxygen. Compared with conventional fuels (e.g. gasoline and diesel) with oxygen contents of less than 1%, biomass commonly contains very high oxygen content of more than 40%, which heavily limits the biomass fuel performance, including its higher heating value (HHV; Peterson et al. 2008). Oxygen in biomass is often removed through two main pathways, that is, dehydration reaction in the form of H_2O and decarboxylation reaction in the form of CO_2. The latter pathway is more favourable because the formation of CO_2 also takes away some carbon atoms, which is beneficial to increasing the H/C ratio (one of the important fuel indexes) of the resulting biofuels. Dehydration and decarboxylation reactions can be influenced by the hydrothermal media (i.e. hot compressed water) and the addition of catalysts (Peterson et al. 2008). The most common woody biomass is composed of three major constituents, which are cellulose, hemicellulose and lignin. They exhibit quite different behaviours in hot compressed water.

6.3 Types of Hydrothermal Processing Technologies

Based on the types of target products and the operating conditions, the hydrothermal technologies for processing biomass can be divided into four main categories: TORWASH, hydrothermal carbonisation (HTC), hydrothermal liquefaction (HTL) and hydrothermal gasification (HTG).

6.3.1 TORWASH

TORWASH is a technology that turns wet, fibrous or saline biomass into high-quality pressed fuel pellets (biocoal) that can be co-fired with coal in power plants or incineration plants to produce heat and power (ECN Company 2013). The raw biomass is processed using water at elevated pressures and temperatures, and the water content in the biomass is pressed out without the evaporation of water from the biomass feedstock. Simultaneously, 99% of the salts contained in the biomass are also extracted, making the 'biocoal' suitable for industrial applications without corrosion and bed agglomeration risks caused by salts (Triqua International Company 2013). A consortium consisting of ECN, LEAF, Averinox and Triqua plans to build a pilot plant for TORWASH processing of biomass.

6.3.2 Hydrothermal Carbonisation

HTC of biomass generally processes the biomass at mild conditions at a temperature equal to 250°C or lower, pressure equal to 2 MPa or lower and residence time of between 1 hour and several days, which aims at producing a charcoal-like carbonaceous fuel material (called 'hydrochar' or 'HTC coal') with a high heating value (Pavlovic et al. 2013). This technology is able to convert as much as 50% to 80% of the feedstock to hydrochar product (Libra et al. 2011). Compared with the raw biomass, hydrochar is hydrophobic and fragile with higher mass and energy densities (Reza 2011). The by-products of water-soluble organic fractions from the HTC process consist of sugars, organic acids and 5-Hydroxymethylfurfural (5-HMF), which are useful in a range of applications. In addition, HTC of biomass can also take place at higher temperatures of 300°C to 800°C (so called 'high-temperature HTC process'), favouring the production of special materials such as carbon nanotubes and graphitic carbon (Hu et al. 2010).

The mechanism of HTC is complex and involves a variety of paralleled reactions including hydrolysis, dehydration, decarboxylation, condensation polymerisation and aromatisation (Funke and Ziegler 2010). Biomass components are hydrolysed to form oligomers and monomers (Mok et al. 1992; Minowa et al. 1998). Soluble extractables undergo degradation reactions mainly including dehydration and decarboxylation. In the meantime, condensation polymerisation reactions proceed and hydrochar is then formed. Beside the above reactions, other reaction pathways have also been proposed, such as transformation reactions, demethylation, pyrolytic reactions and Fischer–Tropsch type reactions (Funke and Ziegler 2010). The HTC process is exothermal because it is dominated by dehydration and decarboxylation reactions (Peterson et al. 2008; Funke and Ziegler 2010).

Owing to the flexible operating conditions and products, besides being used as a solid fuel, hydrochars have also found a variety of promising applications, such as absorbent for processing wastewater, carbon fixation, soil amelioration, catalyst support, medicine and gas sensors (Hu et al. 2010; Jiang et al. 2011; Chen et al. 2012).

There are numerous factors that affect the physical and chemical properties (such as the shape, surface structure and elemental composition) of the produced hydrochar. One factor is the composition and structure of the biomass feedstock. For example, Cao et al. (2013) investigated the carbonisation of two different types of biomass (bark mulch and sugar beet pulp) at operating conditions (i.e. 200°C, 3 h) and found that the aromaticity of bark hydrochars was higher than the sugar beet hydrochars due to the remaining lignin residues in the bark hydrochars. It is believed that lignin is somewhat

stable during low-temperature HTC processing and thus remains in the produced hydrochars (Falco et al. 2011).

Besides, the HTC process and characteristics of hydrochar are highly influenced by the operating conditions including the temperature, pressure and
reaction time (Adnadjevic and Popovic 2009; Cao et al. 2013). Temperature
influences the reaction rate of HTC processes to a great extent. With increasing temperature, the rates of paralleled reactions, such as biomass hydrolysis
and fragment polymerisation, can be enhanced (Funke and Ziegler 2010).
Oxygen content in the produced hydrochar is also decreased at higher temperatures (Reza 2011). With increased pressure, reaction equilibrium shifts
to compressed products of solids and liquids. In the subcritical region, more
substances can be extracted from the biomass due to the increased density
and penetration ability at elevated pressures. Longer reaction times are
believed to increase the hydrochar yield because the polymerisation reaction
time to form solid is prolonged (Funke and Ziegler 2010).

Another factor that affects the hydrochar's properties is the addition of
catalysts. For example, the addition of metal-based catalysts may significantly
affect the shape of the carbon nanomaterials produced under low-temperature
HTC conditions (Yu et al. 2004). The presence of iron ions could lead to both
hollow and massive carbon microspheres, whereas iron oxide nanoparticles
could result in very fine, rope-like carbon nanostructures (Cui et al. 2006).

6.3.3 Hydrothermal Liquefaction

HTL is generally described as the transformation of biomass in hot compressed water with medium temperatures of approximately 180°C to 370°C
and high pressures of 4 to 25 MPa, mainly resulting in a hydrophobic mixture of various organics (bio-oil) with a high heating value of 30 to 36 MJ/kg
and an oxygen content of 10% to 20% (Peterson et al. 2008; Xiu and Shahbazi
2012; Pavlovic et al. 2013). Sometimes, additional reducing gas such as H_2 or
CO is applied with the aim of enhancing the oxygen reduction. When the
temperature increases above the water's critical point (374°C), the gasification
process will become dominant (Toor et al. 2011).

Although different components such as cellulose, lignin, lipids and proteins are contained in biomass, the basic pathways of biomass HTL can be
briefly described as a three-step mechanism (Toor et al. 2011):

   i. Depolymerisation of biomass components into monomers by hydro-
      lysis reactions. For example, cellulose breaks down to mainly form
      glucose, and hemicellulose depolymerises into five-carbon sugar
      xylose and other compounds (Peterson et al. 2008)

  ii. Degradation of monomers into smaller compounds/fragments via
      dehydration, dehydrogenation, deoxygenation and decarboxylation
      (Demirbas 2000)

iii. Rearrangement and recombination of reactive fragments to form bio-oil through condensation, cyclisation and polymerisation (Demirbas 2000)

Compared with fast pyrolysis, which has been extensively researched, biomass HTL is still at the stage of early development. The reaction mechanism and kinetics of biomass HTL are very complicated and not yet sufficiently understood, which is partly ascribed to the complexity of the real biomass (Pavlovic et al. 2013). The relevant fundamental studies are more concentrated on the model compounds of biomass, which are the basic components of real biomass, such as cellulose, hemicelluloses, lignin and proteins (Pavlovic et al. 2013; Ruiz et al. 2013). The modelling of hydrothermal processing has also been reviewed (Ruiz et al. 2013).

The HTL bio-oils are generally composed of the same groups of organic oxygenated compounds as the pyrolytic bio-oils generated from the more commonly used technology of biomass fast pyrolysis. The groups primarily consist of alcohols, phenols, carboxylic acids, furans, aldehydes, esters, ketones and straight and branched aliphatic compounds (Zhang et al. 2008; Biller and Ross 2011).

HTL bio-oils also have similar applications to the pyrolytic bio-oils. For example, they can be utilised as the resources for some specialty chemicals. Catalytic upgrading is required to further remove the heteroatoms (mainly oxygen) to produce liquid transportation fuels (e.g. gasoline and diesel), which has been well reviewed recently (Mortensen et al. 2011; Bridgwater 2012; Xiu and Shahbazi 2012).

Parameters that influence HTL performance (including bio-oil yield, char formation, physical and chemical properties of bio-oil, such as pH value, composition, H/C ratio, oxygen content and HHV) include biomass type and composition, biomass particle size, heating rate, temperature, pressure, residence time, catalyst addition and type.

Biomass type and composition have great influence on HTL performance. HTL processing of a number of biomass materials, from model garbage to bagasse and coconut shells, have been reported, and bio-oils with different yields ranging from 27 to 60 wt% and heating values of more than 30 MJ/kg were obtained (Minowa et al. 1995a,b). Generally speaking, biomass with higher contents of cellulose will be beneficial to higher bio-oil yields (Zhang et al. 2008). On the contrary, lignin content will decrease the bio-oil yield and enhance the char formation (Zhong and Wei 2004). In addition, the aromatic compounds in biomass are relevant to the increased density and viscosity of bio-oil (Yin et al. 2010). For certain types of biomass, such as algae and animal wastes, lipids, protein and carbohydrates are the main components. The conversion efficiency of biomass components into bio-oil exhibits in the order of lipids > protein > carbohydrates, which means that higher amounts of lipids and proteins will lead to higher bio-oil yields (Biller and Ross 2011; Vardon et al. 2011).

Biomass particle size and heating rate have limited effect on HTL performance. As mentioned previously, in SubCW and SCW medium, mass and heat transfers are enhanced, which render the roles of biomass particle size and heating rate in HTL processes not as influential as the role they play in conventional fast pyrolysis (Akhtar and Amin 2011). However, residence time acts as an important parameter. In batch reactors, biomass, water and the liquid products are mixed together and experience the same residence time, which enhances the secondary reactions of the hydrolysis products (e.g. sugars) and thus increases, the char yield (Pavlovic et al. 2013). However, in continuous-flow reactors, the very short residence time (only in seconds) minimises the production of gas and char yields from the secondary reactions (Ehara and Saka 2002).

Reaction temperature is a critical parameter in the biomass HTL process. For the biomass HTL in the subcritical range of temperatures (i.e. $T < 374°C$), increasing the temperature generally results in the increased bio-oil and gas yields as well as the decreased oxygen content in the bio-oil. During this process, the content of water-soluble intermediates declines due to their conversion at higher temperatures. On the contrary, at the supercritical range of temperatures, the increased temperature leads to a decrease in the bio-oil yield. However, the gas yield increases at higher temperatures (Barreiro et al. 2013).

Pressure influences HTL performance through changing the water density. In the subcritical region, as the pressure is increased, the water density is also increased. Water medium with higher density can penetrate into the biomass structure more efficiently, which enhances biomass degradation and increases bio-oil yields. However, in the supercritical region, the increase in pressure has very limited effect on water properties, which thus leads to negligible changes in bio-oil yields (Akhtar and Amin 2011).

The addition of catalysts and their types also play a significant role in the HTL of biomass. Both alkaline and acid catalysts have been employed in previous studies. Generally, the addition of alkaline catalysts (e.g. K_2CO_3, KOH, Na_2CO_3 and NaOH) can enhance the bio-oil yields and suppress char formation (Toor et al. 2011). An important role of alkali during the HTL process is in enhancing the water–gas shift reaction (i.e. $CO + H_2O \leftrightarrow CO_2 + H_2$) via the formation of a formate salt, and the produced H_2 can upgrade the bio-oil through hydrotreating reactions (Sinag et al. 2003, 2004). Acid catalysts, including inorganic acids (e.g. HCl and H_2SO_4) and acid salts (e.g. $AlCl_3$), can increase the formation of water-soluble compounds, such as carboxylic acids and 5-HMF (Pavlovic et al. 2013).

6.3.4 Hydrothermal Gasification

HTG of biomass generally occurs at high temperatures of 400°C to 800°C, and pressures of 4.3 to 50 MPa (typically >20 MPa; Osada et al. 2006) and

TABLE 6.1

Reactions during Cellulose Gasification in Supercritical Water

Reaction No.	Reaction Catalogue	Reaction Name	Formula
1	Hydrolysis	Cellulose hydrolysis	$(C_6H_{10}O_5) + nH_2O \rightarrow nC_6H_{12}O_6$(glucose)
2	Intermediate formation	Glucose decomposition	$C_6H_{12}O_6 \rightarrow C_xH_yO_z$, which represents a range of reactions including isomerisation, dehydration, retro-aldol condensation and hydrolysis
3	Steam-reforming	Steam-reforming I	$C_xH_yO_z + H_2O \rightarrow CO + H_2$
4		Steam-reforming II	$C_xH_yO_z + H_2O \rightarrow CO_2 + H_2$
5	Intermediate decomposition	CO formation	$C_xH_yO_z \rightarrow C_mH_nO_r + CO$
6		CO_2 formation	$C_xH_yO_z \rightarrow C_mH_nO_r + CO_2$
7		CH_4 formation	$C_xH_yO_z \rightarrow C_mH_nO_r + CH_4$
8		H_2 formation	$C_xH_yO_z \rightarrow C_mH_nO_r + H_2$
9	Char formation	Char formation	$C_xH_yO_z \rightarrow$ Char
10	Gas species interconversion	Water–gas shift reaction	$CO + H_2O \leftrightarrow CO_2 + H_2$
11		Methanation of CO	$CO + H_2 \leftrightarrow CH_4 + H_2O$

Source: Resende, F.L.P., and P.E. Savage, *AIChE Journal* 56(9): 2412–2420, 2010.

results in hydrogen-rich or methane-rich gaseous products that mainly consist of H_2, CH_4, CO and CO_2 with some amounts of tars, char and bio-oils as undesirable by-products. In the HTG process, water not only acts as the solvent and reactant but also as a catalyst (Pavlovic et al. 2013).

The mechanism of biomass HTG is complex, which is partly ascribed to the complicated structure of various biomass feedstock. Thus, most efforts have been focussed on modelling the HTG reactions of the biomass compounds, such as cellulose and lignin. For example, for cellulose gasification in supercritical water, the gasification process may involve the reactions, shown in Table 6.1.

According to the target gas product and the operating temperature, biomass HTG can be divided into three catalogues as described below.

6.3.4.1 High-Temperature Gasification

In this case, biomass gasification takes place in supercritical water at the high temperatures of 500°C to 800°C, without catalysts or in the presence of non-metal catalysts, resulting in the hydrogen-rich gas. Free radical reactions and water–gas shift reaction are greatly enhanced, leading to H_2 formation, and thus the addition of catalysts could be avoided.

Temperature has obvious effects on gas yield and composition whereas pressure has very limited influence. The addition of catalysts might affect the chemical reactions, and commonly used catalysts are activated carbon and basic alkali salts (Peterson et al. 2008).

6.3.4.2 Moderate-Temperature Gasification

In this case, biomass is processed in subcritical or supercritical water at temperatures ranging from near-critical (~300°C) to 500°C with the participation of catalysts, aiming at the production of methane-rich gas.

Generally, catalysts are required to enhance the reaction rate and achieve satisfying product selectivity. Catalysts should have the ability to gasify the reactive intermediates (mainly phenols and furfurals) generated from the hydrolysis and dehydration of biomass feedstock at a fast speed to minimise the polymerisation reactions and avoid the formation of tars and chars (Peterson et al. 2008).

6.3.4.3 Low-Temperature Gasification

In this case, biomass is treated in subcritical water at temperatures much lower than the water critical point (374°C) to generate a gas mixture. This work is of great significance because hydrogen can be produced at much lower temperatures compared with conventional studies. For example, the hydrogen produced from the gasification of glucose at the low temperatures of approximately 200°C to 300°C and pressures of 3 to 6 MPa was achieved with the aid of the Pt/Al_2O_3 catalyst (Cortright et al. 2002).

6.3.4.4 Gasification Reactors

Thus far, studies on HTG of biomass have been carried out in different types of reactors, including stirred or unstirred batch reactors (Sinag et al. 2004; Furusawa et al. 2007), tubular flow/continuous fixed-bed reactors (Elliott et al. 1994) and continuous stirred tank reactors (Kruse et al. 2005; Basu and Mettanant 2009). Most experimental studies have been performed in batch reactors due to their simple reactor structure and ease of handling. However, the reaction region in the reactor is not necessarily isothermal. Tubular flow reactors realise the continuous gasification of biomass with major problems of plugging and uneven mixing. Continuous stirred tank reactors overcome these problems, but the structure is more complex and is more energy intensive (Basu and Mettanant 2009). The metals in the reactor wall material may have catalytic effects on the gasification process. To segregate this wall effect, small sealed quartz capillaries (ID = 1 mm) were used in a laboratory environment (Potic et al. 2004).

6.4 Development and Current Status of Hydrothermal Technologies

6.4.1 Hydrothermal Carbonisation

Friedrich Bergius, in 1913, first reported the hydrothermal processing of cellulose with the production of coal-like solids, and HTC technology rapidly underwent development due to the discovery of carbon nanotubes in 1991 (Hu et al. 2010). Today, the primary industrial application of biomass HTC technology is the production of coal-like solids as a fuel.

6.4.1.1 AVA-CO2 Industrial Plants

HTC technology was first commercialised at an industrial scale by the AVA-CO2 company in 2010 in Karlsruhe, Germany. The demonstration plant (HTC-0) can convert wet or dry biomass into CO_2-neutral AVA clean coal or CO_2-negative AVA biochar in a continuous process (AVA-CO2 Company 2013a,b). This plant operates at a temperature range of 220°C to 230°C, pressure range of 2.2 to 2.6 MPa with a hydrochar output of approximately 2660 tons/year. It accepts a variety of biomass types, including sewage sludge, garden wastes and the organic fraction of municipal solid wastes. The feedstock is first preheated in a mixing tank at 160°C and 1.0 MPa, and then fed into the reactor. Afterward, the product flow passes through a buffer tank where the heat is recovered in the solid–liquid separation system (Robbiani 2013). Later, in 2012, the AVA-CO2 company established another industrial-scale plant (HTC-1) with a capacity of approximately 11,000 tons of dry biomass per year, carbon efficiency of more than 90% and net energy efficiency of more than 70% (AVA-CO2 Company 2013a,b).

6.4.1.2 SunCoal Pilot Plant

SunCoal Industries built an HTC pilot plant for developing the CarboREN technology in Ludwigsfelde, Germany. From 2008 to 2010, systematic research was carried out on this plant with the aim of producing dry and solid SunCoal biofuel with high energy yields, using a wide range of biomass materials including wood, leaves and grass as feedstock. Energy management, handling of water from the process and input and output procedures were developed. The biofuel produced possessed similar properties to dry brown coal and could be utilised to produce heat and power in power plants (SunCoal Industries 2013).

6.4.1.3 Nàquera Pilot Plant

Ingelia SL, a company located in Valencia, Spain, started commissioning an HTC pilot plant in August 2010. The plant employs operating parameters of temperature between 180°C and 220°C and pressure between 1.7 and 2.4 MPa, with an annual biomass capacity of 1100 tons. Patented 'pressure and temperature control system' and 'inverted flow reactor' were adopted in the plant. Hydrochar products with a gross caloric value of more than 24 MJ/kg, carbon content of more than 60% and bulk density of more than 950 kg/m^3 were obtained (Ingelia SL 2011).

6.4.2 Hydrothermal Liquefaction

In 1971, the U.S. Bureau of Mines speculated on the possibility of converting cellulose, starch and other carbohydrates into oil products by treatment with increased temperature and pressure in the presence of water, carbon monoxide and alkaline salts (White et al. 1987). Then, in the early 1970s, the Bureau of Mines confirmed that the cellulosic materials, wood wastes, urban wastes, sewage sludge and others could be converted into oil with H_2O and CO. Additionally, in the 1970s (Appell et al. 1971; Appell et al. 1975), sponsored by the U.S. Department of Energy, Battelle Pacific Northwest Laboratories carried out a fundamental study on biomass liquefaction using pure cellulose in a series of autoclaves. It was found that the nonvolatile fraction of the produced oil contained 44% aromatic carbon and 7% aromatic hydrogen, whereas the volatile fraction was composed of furans, cyclic ketones, alkene and phenols (White et al. 1987).

In the following sections, some representative biomass liquefaction plants at the pilot or demonstration scale are briefly reviewed.

6.4.2.1 Albany Biomass Liquefaction Experimental Facility

Some pioneering work on biomass liquefaction was conducted by Appell and coworkers at the Pittsburgh Energy Research Center (PERC) in the 1970s, and a pilot plant (Biomass Liquefaction Experimental Facility in Albany, OR) with a design capacity of 1 ton/day was subsequently set up (Elliott 2011). This continuous processing flow (known as the PERC process) employed recycled oil as the reaction media rather than water phase. The wood flour was blended with recycled oil and then preheated by a scraped surface preheater (later replaced with a fired tubular preheater). Afterward, the reaction took place in a stirred-tank reactor, which was later replaced with a standpipe reactor. The effluent stream then passed through an air cooler and a flash tank, and was finally processed with a vacuum distillation tower to extract the distillate of bio-oil products (Elliott 2011). The biomass was processed at temperatures between 300°C and 370°C, pressure of 20 MPa and residence time of 10 to 30 min in the presence of 10% (on feedstock basis) alkaline catalyst (Peterson et al. 2008; Toor et al. 2011). Syngas with a composition of 60% CO and 40% H_2 was added as reducing gas. Oil yield of approximately 53% (on feedstock basis) was obtained. This facility stopped operating in the 1980s due to the drop in petroleum prices and a shift in research interests (Peterson et al. 2008; Elliott 2011).

6.4.2.2 Lawrence Berkeley Laboratory

A derivative technology known as the LBL process was developed by the Lawrence Berkeley Laboratory and was demonstrated in the Albany facility. In this process, wood flour was first prehydrolysed by acid. The produced wood slurry then successively went through a stirrer with the addition of alkali catalyst, a pulp refiner, a fired tubular preheater, an air cooler, flash tank and a gravity separator (Elliott 2011).

6.4.2.3 HTU Process

Another demonstration called the hydrothermal upgrading (HTU) process was carried out by Shell in the 1980s and then abandoned. This system, with a design capacity of 0.1 ton/h, used a wide variety of wet agriculture wastes (e.g. sugar beet pulp and onion waste) as the feedstock and produced approximately 560 L of oil (Elliott 2011). A Dutch consortium with Shell Netherlands and Stork Engineers & Contractors as the main partners resumed the HTU process in 1997, applying heating temperatures of approximately 300°C to 350°C, pressure of 12 to 18 MPa and residence time of 5 to 20 min, and produced bio-oils with a heating value of approximately 30 to 35 MJ/kg and oxygen content of approximately 10% (Goudriaan et al. 2001; Peterson et al. 2008; Toor et al. 2011; Pavlovic et al. 2013).

6.4.2.4 CatLiq Process

A CatLiq process with a capacity of 480 L/day has been developed by SCF Technologies. This pilot-scale facility is located in Herlev outside Copenhagen, Denmark and started running in 2007 (SCF Technologies A/S 2010). It converts wet biomass and organic waste into bio-oil with the addition of K_2CO_3 and zirconia catalysts under the conditions of 280°C to 350°C and 22 to 25 MPa. Bio-oil yield of around 30% to 35% was achieved (Toor et al. 2011). In 2009, engineering and feasibility studies were performed to investigate the next stage of building an industrial-scale demonstration plant (SCF Technologies A/S 2010).

6.4.2.5 Other Related Processes

Other processes, such as treatments of sewage sludge and food-processing wastes, are also related to the biomass hydrothermal processing technologies. In 1980s, a slurry-to-oil reactor system (STORS) in Cincinnati, OH was developed by the Water Engineering Research Laboratory of the U.S. Environmental Protection Agency. It could process 30 L/h of municipal sewage sludge at 300°C, and bio-oil product with a heating value of 36 MJ/kg was obtained (Toor et al. 2011). Changing World Technologies, Inc. activated a large commercial plant based on a thermal conversion process in Carthage, Missouri in 2004. It could convert 250 tons/day of turkey offal and fats into 60,000 L of oil product at 200°C to 300°C and 4 MPa, and the oil product was mainly composed of linear hydro-carbons (Adams and Appel 2004; Roberts et al. 2004; Toor et al. 2011).

6.4.3 Hydrothermal Gasification

In the 1970s, Model and co-workers proposed the conversion of biomass into useful gas products in supercritical water and carried out some pioneering work (Modell et al. 1978). Afterward, several research groups joined this topic and contributed to the development of the biomass HTG. Today, there are a few pilot-scale plants in operation, which are listed below.

6.4.3.1 VERENA

The VERENA pilot plant (a German acronym for 'experimental plant for the energetic use of agricultural materials') was built by the Institut fur Technische Chemie, Forschungszentrum Karlsruhe in Germany. This facil-ity for biomass treatment in SCW started the operation in 2003 and is still in use with a total throughput of 100 kg/h with a maximum design tem-perature of 700°C and pressure of 35 MPa (Institute of Catalysis Research and Technology [IKFT] 2013). The gasification efficiency was reported to be as high as 90% to 98% (Pavlovic et al. 2013). The whole flow can be divided into three main parts, that is, the feed system, the reaction system and the separation system as described below (Boukis et al. 2007). In the feed system, the particle size of the raw biomass particles is reduced to less than 1 mm by a cutting mill followed by a colloid mill. After the biomass power is mixed with a suitable amount of water to form a homogeneous phase, it is pumped into the reaction system by a mass flow–controlled high-pressure metering pump. After preheating, the feed is then introduced into a down-flow reac-tor, which is made up of a vessel with a volume of 35 L. In the separation system, gas–liquid separators and a CO_2 scrubber are installed.

6.4.3.2 Thermochemical Environmental Energy System

The Pacific Northwest National Laboratory, US developed the Thermo-chemical Environmental Energy System (TEES; a registered trademark of Onsite*Ofsite, Inc., Duarte, CA) with the target of catalytical gasification of organic feedstock to methane-rich, medium-Btu fuel gases at temperatures of 250°C to 350°C and pressure of 15 to 20 MPa (Elliott et al. 1993; Sealock et al. 1996). There are optional reactor system designs for the TEES continu-ous pilot-scale operation, including tubular reactors and approximately 38 L/h dual-shell reactor (material: Cr-Mo/Ti). The main components of the process include a mixer/feeder, a homogeniser, a high-pressure pump, a heat exchanger, catalytic reactors, an auxiliary heater, a gas–liquid separa-tor and a membrane separator. This system can process a wide variety of biomass feedstock from high-moisture crops and food processing wastes to wastewater. A product gas with a typical composition of CH_4 of 45% to 60%, CO_2 of 35% to 50%, H_2 of less than 5%, C_2H_6 of less than 2%, C_2H_4 or CO of less than 0.1% and low concentrations of higher hydrocarbons (Sealock et al. 1996).

There are also other pilot plants available, such as the Energia Co. plant in Japan (Matsumura 2005) and the Osaka Gas plant for wastewater treatment (Osaka Gas Company 2013).

6.5 Engineering Obstacles and Challenges

Although hydrothermal technologies for processing biomass have many potential benefits, these technologies still remain at the research and development and pilot/demonstration stage, and are not widely commercialised. There are many reasons for this.

6.5.1 Reactor Designs

Hydrothermal processing of biomass requires a water medium with high pressure and certain temperatures. It is essential that the structure and material of the reactor and other components of the system are specially designed. Although this factor is no longer a technical obstacle, it is the main barrier that is responsible for the high capital cost of biomass hydrothermal plants.

A substantial difficulty is associated with the design and safety considerations due to various corrosion phenomena that can occur in subcritical and supercritical water conditions (Bermejo and Cocero 2006). For example, during biomass gasification in supercritical water, corrosion will take place via active dissolution of metals in the reactor material due to the low electrochemical potentials of the metal oxide film. Metals including Ni, Mo and Cr can suffer from the dealloying due to their reactions with alkaline, acidic chloride or sulphide (Marrone and Hong 2009). Ni alloys (e.g. Inconel 625 and Hasteloy C-276) are mostly used as reactor materials due to their good corrosion resistance and mechanical strength (Toor et al. 2011).

6.5.2 Biomass Loading in the Feed

The biomass loading in the slurry feed is usually at low levels to avoid feeding obstacles, such as a blockage. In scaled-up facilities, biomass loadings of more than 15% to 20% in the feed are required to achieve practical economy. In the case of lower biomass loadings that lead to lower product outputs, the cost related to capital investment, power consumption and heat loss will make the hydrothermal processing economically unviable. Increasing biomass loading in the slurry feed may cause feeding difficulties. Various approaches have been used to resolve this issue, such as using the prehydrolysed feedstock and starch gels with cement pumps (Peterson et al. 2008).

6.5.3 Salt Precipitation

The biomass feedstock used in industrial applications are highly complex, containing a variety of components, including impurities such as inorganic salts. Under atmospheric pressure conditions, water is a good solvent for most salts. However, the solubility of most salts becomes very low (typically 1–100 ppm) in low-density SCW (Armellini and Tester 1991; Armellini et al. 1994; Rogak and Teshima 1999). This results in the precipitation of salts on the reactor walls, causing clogging of the reactor and plugging of catalyst pores even at high flow rates (Kritzer and Dinjus 2001; Peterson et al. 2008). This issue can be addressed by the introduction of a mobile surfaces where salts can settle (Whiting and Metha 1996), increasing the pressure to increase the solubility of salts (Kritzer and Dinjus 2001) and changing the reactor designs (e.g. a reverse flow tank reactor with a brine pool; Marrone et al. 2004).

6.5.4 Catalyst Problems

Heterogeneous catalysts are often used to catalyse the hydrothermal process. Similar to other industrial processes that apply catalysts, these heterogeneous catalysts also undergo the deactivation due to coking, salt plugging at the active pores and poisoning by the sulphate. Maintaining the catalysts' activity throughout the long duration time and regeneration of the deactivated catalysts in scaled-up plants needs to be effectively managed to achieve sustainable long-term operation.

The deactivation problem will not take place if homogeneous catalysts are used. However, the recovery of catalysts from the effluent stream is a challenge (Peterson et al. 2008). Otherwise, the process tends to be less economical, and some environmental problems may be associated with the discharge of liquid waste.

The high nickel content in the commonly used inconel and hastelloy reactor materials often acts as an additional catalyst in the hydrothermal process. A better understanding of the catalytic effect of the reactor wall on the hydrothermal reactions in scaled-up reactors is needed (Peterson et al. 2008).

References

Adams, T. N. and B. S. Appel (2004). Converting turkey offal into bio-derived hydrocarbon oil with the CWT thermal process. *Power-Gen Renewable Energy Conference*. Las Vegas, Nevada.

Adnadjevic, B. and A. Popovic (2009). Hydrothermal transformation of sawdust into synthetic coke-mechanism and influence of experimental parameters. *Energy Sources Part A—Recovery Utilization and Environmental Effects* **31**(10): 807–813.

Akhtar, J. and N. A. S. Amin (2011). A review on process conditions for optimum bio-oil yield in hydrothermal liquefaction of biomass. *Renewable & Sustainable Energy Reviews* **15**(3): 1615–1624.

Appell, H. R., Y. C. Fu et al. (1971). Converting Organic Wastes to Oil: A Replenishable Energy Source. Report of Investigations 7560. Pittsburgh Energy Research Center, Pittsburgh, PA, USA.

Appell, H. R., Y. C. Fu et al. (1975). Conversion of Cellulosic Wastes to Oil. Report of Investigations 8013. Pittsburgh Energy Research Center, Pittsburgh, PA, USA.

Armellini, F. J. and J. W. Tester (1991). Experimental methods for studying salt nucleation and growth from supercritical water. *Journal of Supercritical Fluids* **4**: 254.

Armellini, F. J., J. W. Tester et al. (1994). Precipitation of sodium-chloride and sodium-sulfate in water from sub- to supercritical conditions—150 to 550-degrees-C, 100 to 300 bar. *Journal of Supercritical Fluids* **7**(3): 147–158.

AVA-CO2 Company (2013a). Hydrothermal carbonization (HTC): Simply impressive. Retrieved October 20, 2013, from http://www.ava-co2.com/web/pages/en/technology.php.

AVA-CO2 Company (2013b). Hydrothermal carbonization, how to convert wet biomass to energy? Retrieved October 24, 2013, from http://www.ibc-leipzig.de/typo3/fileadmin/templates/IBC2013/presentation/Klaeusli_AVA_CO2.pdf.

Barreiro, D. L., W. Prins et al. (2013). Hydrothermal liquefaction (HTL) of microalgae for biofuel production: State of the art review and future prospects. *Biomass & Bioenergy* **53**: 113–127.

Basu, P. and V. Mettanant (2009). Biomass gasification in supercritical water—A review. *International Journal of Chemical Reactor Engineering* **7**: 1–61.

Bermejo, M. D. and M. J. Cocero (2006). Supercritical water oxidation: A technical review. *AIChE Journal* **52**(11): 3933–3951.

Biller, P. and A. B. Ross (2011). Potential yields and properties of oil from the hydrothermal liquefaction of microalgae with different biochemical content. *Bioresource Technology* **102**(1): 215–225.

Boukis, N., U. Galla et al. (2007). Biomass gasification in supercritical water. Experimental progress achieved with the VERENA pilot-plant. *15th European Biomass Conference and Exhibition*. Berlin, Germany, 1013–1016.

Bridgwater, A. V. (2012). Review of fast pyrolysis of biomass and product upgrading. *Biomass & Bioenergy* **38**: 68–94.

Cao, X., K. S. Ro et al. (2013). Effects of biomass types and carbonization conditions on the chemical characteristics of hydrochars. *Journal of Agricultural and Food Chemistry*.

Carr, A. G., R. Mammucari et al. (2011). A review of subcritical water as a solvent and its utilisation for the processing of hydrophobic organic compounds. *Chemical Engineering Journal* **172**(1): 1–17.

Chen, J. Z., Z. H. Chen et al. (2012). Calcium-assisted hydrothermal carbonization of an alginate for the production of carbon microspheres with unique surface nanopores. *Materials Letters* **67**(1): 365–368.

Cortright, R. D., R. R. Davda et al. (2002). Hydrogen from catalytic reforming of biomass-derived hydrocarbons in liquid water. *Nature* **418**(6901): 964–967.

Cui, X. J., M. Antonietti et al. (2006). Structural effects of iron oxide nanoparticles and iron ions on the hydrothermal carbonization of starch and rice carbohydrates. *Small* **2**(6): 756–759.

Demirbas, A. (2000). Mechanisms of liquefaction and pyrolysis reactions of biomass. *Energy Conversion and Management* **41**(6): 633–646.

Demirbas, A. (2009). Hydrocarbon-rich products from sunflower oil by alkali catalytic pyrolysis. *Energy Sources Part A—Recovery Utilization and Environmental Effects* **31**(6): 546–552.

ECN Company (2013). Waste flows are turned into fuel by TORWASH. Retrieved October 29, 2013, from https://www.ecn.nl/newsletter/english/2012/september/waste-flows-are-turned-into-fuel-by-torwash/.

Ehara, K. and S. Saka (2002). A comparative study on chemical conversion of cellulose between the batch-type and flow-type systems in supercritical water. *Cellulose* **9**(3–4): 301–311.

Elliott, D. C. (2011). Hydrothermal processing. In *Thermochemical Processing of Biomass: Conversion into Fuels, Chemicals and Power*, R. C. Brown ed. The Atrium, United Kingdom, John Wiley & Sons Ltd.

Elliott, D. C., M. R. Phelps et al. (1994). Chemical-processing in high-pressure aqueous environments. 4. Continuous-flow reactor process-development experiments for organics destruction. *Industrial & Engineering Chemistry Research* **33**(3): 566–574.

Elliott, D. C., L. J. Sealock et al. (1993). Chemical-processing in high-pressure aqueous environments. 2. Development of catalysts for gasification. *Industrial & Engineering Chemistry Research* **32**(8): 1542–1548.

Falco, C., N. Baccile et al. (2011). Morphological and structural differences between glucose, cellulose and lignocellulosic biomass derived hydrothermal carbons. *Green Chemistry* **13**(11): 3273–3281.

Funke, A. and F. Ziegler (2010). Hydrothermal carbonization of biomass: A summary and discussion of chemical mechanisms for process engineering. *Biofuels Bioproducts & Biorefining* **4**(2): 160–177.

Furusawa, T., T. Sato et al. (2007). Hydrogen production from the gasification of lignin with nickel catalysts in supercritical water. *International Journal of Hydrogen Energy* **32**(6): 699–704.

Goudriaan, F., B. van de Beld et al. (2001). Thermal efficiency of the HTU® process for biomass liquefaction. In *Progress in Thermochemical Biomass Conversion*, A. Bridgwater ed. Tyrol, Austria, Blackwell Science, 1312–1325.

Hu, B., K. Wang, et al. (2010). Engineering carbon materials from the hydrothermal carbonization process of biomass. *Advanced Materials* **22**(7): 813–828.

Ingelia SL (2011). Solid HTC biofuel from hydrothermal carbonisation. Retrieved October 24, 2013, from http://www.rhc-platform.org/fileadmin/user_upload/Structure/Biomass/Download/17.-_Marisa_HERNANDEZ.pdf.

Institute of Catalysis Research and Technology (IKFT) (2013). VERENA pilot plant. Retrieved October 28, 2013, from http://www.ikft.kit.edu/english/138.php.

Jiang, W., X. J. Zhang et al. (2011). Preparation and mechanism of magnetic carbonaceous polysaccharide microspheres by low-temperature hydrothermal method. *Journal of Magnetism and Magnetic Materials* **323**(22): 2741–2747.

Jin, F. M. and H. Enomoto (2009). Hydrothermal conversion of biomass into value-added products: Technology that mimics nature. *Bioresources* **4**(2): 704–713.

Kritzer, P. and E. Dinjus (2001). An assessment of supercritical water oxidation (SCWO)—Existing problems, possible solutions and new reactor concepts. *Chemical Engineering Journal* **83**(3): 207–214.

Kruse, A. and E. Dinjus (2007a). Hot compressed water as reaction medium and reactant—Properties and synthesis reactions. *Journal of Supercritical Fluids* **39**(3):362–380.

Kruse, A. and E. Dinjus (2007b). Hot compressed water as reaction medium and reactant—2. Degradation reactions. *Journal of Supercritical Fluids* **41**(3): 361–379.

Kruse, A., A. Krupka et al. (2005). Influence of proteins on the hydrothermal gasification and liquefaction of biomass. 1. Comparison of different feedstocks. *Industrial & Engineering Chemistry Research* **44**(9): 3013–3020.

Libra, J. A., C. Kammann et al. (2011). Hydrothermal carbonization of biomass residuals: A comparative review of the chemistry, processes and applications of wet and dry pyrolysis. *Biofuels* **2**(1): 89–124.

Marrone, P. A., M. Hodes et al. (2004). Salt precipitation and scale control in supercritical water oxidation—Part B: Commercial/full-scale applications. *Journal of Supercritical Fluids* **29**(3): 289–312.

Marrone, P. A. and G. T. Hong (2009). Corrosion control methods in supercritical water oxidation and gasification processes. *Journal of Supercritical Fluids* **51**(2): 83–103.

Matsumura, Y. (2005). Biomass conversion using supercritical water and hydrothermal treatment. Retrieved October 31, 2013, from http://www.biomass-asia-workshop.jp/biomassws/01workshop/material/Yukihiko-matsumura.pdf.

Minowa, T., Z. Fang et al. (1998). Decomposition of cellulose and glucose in hot-compressed water under catalyst-free conditions. *Journal of Chemical Engineering of Japan* **31**(1): 131–134.

Minowa, T., M. Murakami et al. (1995a). Oil production from garbage by thermochemical liquefaction. *Biomass & Bioenergy* **8**(2): 117–120.

Minowa, T., S. Yokoyama et al. (1995b). Oil production from algal cells of dunaliella-tertiolecta by direct thermochemical liquefaction. *Fuel* **74**(12): 1735–1738.

Modell, M., R. C. Reid et al. (1978). Gasification Process. U.S. Pat. No. 4,113,446.

Mok, W. S. L., M. J. Antal et al. (1992). Formation of charcoal from biomass in a sealed reactor. *Industrial & Engineering Chemistry Research* **31**(4): 1162–1166.

Mortensen, P. M., J. D. Grunwaldt et al. (2011). A review of catalytic upgrading of bio-oil to engine fuels. *Applied Catalysis A-General* **407**(1–2): 1–19.

Osada, M., T. Sato et al. (2006). Catalytic gasification of wood biomass in subcritical and supercritical water. *Combustion Science and Technology* **178**(1–3): 537–552.

Osaka Gas Company (2013). Energy-creating wastewater treatment process: Hydrothermal gasification process. Retrieved October 31, 2013, from http://www.osakagas.co.jp/en/rd/technical/1198912_6995.html.

Pavlovic, I., Z. Knez et al. (2013). Hydrothermal reactions of agricultural and food processing wastes in sub- and supercritical water: A review of fundamentals, mechanisms, and state of research. *Journal of Agricultural and Food Chemistry* **61**(34): 8003–8025.

Peterson, A. A., F. Vogel et al. (2008). Thermochemical biofuel production in hydrothermal media: A review of sub- and supercritical water technologies. *Energy & Environmental Science* **1**(1): 32–65.

Potic, B., S. R. A. Kersten et al. (2004). A high-throughput screening technique for conversion in hot compressed water. *Industrial & Engineering Chemistry Research* **43**(16): 4580–4584.

Resende, F. L. P. and P. E. Savage (2010). Kinetic model for noncatalytic supercritical water gasification of cellulose and lignin. *AIChE Journal* **56**(9): 2412–2420.

Reza, M. T. (2011). *Hydrothermal Carbonization of Lignocellulosic Biomass*. University of Nevada, Reno, Nevada.

Robbiani, Z. (2013). *Hydrothermal Carbonization of Biowaste/Fecal Sludge: Conception and Construction of a HTC Prototype Research Unit for Developing Countries*. Swiss Federal Institute of Technology, Zurich, Switzerland.

Roberts, M., J. Williams et al. (2004). Animal waste to marketable products. *Natural Gas Technologies Conference*. Phoenix, Arizona.

Rogak, S. N. and P. Teshima (1999). Deposition of sodium sulfate in a heated flow of supercritical water. *AIChE Journal* **45**(2): 240–247.

Ruiz, H. A., R. M. Rodriguez-Jasso et al. (2013). Hydrothermal processing, as an alternative for upgrading agriculture residues and marine biomass according to the biorefinery concept: A review. *Renewable & Sustainable Energy Reviews* **21**: 35–51.

SCF Technologies A/S (2010). SCF Technologies A/S-Summary March 2010. Retrieved October 20, 2013, from www.scf-technologies.com/file.asp?id=472.

Sealock, L. J., D. C. Elliott et al. (1996). Chemical processing in high-pressure aqueous environments. 5. New processing concepts. *Industrial & Engineering Chemistry Research* **35**(11): 4111–4118.

Sinag, A., A. Kruse et al. (2003). Key compounds of the hydropyrolysis of glucose in supercritical water in the presence of K2CO3. *Industrial & Engineering Chemistry Research* **42**(15): 3516–3521.

Sinag, A., A. Kruse et al. (2004). Influence of the heating rate and the type of catalyst on the formation of key intermediates and on the generation of gases during hydropyrolysis of glucose in supercritical water in a batch reactor. *Industrial & Engineering Chemistry Research* **43**(2): 502–508.

SunCoal Industries (2013). Hydrothermal carbonization pilot plant. Retrieved October 24, 2013, from http://www.suncoal.de/en/technology/htc-pilot-plant.

Toor, S. S., L. Rosendahl et al. (2011). Hydrothermal liquefaction of biomass: A review of subcritical water technologies. *Energy* **36**(5): 2328–2342.

Triqua International Company (2013). Triqua participates in energy from biomass project in The Netherlands. Retrieved October 29, 2013, from http://www.triqua.eu/triqua/fs3_site.nsf/htmlViewDocuments/5D2C2AFAC16F23F7C12 5791F003322AA.

Vardon, D. R., B. K. Sharma et al. (2011). Chemical properties of biocrude oil from the hydrothermal liquefaction of Spirulina algae, swine manure, and digested anaerobic sludge. *Bioresource Technology* **102**(17): 8295–8303.

White, D. H., D. Wolf et al. (1987). Biomass liquefaction utilizing extruder-feeder reactor systems. *American Chemical Society, Division of Fuel Chemistry Preprints*. **32**: 106–116.

Whiting, P. and A. H. Metha (1996). Supercritical water oxidation of organics using a mobile surface. US Patent 5,543,057.

Xiu, S. N. and A. Shahbazi (2012). Bio-oil production and upgrading research: A review. *Renewable & Sustainable Energy Reviews* **16**(7): 4406–4414.

Yin, S. D., R. Dolan et al. (2010). Subcritical hydrothermal liquefaction of cattle manure to bio-oil: Effects of conversion parameters on bio-oil yield and characterization of bio-oil. *Bioresource Technology* **101**(10): 3657–3664.

Yu, S. H., X. J. Cui et al. (2004). From starch to metal/carbon hybrid nanostructures: Hydrothermal metal-catalyzed carbonization. *Advanced Materials* **16**(18): 1636–1640.

Zhang, B., M. von Kcitz et al. (2008). Maximizing the liquid fuel yield in a biorefining process. *Biotechnology and Bioengineering* **101**(5): 903–912.

Zhong, C. L. and X. M. Wei (2004). A comparative experimental study on the liquefaction of wood. *Energy* **29**(11): 1731–1741.

7

Anaerobic Digestion

Annette Evans, Vladimir Strezov and Tim J. Evans

CONTENTS

7.1 Introduction

Anaerobic digestion is the fermentation of organic wastes in the absence of free oxygen (Abbasi et al. 2012). The products of anaerobic digestion are an energy-rich biogas (methane and carbon dioxide) and nutrient-rich digestate (waste liquor and solid waste), which is typically applied as a fertilizer. A typical anaerobic digestion facility using municipal solid waste (MSW) as its feedstock will produce 15% biogas, 42.5% digestate liquor and 42.5% digestate solids by mass (Ostrem et al. 2004).

Anaerobic digestion provides a solution for converting waste into energy, compost and nutrient recovery whilst preventing pollution (Wellinger 2007). Aerobic composting is increasingly being replaced by anaerobic digestion because it enables better odour management and hygiene (Weiland 2005). The production of biogas is one of the most efficient and environmentally beneficial methods of extracting energy from biomass (Weiland 2010). It is also significantly less water intense, with the lowest process water requirement of all biofuels (Al Seadi et al. 2008). Anaerobic digestion is more cost-effective over the course of its life cycle compared with other waste treatment options. Approximately 90% of the energy from degraded biomass is retained as methane (IEA 2005).

7.1.1 History

Anaerobic digestion is an established waste treatment option that has been operated over several centuries. In the developing world, animal wastes, weeds and agricultural wastes are used to generate energy. In the developed world, it has traditionally been used more as a wastewater treatment technology, with any energy generated from the biogas seen as a bonus rather than as a desired product.

Historically, biogas has been a more valuable resource in developing and Eastern countries where access to energy is limited and highly prized. In such countries, small biogas systems produce methane from mostly animal wastes for localised cooking and heating. Up to 18 million rural household biogas digesters were operating in China in 2006, with the total Chinese biogas potential estimated at around 145 billion m³, whereas India had approximately 5 million small-scale biogas plants operating in 2008 (Al Seadi et al. 2008).

The focus in developed countries has been different, as the primary purpose of anaerobic digestion has previously only been on the cost-effective, sanitary decomposition of wastes. Recent renewable energy policy incentives and the push toward waste and greenhouse gas reductions have seen dramatic increases in the uptake of anaerobic technologies in the developed world. Accordingly, biogas production has seen significant growth in recent years, as shown in Figure 7.1.

There has been a big increase in the installation rates of MSW anaerobic digestion plants in Europe in recent years, with more than 120 plants installed between 2001 and 2010 (Weiland 2005). The most significant growth in the industry has been in the United States and Germany, which are now the world's largest biogas producers. Together, these two countries account for more than 50% of the biogas production in 2008, as shown in Figure 7.2. One of the primary influences on this has been the scale of new plants. In 1985, the largest plants had a capacity of 25,000 tonnes/year, current capacities now exceed 500,000 tonnes/year feed capacity (Arsova et al. 2010). Germany has many of the largest installations worldwide, including 'Klarsee' at Penkun, with more than 20 MW installed capacity, or more than 1.5 GW of biogas-based electricity production in the energy park, made up of 40 standardised 500-kW modules (EnviTec Biogas 2006). The main feed substrates are maize, corn and wheat, with manure contributing less than 50% of the feed. Most new plants have electrical capacities of approximately 400 to 800 kW (Abbasi et al. 2012).

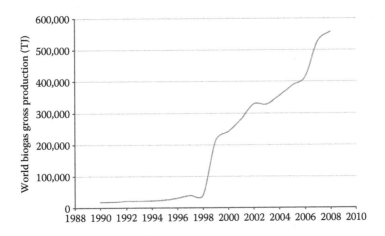

FIGURE 7.1
Historical world biogas gross production. (From UNDP 2012.)

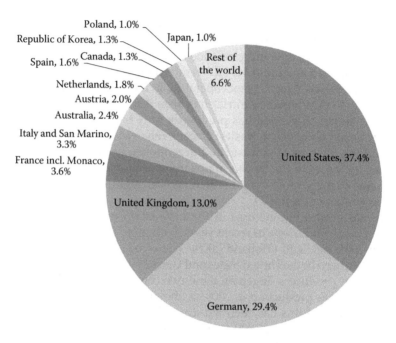

FIGURE 7.2
Worldwide biogas generation distribution by country, 2008. (From UNDP 2012.)

Anaerobic digesters were originally designed for treating sewage sludge and animal manure. Biogas is now produced from manure, sewage, bio-wastes, landfill, energy crops and industrial and municipal wastes. Almost any putrescible material may be digested; however, woody wastes are largely unaffected by digestion as most anaerobes are unable to digest lignin. Lignin will not degrade and can prevent the degradation of fats, carbohydrates and proteins in plant materials (Abbasi et al. 2012). The recent uptake in the western world has also seen a change in focus, with anaerobic digestion no longer just a waste treatment option. Now energy crops are being grown specifically for processing in anaerobic digestion. Common examples of energy crops include maize, miscanthus, sorghum and clover (Al Seadi et al. 2008). These crops typically benefit from pretreatment, and methane yields are improved when codigested with manures (Lehtomäki et al. 2007; Wu et al. 2010).

The advantages of anaerobic digestion over aerobic digestion (composting) include a faster rate of degradation, more stable waste, larger percentage of organics converted into gases, biogas capture, reduced odour emissions and lower sludge production (Walker et al. 2009). Anaerobic digestion is the most efficient and cost-effective means of treating and generating energy from wastes containing less than 30% solids (OECD 2010; Wellinger 2007). Unlike composting, very little heat is generated in anaerobic digestion, instead, the energy, chemically bound in the substrate, remains mainly in the product gas as methane (Al Seadi et al. 2008). Typical conversion efficiencies are between 30% and 60% biomass to biogas, with higher efficiencies at longer residence times. In many cases, biogas is utilised in combined heat and power plants, in which electrical efficiencies are typically 33% and thermal efficiencies are 45% (Appels et al. 2011).

Anaerobic digesters may operate as batch or continuous systems, under mesophilic, thermophilic or psychrophilic conditions. Mesophilic digestion is in the range of 20°C to 45°C, with optimal digestion between 30°C and 38°C. Thermophilic digestion occurs up to 70°C, with optimal digestion between 47°C and 57°C. Psychrophilic digestion occurs at low temperatures (<20°C), with optimal temperatures between 15°C and 20°C. The stability of the reactor is inversely proportional to the digestion temperature, with low temperatures offering the greatest stability. Reactor size has the same relationship to temperature, such that lower temperatures require larger digestion tanks due to the slower rate of digestion. Therefore, mesophilic digestion is considered more stable and is more tolerant of changes than thermophilic digestion, but requires longer residence times, and hence larger digesters. Thermophilic digestion requires a higher energy input than mesophilic digestion; however, more energy is removed from the biomass, with faster reaction rates and greater sterilisation of the product digestate (OECD 2010). Psychrophilic digestion gives overall methane yields comparable to mesophilic digestion; however, production rates are so slow that digester sizes are typically too large to be economical (Safley and Westerman 1990).

Mesophilic digesters are the most common due to the above reasons, but also because mesophilic bacteria are the most prominent and commonly found naturally occurring bacteria in most feed materials. Conversely, thermophilic and psychrophilic bacteria are quite rare; therefore, they typically must be seeded into the digester (Schanbacher 2009).

7.2 Anaerobic Digestion Process

The process of anaerobic digestion occurs over four reaction stages. The reactions can be described as the following:

1. *Hydrolysis.* Complex molecules (large protein macromolecules, fats, cellulose and starch) are converted into simple sugars, long-chain fatty acids and amino acids. Polymers are converted into monomers and oligomers. Hydrolysis is catalysed by the enzymes excreted from the bacteria. The rate of hydrolysis depends on the complexity

of the feedstock, carbohydrates convert quite rapidly, whereas raw cellulosic waste is converted slowly (Ostrem and Themelis 2004). The main reactions and bacteria are the following (Al Seadi et al. 2008):

$$lipids \xrightarrow{lipase} fatty\ acids,\ glycerol$$

$$polysaccharide \xrightarrow{cellulase,\ cellobiase,\ xylanase,\ amylase} monosaccharide$$

$$proteins \xrightarrow{protease} amino\ acids$$

The hydrolysis reaction is given in Equation 7.1

$$C_6H_{10}O_4 + 2H_2O \rightarrow C_6H_{12}O_6 + 2H_2 \qquad (7.1)$$

2. *Acidogenesis or fermentation.* Bacteria convert the products of hydrolysis into volatile fatty acids (VFAs; mainly lactic, propionic, butyric and valeric acid), acetates, alcohols, ammonia, carbon dioxide and hydrogen sulphide, as shown in Equations 7.2 and 7.3

$$C_6H_{12}O_6 \leftrightarrow 2CH_3CH_2OH + 2CO_2 \qquad (7.2)$$

$$C_6H_{12}O_6 + 2H_2 \leftrightarrow 2CH_3CH_2COOH + 2H_2O \qquad (7.3)$$

3. *Acetogenesis.* Further digestion produces acetic acid, carbon dioxide and hydrogen via the routes shown in Equations 7.4 through 7.7

$$CH_3CH_2COO^- + 3H_2O \leftrightarrow CH_3COO^- + H^+ + HCO_3^- + 3H_2 \qquad (7.4)$$

$$C_6H_{12}O_6 + 2H_2O \leftrightarrow 2CH_3COOH + 2CO_2 + 4H_2 \qquad (7.5)$$

$$CH_3CH_2OH + 2H_2O \leftrightarrow CH_3COO^- + 2H_2 + H^+ \qquad (7.6)$$

$$2HCO_3^- + 4H_2 + H^+ \leftrightarrow CH_3COO^- + 4H_2O \qquad (7.7)$$

4. *Methanogenesis.* Methane, carbon dioxide and water are produced by acetotrophic (primary), hydrogenotrophic and methylotrophic bacteria (Abbasi et al. 2012; Al Seadi et al. 2008). The main reactions and bacteria are the following:

$$acetic\ acid \xrightarrow{methanogenic\ bacteria} methane + carbon\ dioxide$$

$$hydrogen + carbon\ dioxide \xrightarrow{methanogenic\ bacteria} methane + water$$

Detailed reactions occurring during methanogenesis are given in Equations 7.8 through 7.11

$$2CH_3CH_3OH + CO_2 \leftrightarrow 2CH_3COOH + CH_4 \qquad (7.8)$$

$$CH_3COOH \leftrightarrow CH_4 + CO_2 \qquad (7.9)$$

$$CH_3OH + H_2 \leftrightarrow CH_4 + H_2O \qquad (7.10)$$

$$CO_2 + 4H_2 \leftrightarrow CH_4 + 2H_2O \qquad (7.11)$$

Other important side reactions are given in Equations 7.12 and 7.13:

$$CH_3COO^- + SO_4^{2-} + H^+ \rightarrow 2HCO_3 + H_2S \qquad (7.12)$$

$$CH_3COO^- + NO^- + H_2O + H^+ \rightarrow 2HCO_3^- + NH_4^+ \qquad (7.13)$$

A simplified generic equation for the entire process is shown in Equation 7.14:

$$C_6H_{12}O_6 \rightarrow 3CO_2 + 3CH_4 \qquad (7.14)$$

The acetotrophic methanogenic reaction shown in Equation 7.9 is the primary methanogenic route, hence theoretical calculations are typically made using this pathway (Abbasi et al. 2012).

Although the anaerobic digestion process can be broken down into four separate stages, realistically, all processes occur simultaneously and synergistically, in that the first group must perform its action before the second reaction can proceed, and so on (Ostrem et al. 2004).

As shown in Equations 7.12 and 7.13, some hydrogen sulphide and ammonia are generated in the process. Therefore, the digestate requires ageing in an aerobic composting to break the ammonia down into nitrates and reduce any odour before application as a fertiliser. It is best to operate the composting under negative pressure to capture and treat waste gases to avoid odour pollution.

According to Bajpai (2001), hydrolysis has a slow rate and is typically the rate-limiting step. This point is clarified by Ostrem et al. (2004), who explain that the rate of hydrolysis is dependent on the molecular complexity of the feedstock, with carbohydrates hydrolysed quite quickly and more complex cellulosic feedstocks hydrolysed quite slowly. Ostrem also states that methanogens have a much slower rate of growth than acidogens and so methanogenesis is typically the rate-controlling step, such that the kinetics of methanogenesis describe the kinetics of the entire process (Davis and Cornwell 1998).

TABLE 7.1

Microorganisms Involved in Anaerobic Digestion

Stage	Reaction	Bacteria
2	Hydrolysing and fermenting	*Bacteroides, Clostridium, Butyrivibrie*
2	Hydrolysing and fermenting	*Eubacterium, Bifodobacterium, Lactobactillus*
3	Acetogenic	*Desulfovibrio, Syntrophobacter wolinii*
3	Acetogenic	*Syntrophomonas*
4	Methanogenesis	*Methanobacterium formicium, M. ruminantium*
4	Methanogenesis	*M. bryantii, Methanobrevibacter*
4	Methanogenesis	*Methanobrevibacter arboriphilus*
4	Methanogenesis	*Methanospirilum hungatei, Methanosarcina barkeri*

Source: Abbasi, T. et al., *Biogas Energy.* SpringerLink ebooks—Engineering, 2012.

7.2.1 Bacteria

The presence of adequate bacterial colonies is essential for efficient digestion. Optimal sources of bacteria include animal manure, slaughterhouse wastes and sewage. For this reason, reactors may be seeded with these materials. There are three groups of bacteria involved in anaerobic digestion, as shown in Table 7.1.

Facultative anaerobes such as Streptococci and Enterobacteriaceae also take part in the hydrolysis and fermentation (Weiland 2010). Although most of the bacteria involved in the process are strict anaerobes such as bacteriocides, clostridia and bifidobacteria (Weiland 2010), strictly speaking, it is only the final methanogenic stage that is truly anaerobic; other cellulolytic, acidogenic and acetogenic bacteria are aerobic or facultative (Abbasi et al. 2012). Methanogenic bacteria occur naturally in deep sediments or in the rumen of herbivores (Ostrem et al. 2004).

7.2.2 Factors Affecting Biogas Production

The most important factors to consider when choosing a biomass feed for anaerobic digestion biogas production are the total solids content, percentage volatile solids, carbon to nitrogen ratio (C/N) and biodegradability of the feedstock. The biogas yield is most strongly a function of volatile solids, organic composition and bioavailability. Gas yield is also a function of the hydraulic and solids retention times, pH, temperature of fermentation, loading rate, inhibitory effects of substrate compounds and intermediate products (e.g. ammonia, VFAs, hydrogen sulphide), toxicity of any feed or reaction products, degree of mixing/agitation and the presence of any pathogens (Abbasi et al. 2012). The effects of each parameter are discussed below.

- *Solids content and dilution*: Solids should be diluted as needed to form an appropriate slurry that can be stirred and allows for gas to flow upwards, but not too thin that particles settle. Each value is reactor specific, but generally 10% to 25% solids.
- *C/N*: A carbon to nitrogen ratio of 20:30 is typically optimal. If the ratio is too high, nitrogen is rapidly consumed by methanogens for protein formation and insufficient nitrogen remains to react with leftover carbon material. If the ratio is too low, nitrogen is liberated and accumulates as ammonia, which increases the pH and exerts a toxic effect on methanogenic bacteria. To maintain an optimal C/N, materials can be mixed as each material has its own inherent C/N.
- *pH*: The optimal input pH value is between 6 and 7. Initially, during digestion, the pH decreases and then increases as the reaction proceeds due to ammonia production. When methane production stabilises, the pH is typically 7.2 to 8.2. Methanogenic bacteria prefer a neutral to slightly alkaline environment and cannot survive at a pH of less than 6 (Ostrem et al. 2004). Running a digester on plant material in which the digester operates in batch mode may require the addition of lime for pH adjustment.
- *Temperature*: Large-scale anaerobic digestion is generally mesophilic, with less thermophilic and much less psychrophilic digestion. Thermophilic digestion is generally more efficient than mesophilic digestion, with a faster digestion rate and consequently smaller digester, but it is more difficult to control, the bacteria are rarer and so typically need to be seeded into the reactor, investment costs are higher and it requires extra energy inputs to maintain the required temperature. Psychrophilic anaerobic digestion is very rare due to the extremely slow rate of digestion at such low temperatures.
- *Loading rate*: The organic loading rate is a measure of the biological conversion capacity of the system. It determines the amount of volatile solids that a system can tolerate. Overloading quickly leads to system failure through inadequate mixing, increased VFA content and decreased pH.
- *Retention time*: The duration of contact in the digester of organic material (substrate) and microorganisms (solids) needed to achieve the desired degradation is the retention time. Reactor efficiency increases and necessary reactor volumes are reduced as the retention time required is lowered. Achieving low substrate retention times requires high simultaneous microorganism (solids) retention time.
  - Hydraulic residence time (HRT). Time that an organic material spends in a digester from entry to exit
  - Solids residence time (SRT or ST). The duration of time active microorganisms spend in the digester. 'Solids' is used to denote

microorganisms in a digester; however, this is not a precise term because most digester feed contains suspended solids, not necessarily made up of live biomass. It is only the volatile solids (VS) content that is involved in anaerobic digestion, nonvolatile or 'refractory' organics are not. In high solids digestion or solid feed digestion, 'solids' is not meant to denote microorganisms

- The relationship between HRT and SRT, and the importance of the 'food to microorganism ratio' (F/M), is such that the ratio of the quantity of substrate to the quantity of bacteria available to consume that substrate (the F/M) is the controlling factor in all biological treatment. The only way to keep the F/M adequately low, whilst reducing the HRT (increasing efficiency) and keeping the SRT high, is to find a way to pass the substrate through quickly and for the microorganisms to pass through much more slowly

- *Toxicity*: Mineral ions, especially of heavy metals and detergents, inhibit normal bacterial growth. Small amounts of minerals such as sodium, potassium, calcium, magnesium, ammonia and sulphur stimulate bacterial growth but higher concentrations are toxic. Heavy metals such as copper, nickel, cobalt, chromium, zinc and lead are essential for bacterial growth in very small quantities but, at higher quantities, are toxic and will prevent the use of the digestate as a fertiliser. Detergents (soap), antibiotics and organic solvents inhibit bacteria. Recovery following toxic inhibition can only be achieved by stopping and flushing or diluting contents to push below the toxic level.

- *Mixing/agitation*: Some form of mixing or agitation is required to maintain fluid homogeneity, thereby producing process stability. The objectives of mixing are to combine incoming material with bacteria, stop scum formation and avoid pronounced temperature gradients within the digester. Rapid mixing can disrupt bacterial communities whereas mixing too slow can cause short-circuiting.

- *Pathogens*: Certain pathogenic bacteria and viruses in MSW can pose a risk of infection to workers. At-risk material needs pretreatment at 70°C for at least 1 h.

7.2.3 Biogas Yields from Different Feedstock

As previously outlined, there is a wide variety of feedstock suitable for anaerobic digestion. Historically, digestion has only used wastes as a feedstock; however, with the increasing uptake of biogas generation in the western world has come an increase in the number of energy crops. Traditional feeds like manure and wastewater give lower methane yields compared with energy-dense crops and slaughterhouse waste. Fats and proteins generate significant amounts of hydrogen and hence provide the highest biogas yield, but unsaturated long-chain fats have poor bioavailability. Short train fats and carbohydrates have the fastest conversion rates but their yield is significantly lower (Abbasi et al. 2012). Under certain conditions, intermediates can be converted into different reaction products than methane, and so the overall biogas yield and methane content vary according to the substrate, biological colonies and reactor conditions used. The typical methane content of biogas is 55% to 65% by volume, but can vary up to between 40% and 70% by volume (Abbasi et al. 2012). The methane yield of a wide variety of substances have been published extensively (e.g. Appels et al. 2011; Qiao et al. 2011).

Animal wastes have several advantages over other anaerobic digestion feedstocks, including the naturally occurring bacterial content, high water content, cheap price and high availability (Al Seadi et al. 2008). However, animal wastes typically have a low methane yield, which can be improved by codigestion with food or agricultural wastes (Al Seadi et al. 2008). When agricultural crops are digested without the addition of stabilising manure, greater process control is required (Weiland 2005). It is typically found that the codigestion of different substances together increases the overall methane yield, compared with single substances digested alone. For example, Macias-Coral et al. (2008) found that, digested alone, the organic fraction of MSW and cow manure gave yields of 0.03 and 0.08 m^3 CH_4 kg^{-1} VS added, respectively. When the two were digested together, the yield increased to 0.1 m^3 CH_4 kg^{-1} VS added. This increase is attributable to the improved carbon to nitrogen ratio and bacteria to food balance seen when mixing substances.

Methane yields are often reported in cubic metres per tonne of volatile solids in the feedstock (m^3/t VS). Because 1 tonne of volatile solid has an energy content of 19 GJ, and 1 m^3 of methane has an energy content of 38 GJ, the maximum theoretical yield of methane is 500 m^3/t VS (Murphy et al. 2011). Alcohols and acids may be present in some silage material, which allows for methane production in excess of the volatile solids limit. According to data from Murphy et al. (2011), the highest yielding feedstocks in terms of methane yield per tonne of volatile solids are barley, triticale, alfalfa and fodder beet at 658, 555, 500 and 500 m^3/t VS, respectively. Murphy et al. (2011) also compared the total energy inputs against outputs for these crops and found that fodder beet gave the best net energy gain, with 4.7 times more energy output than input, followed by potatoes at 4.6 and maize at 4.3.

Although reporting in terms of yield from mass volatile solids input gives information about the extent of volatile solids conversion (efficiency) of the process, it is also important to know the yield of methane per crop growing area when discussing energy crops. Table 7.2 shows the typical methane yield per hectare of typical energy crops. The highest yielding crops per hectare include wheat, sorghum and maize. As with the yields reported in terms of volatile solids, the most productive feedstocks are common food staples in most countries, which raises concerns about competition for agricultural land between energy and food crops.

TABLE 7.2

Methane Yield per Hectare of Different
Energy Crops

Crop	Methane Yield (m³/ha)
Sugar beet	3600–6600
Fodder beet	6400–10000
Maize	8100–14000
Corn cob mix	2400–3800
Wheat	9500–17000
Triticale	7000–9000
Sorghum	6300–14000
Grass	3100–5000
Red clover	1300–2200
Sunflower	2100–3800
Wheat grain	1900–3400
Rye grain	1000–2400

Source: Appels, L. et al., *Renewable and Sustainable Energy Reviews* 15, 4295–4301, 2011.

Amon et al. (2007) compared the methane yield per hectare of several crops grown for the purpose of energy production and found maize to have the highest yield, more than double the possibility of the other crops studied. They also suggest a sustainable crop rotation that integrates food, feed and energy crops by planting a succession of different crops and utilising different components for energy, varying from whole crop to straw and leaf silage.

Current research and development investigations into the physical and chemical pretreatment of lignocellulosic biomass will in time enable efficient enzymatic hydrolysis in the digestion of crops and waste containing lignocelluloses (Mosier et al. 2005; Hendriks and Zeeman 2009). Methods under development include steam, liquid hot water, ammonia and lime pretreatment options.

7.2.4 Applications for Digestate

As well as valuing the energy-rich biogas, attention must be given to the value of the digestate, which is rich in nitrogen, phosphorus and potassium. Tambone et al. (2010) compared the properties of digestate with the raw feed materials (ingestates) and compost. They found that the properties of the digestate differed considerably from both ingestates and compost, with the starting organic mix influencing the final digestate characteristics. They conclude that digestate has excellent fertiliser properties, as it is an abundant source of available nitrogen, phosphorus and potassium, suitable for replacing chemical fertilisers. Soil benefits were also enhanced by the concentrating effect of anaerobic digestion on lignin-like materials, complex lipids and steroids, which have been reported to be humus precursors. Tambone et al. (2009) also found a high degree of biological stability in the digestate, with the oxygen uptake rate being reduced significantly during the process, to a final value typical of that of mature composts.

Another avenue explored for digestate application has been biochar. Inyang et al. (2010) compared the properties of raw (undigested) bagasse with anaerobically digested bagasse digestate, after pyrolysis under the same conditions. They found that the digestate gave a biochar that was superior to the raw bagasse for the purpose of soil amelioration, contaminant remediation or wastewater treatment. They recommend that digestate may be an economical source of producing an environmentally friendly and high-quality biochar. Further work by Inyang et al. (2012) showed that biochars produced from digestate are successful at removing heavy metal impurities from wastewater.

7.2.5 Obstacles to Further Development of Anaerobic Digestion

To facilitate increased development and uptake of anaerobic digestion worldwide, there are some key challenges that need to be overcome. These include issues of

- Reliability
  - Controlled digestion requires sustaining somewhat delicate microbial ecosystems
  - Digesters must have carefully controlled temperatures
  - Inorganic and/or nondigestible waste can damage systems
  - Questions about long-term stability remain
- Investment uncertainty
  - Costly capital but payback times of only 3 to 7 years
- Interconnection with the electricity grid (Mullins and Tikalsky 2012)

7.3 Types of Anaerobic Digestion

7.3.1 Single or Multistage

The anaerobic digestion reactions may be carried out in single-stage or multiple-stage digesters. Single-stage reactors have lower construction costs, but also less control as each reaction stage has a different bacterial mix and requires a specific pH for optimal operation, with reaction stages one to three requiring a low pH and stage four between 6.5 and 8. The biological reactions of different species can be in direct competition with each other. Therefore, acidogenic bacteria lowering the pH can inhibit the critical methanogenic stage and it can be beneficial to separate digestion into two stages. In two-stage reactors, the first three reaction stages occur in one vessel and are then transferred to the second vessel for methanogenesis. Some methane is produced in the first stage (Abbasi et al. 2012).

7.3.2 Low-Rate and High-Rate

Most biogas digesters in China, India and developing countries are low-rate. In the simplest example, water mixed with animal dung is fed into one side of the reactor, spends approximately 40 to 50 days residence time, before the digested slurry and biogas exit at the other end. The reactor represents 70% to 80% of the cost, with operation and maintenance only 20% to 30%. For cost reduction, the reactor size must be reduced, which can only be achieved by increasing efficiency, by lowering the HRT.

The anaerobic-activated sludge process was developed as a high-rate, first-generation process, but it is still slow at 10 to 15 days. A breakthrough was the development of the anaerobic filter (1969), which utilises a means of retaining an active mass of microorganisms in the reactor despite a faster rate of substrate processing and enables low HRTs with high SRTs.

In low-rate digestion, the HRT is the same as the SRT. In high-rate digestion, the retention of active microorganisms means that the HRT is significantly lower than the SRT (Abbasi et al. 2012).

7.3.3 Low-Rate Digestion

Low-rate digesters are suited to animal waste at a low scale, dispersed manner. They are economically viable, net energy producers even at small scale, whereas high-rate digesters would not be viable at this scale.

The major limitations of low-rate digesters are that they lack a provision for stirring; that microbes are removed with the exiting slurry and some of the active microbial populations are washed out, hampering digester performance; and that the bacteria, optimal conditions, kinetics and sensitivity of the last two phases are very different so that the overall yield suffers from the lack of control of each step (Abbasi et al. 2012).

7.3.3.1 Floating Dome

The floating dome reactor, as shown in Figure 7.3, consists of two major parts, the digester and the gas holder. As biogas is produced, it exerts upward pressure on the gas holder, causing it to rise. There is no need for any safety valve as the dome is free to rise under pressure; therefore, there is never extensive pressure buildup. If the digester is greater than 1.5 m in diameter, a vertical partition wall is installed in the middle to prevent short-circuiting and

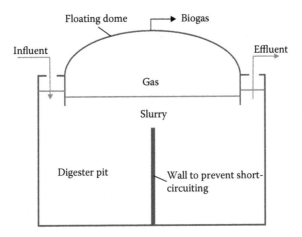

FIGURE 7.3
Floating-dome digester.

encourage complete digestion. Capacities typically range from 1 to 8 m³, but may be as large as 100 m³, processing a slurry with total solids content of approximately 9%, with an HRT of 40 to 55 days (Abbasi et al. 2012).

7.3.3.2 Fixed Dome

As with the floating dome, this reactor consists of two major parts, the digester and the gas holder. Based on the Chinese drumless model shown in Figure 7.4, the difference is that the dome is fixed in place and cannot move. Fixed-dome reactors are cheaper on a volumetric throughput basis compared with floating-dome reactors.

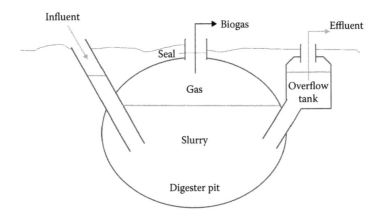

FIGURE 7.4
Fixed-dome digester.

Gas accumulation exerts pressure on the slurry, displacing it to inlet and outlet tanks. Digested slurry that is more than 50 days old is lighter than fresh slurry so that it forms a layer between the gas and the fresh slurry, which is displaced by the pressure, forcing it out of the digester. The feed slurry in fixed-dome reactors typically have solids contents of between 4% and 8%. The most common reactor size and HRT is 2 m^3 and 50 to 66 days, respectively (Abbasi et al. 2012). Digesters are limited to less than 20 m^3 due to the pressure buildup from biogas, and the risk of cracks forming if pressures are exceeded.

7.3.3.3 Balloon Digester

A balloon digester is constructed from an inflatable rubber or plastic, such that the upper portion inflates as it collects biogas, as shown in Figure 7.5. These particular digesters are popular in China due to their immense simplicity and wide range of feeds that may be used, even water hyacinths (Austin and Morris 2012).

Advantages of balloon digesters include their low cost (amongst the lowest of all manure digesters), ease of transport, construction and attaining temperature, as well as the uncomplicated nature of emptying, cleaning and maintenance. However, drawbacks of these systems include their short life (typically 5 years or less), they are easily damaged and there is limited potential for repairs once damage occurs (Abbasi et al. 2012). There is also a very limited amount of gas storage available in a balloon digester (Austin and Morris 2012).

7.3.4 Large-Scale, Low-Rate Digesters

Plug-flow/complete mix digesters are the most common in developed countries, accounting for more than 73% of large-scale manure digesters.

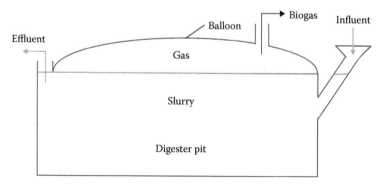

FIGURE 7.5
Balloon digester.

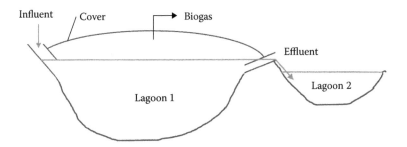

FIGURE 7.6
Covered lagoon digester.

7.3.4.1 Covered Lagoon

The covered lagoon, shown in Figure 7.6, is the simplest form of anaerobic digester. It consists of an anaerobic pond enclosed by an impermeable cover. Best operated with liquid manure at less than 2% solids content. The rate of methane production is a function of the ambient temperature; therefore, it is not efficient at cold temperatures. They are less expensive than other digesters and are effective at reducing odours, but require large areas of land and have poor process control. Due to the slow rate of biogas production, covered lagoons have long residence times and large volumes.

7.3.4.2 Plug-Flow

Plug-flow reactors, pictured in Figure 7.7, are long, tunnel-like or rectangular concrete tanks with airtight corners. Typically, feed enters at one side and exits at the opposite side, but they may also be U-shaped, with the entry and exit at the same end. They can be heated to mesophilic or thermophilic temperatures, with optimal digestion under thermophilic conditions giving an HRT of 15 to 20 days. Optimal solids loading is in the range of 11% to 14%.

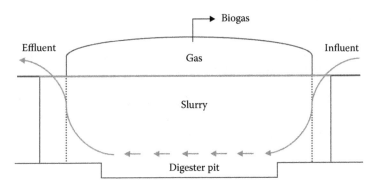

FIGURE 7.7
Plug-flow digester.

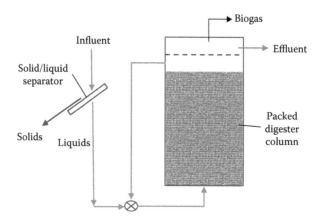

FIGURE 7.8
Fixed-film digester.

7.3.4.3 Fixed Film

A fixed-film digester, as shown in Figure 7.8, is a column packed with media (e.g. wood chips) on which methane-forming bacteria grow and remain anchored. Microorganisms digest the substrate as manure liquid passes through the media. This enables the retention of microorganisms as substrate is passed through the digester, allowing for HRT of less than 5 days and, consequently, small digester volumes. Effluent is typically recycled to maintain a constant upward flow.

Manure solids can plug the media; therefore, solids separation is required predigestion to reduce the solids loading to between 1% and 5%. The efficiency of the system is a function of the efficiency of solids separation. Removing solids predigestion results in some potential biogas loss.

7.3.4.4 Suspended Media

Suspended media digestion relies on manure particles, or granules derived from them, to provide attachment surfaces for microorganisms. There are two common types of suspended media reactors, upflow anaerobic sludge blankets (UASB) and induced blanket reactors (IBR). The primary difference between the two is that UASB are better at digesting dilute waste with less than 3% solids, whereas IBR, shown in Figure 7.9, operate most efficiently with more concentrated wastes, between 6% and 12% total solids. UASB are further explained in high-rate digesters.

7.3.4.5 Anaerobic Sequencing Batch Reactor

The anaerobic sequencing batch reactor (ASBR), shown in Figure 7.10, operates in a cycle of four phases: fill, react, settle and decant. The cycle is repeated

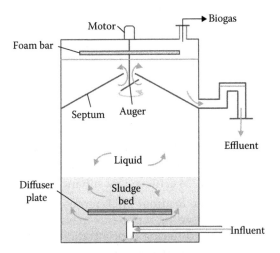

FIGURE 7.9
Induced blanket reactor.

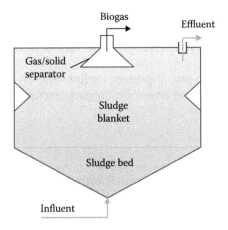

FIGURE 7.10
Anaerobic sequencing batch reactor.

up to four times per day for nearly constant gas production. Liquid retention times can be as short as 5 days. This reactor is well suited to manures in a wide range of concentrations but operates best at very dilute concentrations, less than 1% total solids. If the reactor is filled with active microbes during start-up, it can even produce biogas with completely soluble organic liquids. It is necessary to periodically remove sludge from the reactor.

7.3.5 High-Rate Anaerobic Digesters

High-rate digesters aim to minimise HRT by minimising reactor volumes and maximising flow rates, whilst maximising SRT by retaining microorganisms in the reactor. This is achieved;

1. In attached growth systems by anchoring microorganisms on solid support systems
2. In suspended growth systems, like UASB, by developing highly active sludge of good settling and providing means that sludge doesn't get washed out with exiting treated influent
3. By minimising food, F/M achieved by enhancing SRT/HRT
4. By enhancing digester loading. HRT represents volumetric loading whereas digester loading represents mass loading. As different digester feeds contain differing concentrations of digestible organics, the same HRT but increased substrate concentration provides increased microorganisms and increased biogas

Whereas low-rate digesters have been developed in poorer nations, high-rate digesters have been developed in economically advanced countries. The main objective of high-rate digestion differs accordingly because the focus is not on energy production, but instead on treating biodegradable wastewaters efficiently and economically. These digesters rarely have a positive energy balance.

First generation high-rate digesters include the anaerobic continuously stirred reactor (ACSTR) and anaerobic contact reactor (ACR).

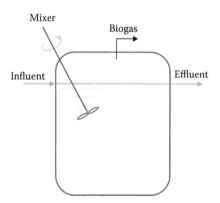

FIGURE 7.11
Anaerobic continuously stirred reactor.

7.3.5.1 Anaerobic Continuously Stirred Reactor

The CSTR, shown in Figure 7.11, is characterised by the provision for mixing continuously or periodically. Mixing can be mechanical, hydraulic or pneumatic, using the compression and sparging of biogas. Gas mixing is preferred in larger reactors. They are operated continuously or semicontinuously by controlling the feed. By insulating and stirring, very large capacities are possible, up to 500 m³ (Walfer 2008). HRTs are around 15 to 20 days. These reactors are well suited to animal wastes.

Advantages of CSTRs include a significant level of experience at operation and the wide range of total solids that can be successfully processed. The main drawback of these systems is that there is no biomass retention, so that microbes are washed away with the effluent.

7.3.5.2 Anaerobic Contact Reactor

The ACR, shown in Figure 7.12, was developed to improve CSTR by retaining microbes. SRT is enhanced as the HRT is lowered. Microbes from the effluent stream are separated and recycled back into the reactor. There is a settling tank in which effluent passes through a portion of activated settled sludge for filtration. The settled sludge and bacterial flocculent are recycled and mixed thoroughly with the feed.

Performance is a function of the microbe efficiency and solids settling. ACRs are best suited to dairy and sugar beet waste. Difficulty is often

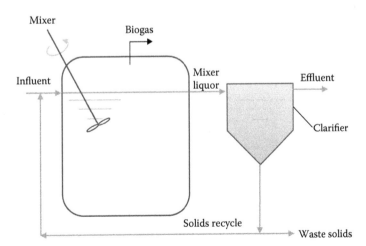

FIGURE 7.12
Anaerobic contact reactor.

encountered in good settling, and in large reactors, it can be difficult to achieve adequate mixing.

7.3.6 Second Generation High-Rate Digesters

Attention in second generation high-rate reactors has focused on the retention of active microflora independent of the HRT and without recycling procedures. These retained biomass reactors include upflow anaerobic filter (UAF), UASB, downflow stationary fixed film (DFSFF) and fluidised bed/expanded bed (FB/EB). In the UAF, DFSFF and FB/EB digesters, there is a reliance on the propensity of bacteria, particularly methanogens, to attach to surfaces of inert support materials to ensure their retention in the reactor (Evans et al. 2011). UASB depends on the aggregation of active flora into dense granules retained in the reactor for extremely long periods by an efficient gas–liquid separator (Lettinga et al. 1981).

7.3.6.1 Upflow Anaerobic Filter

An UAF (Figure 7.13) is a vertical packed column filled in a random fashion with inert support material (e.g. stone, plastic, ceramic or fired clay). The feed distribution header is located in the bottom of the reactor, creating upward flow through submerged support material. Dispersion rings placed at intervals prevent short-circuiting. After wastewater is introduced, active microbial flora gradually develops and become attached as a biofilm to support material surfaces. Microbes are also retained in flocculent form in the interstitial spaces between matrix particles. These digesters are suitable for dilute soluble wastes and wastes with easily degradable suspended material.

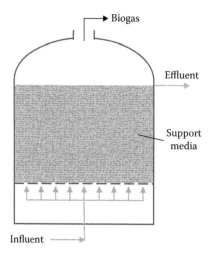

FIGURE 7.13
Upflow anaerobic filter.

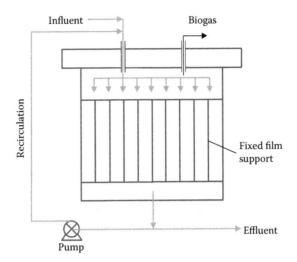

FIGURE 7.14
Downflow stationary fixed-film digester.

7.3.6.2 Downflow Stationary Fixed Film

The DFSFF digesters, as shown in Figure 7.14, have been developed to avoid the problems encountered in UAF of the accumulation of solids and consequent plugging. A DFSFF contains solid packing material like UAF, but operates in downflow mode. Another advantage of DFSFF over UAF is the dispersion of downflowing waste by gas flowing up. The formation and stability of an active biomass film on the support material is vital. These digesters are capable of treating a wide variety of wastes, from dilute to fairly concentrated (Abbasi et al. 2012).

7.3.6.3 Upflow Anaerobic Sludge Blanket

The UASB digesters (Figure 7.15) also seek to overcome plugging issues seen in UAF, by replacing solid packing material with a simple gas collection device. Active microbial biomass forms dense granules that are highly settleable (Abbasi and Abbasi 2011). This achieves a very high concentration of active biomass per unit of working volume.

These digesters are able to operate at very high chemical oxygen demand (COD) loading rates and provide adequate treatment at lower HRTs than is possible in UAF. UASB operate in upflow mode, with feed entering at the bottom on the digester, passing through an active granular sludge and then a gas–liquid–solid separation device. Only liquid effluent flows out of the reactor, the solid sludge settles back in whilst gas is collected in a gas collector. According to Bunger (2005), the UASB is the most widespread system for wastewater treatment in the world.

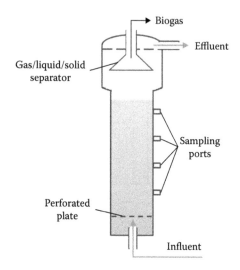

FIGURE 7.15
Upflow anaerobic sludge blanket.

As in UAF, the efficient operation of the system is dependent on suspended growth and the same types of waste are suited. The key to the good performance of the UASB is the quality of the sludge granules (Durai and Rajasimman 2011). Some wastes readily form granular sludge (e.g. sugar wastes and highly volatile acid wastes), others develop it slowly or not at all. This is the major challenge of UASB. Inoculation with large amounts of sludge from a well-functioning UASB often helps. Sludge characteristics may change with different waste types (Ward et al. 2008).

7.3.6.4 Fluidised Bed/Expanded Bed

FB/EB digesters, as shown in Figure 7.16, are similar to suspended growth reactors but use small, inert particles like fine sand or alumina kept in suspension by rapid but even upflow for active biomass growth and attachment. The rate of liquid flow and resulting bed expansion determine whether the bed is fluidised (15%–25% expansion) or expanded (10%–15%). Preferred waste substrates are soluble or easily degradable such as whey, whey permeate, black liquor condensate and others. FB/EB can also treat raw sewerage at fairly high loading rates with high COD removal.

7.3.7 Third Generation High-Rate Digesters

Third generation high-rate digesters were developed to overcome problems of clogging and washout of microbes, to enhance mixing and settling of microbe granules and to treat a larger variety of wastewaters than previous

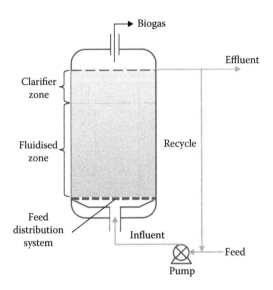

Biogas

Effluent

Clarifier
zone

Fluidised
zone

Recycle

Feed
distribution
system

Influent

Feed

Pump

FIGURE 7.16
Fluidised bed/expanded bed.

digesters. A large number of new digesters have evolved, and these are often hybrids of second generation digesters.

7.3.7.1 UASB-UAF Hybrids

7.3.7.1.1 Upflow Sludge-Bed Filters

The UBF hybrid design, as shown in Figure 7.17, maximises both the biomass retention (characteristic of UAF) and good contact between the biomass and the substrate (characteristic of UASB). These upflow sludge-bed filters generally have a higher efficiency than UAF or UASB.

The general configuration contains two vertical compartments, the upper section operating as a UAF and typically occupying one-third of the reactor volume, the lower section operating as a UASB. The UAF section acts as both a means of retaining biomass and as a solid–liquid–gas separator. Hybrid use has been extended to carbon dioxide sequestration using algae and cyanobacteria (Kumar et al. 2011).

7.3.7.1.2 Modified UASB Reactors

As the UASB is the most used worldwide of all high-rate reactors, it is unsurprising that many modified operations and designs have been developed for different wastes. This includes some that interrupt continuous upflow, increasing performance by providing a better substrate for biomass distribution. Examples include multiplate anaerobic reactor (MPAR; El-Mamouni et al. 1995) and the Biopaq UASB reactor (PAQUES 2012).

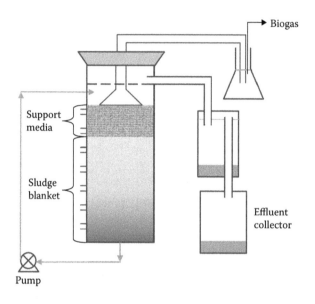

FIGURE 7.17
Upflow sludge-bed filters.

7.4 Biogas Capture from Solid Waste by Solid-State Digestion

Solid-state digestion is the digestion of high solids waste, with feed solids concentrations exceeding 23%, up to 40% solids in the feed (Li et al. 2011). According to Abbasi and Abbasi (2010), problems in anaerobic digestion from solid waste mean that more energy needs to be invested in the process than is gained in biogas. However, the existence of many commercial solid-state anaerobic digesters, including Valorga, Kompogas and Dranco SS-AD, would imply that the process can be made economically viable when correctly applied. Biogas yields of between 0.3 and 0.5 m³ CH₄/kg VS are common (Rapport et al. 2008). There has been a steady increase in dry installation in Europe in the last 5 years due to increasing partial stream digestion and development of increasingly efficient dry fermentation systems (Weiland 2005). Thermophilic digestion is better suited to solid-state digestion than mesophilic digestion as more biogas can be produced at thermophilic temperatures and the start-up period is shortened without significant increases to energy consumption for heating requirements (Li et al. 2011).

Advantages of solid-state digestion over wet digestion include the following:

1. Smaller reactor capacity requirements
2. Less energy used for heating

3. No processing energy needed for stirring

4. The digestate is easier to handle due to the lower water content (Li et al. 2011)

Complications of solid-state digestion include the following:

1. Solid waste cannot be fed to conventional low-rate digesters due to accumulation leading to clogging

2. CSTRs can be used only after shredding to fine pieces and making a slurry, which adds significant energy consumption to the process

3. Food waste and weeds often have less than 4% volatile solids and total solids less than 7%, with 93% to 95% of phytomass as water. This makes them a lean source of energy, with a poor energy yield per unit digester volume, less than is economically viable (Abbasi and Abbasi 2010)

4. Larger amounts of inocula required than for wet systems

5. Much longer retention time needed than wet digestion (Li et al. 2011)

The operation of different solid-state digesters is described in the following subsections.

7.4.1 Multiphase Digestion

Phase separation involves operating anaerobic digestion in distinct phases. Operating all three phases separately is 'three phase', 'three stage', or 'triphasic'. Sometimes, the first and second phases are operated together whereas the methanogenesis phase is run separately. This is known as 'two phase', 'two stage', or 'diphasic'. The products of the first two stages are VFAs, soluble acids used as feed in high-rate digesters (e.g. UAF and UASB).

Phase separation is useful for phytomass as VFAs can be extracted in liquid (aqueous solution) form, making it easy to convert VFAs to biogas in any low-rate or high-rate anaerobic digestion (Sankar Ganesh et al. 2008; Abbasi and Abbasi 2010).

The popularity of two-phase digestion declined sharply between the 1990s and 2010, as it was seen that the advantages of two-phase digestion did not make up for the extra costs and advancements in single-phase digestion, which are making it increasingly efficient (Weiland 2005).

7.4.2 Solid Feed Anaerobic Digestion

Biodegradable solid waste can be fed in solid-state in either chopped pieces or air-dried in specially designed solid feed anaerobic digesters (SFADs). By feeding in larger pieces, some energy is saved that would have been used in shredding. There are two primary designs for SFAD, which are SFAD-1, pictured in Figure 7.18, and SFAD-2, pictured in Figure 7.19. The primary difference between SFAD-1 and SFAD-2 is the separation of liquid from solids, with SFAD-1 separating within the digester and SFAD-2 adding this function as a separate unit.

The term 'solids retention time' here denotes 'solids' as the substrate to be degraded. It is important to differentiate between 'solid feed anaerobic digestion' in which the feed is weeds or phytomass with a volatile solids

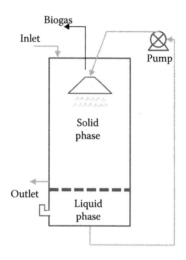

FIGURE 7.18
SFAD-1.

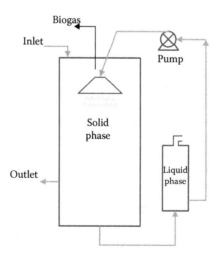

FIGURE 7.19
SFAD-2.

concentration of less than 15%, and 'high-solids anaerobic digestion', which typically works with thick slurries in which volatile solids content exceeds 15%.

The SFAD units depicted above produce VFA-rich leachate, which is converted to biogas in an UAF. SFADs generate some biogas but attaching UAF greatly enhances the yield. These reactors can generate up to 2 m^3 of biogas per cubic metre of reactor volume, making them economically viable. SFAD have steady performance (Abbasi et al. 2012).

7.4.2.1 High-Solids Anaerobic Digestion

The key challenge in biogas is producing a product gas that is economically competitive with natural gas. Major hurdles include the following:

1. Reactor capital costs are a significant economic burden due to large reactor volumes in current processes, operated at low solids levels, typically 3% to 5% solids
2. Reducing reactor volume would improve financial prospects, for example, by increasing the solids load
3. Nonmixed systems tend to have lower rates of gas production than mixed systems
4. High-solids systems are typically focused on batch, nonmixed generation with circulation of effluent
5. Retention times are long, from several weeks at thermophilic temperatures to several months at mesophilic temperatures

Given the economies of scale involved in treating MSW, only large facilities are typically installed, meaning that high tonnages must be processed to obtain reasonably low treatment costs per tonne (Abbasi et al. 2012).

7.4.3 Treating MSW by Anaerobic Digestion

The use of anaerobic digestion to treat MSW is, per tonne of waste, much costlier than landfill, but is still commonly used in developed countries due to the following:

1. The enclosed system allows biogas capture; in landfills, only 30% to 40% is captured, if any at all
2. The end product is a soil conditioner, mixing with animal dung increases the efficiency, allowing for a simpler design and improving economic viability due to a better C/N
3. Diverting easily digestible organic waste to anaerobic digestion over landfill means that better methane capture is possible

Downsides of treating MSW by anaerobic digestion include the following:

1. The nature of organic waste varies; consequently, the C/N and rate of methane production are also variable
2. Inadequate mixing can affect efficiency
3. Large pieces block pipes, which is common in continuous systems (Weiland 2005)

7.4.3.1 Examples of Anaerobic Digestion for Treating MSWs

7.4.3.1.1 Single-Stage Wet Systems

The evolution of MSW/anaerobic digestion began with the adaptation of water-based anaerobic digestion technologies to MSW, for example, the Waasa system.

The Waasa system contains a vertical pulper that homogenises incoming MSW and removes floating debris from the surface and sunken grit from the bottom. Density-fractioned MSW is pumped into the prechamber of a CSTR to alleviate short-circuiting, and an inoculation loop ensures that incoming waste is exposed to microorganisms to minimise acid buildup. The process produces 100 to 150 m³ of biogas per tonne of wet source separated waste. The relatively high yield of biogas indicates high digestibility and good conversion efficiency (Weiland 2005). Installed operating plants have capacities of 3000 to 8500 tons/year and operate either at mesophilic temperatures with a residence time of 20 days or at thermophilic temperatures with a residence time of 10 days (Vandevivere 1999). The strength of this process is its simplicity and longer operating history compared with high-solids systems; however, heavier fractions tend to form a layer at the bottom of the reactor and lighter fractions float to the top and form a scum, which require periodic removal and lower the biogas potential of the unit. Also, maintaining 15% solids content in the reactor requires the addition of significant quantities of water, which increases the digester volume and heating cost, and adds to postdigestion dewatering requirements. These effects offset the gains of the low-cost slurry handling equipment (Verma and Themelis 2002).

7.4.3.1.2 Single-Stage Dry Systems

'Dry' or high-solids systems consists of a feed with a total solids content of 15% or higher, employing special devices to enable the smooth introduction of feed into digesters, for example, screw or piston and screw feeds. Examples include the Dry Anaerobic Composting (Dranco), Kompogas and Valorga processes (Rapport et al. 2008).

The Dranco process is a thermophilic process (50°C–58°C), which uses a vertical silo with feed entering at the top and a conical-shaped bottom auger discharge. There is no internal mixing mechanism, as the fresh feed is mixed with recycled digestate outside the digester at a ratio of one part fresh feed to up to six parts recycled digestate (Rapport et al. 2008; Martin et al. 2003). Typical solids loading in the reactor is 20% to 40% (De Baere 2008). Operating plants typically have capacities of 10,000 to 120,000 tons/year, with retention times of approximately 20 days and average biogas production of 100 to 200 Nm^3/mg of feed (Arsova et al. 2010). According to a study by Erkut et al. (2008), the Dranco process is the best anaerobic digestion technology available in terms of greenhouse gas emissions, energy recovery, material recovered and operating costs.

The Kompogas process uses a horizontal steel tank, fitted with slowly turning axial mixers that help move the material along from the feed chute to the outlet, keep heavy solids entrained in the thick suspension and remove gas as digestion takes place. Inoculation occurs via a recycle loop of digestate added into the feed, where process water may also be added to control the solids content to between 23% and 28% in the reactor (Li et al. 2011). Before entering the digester, feed is mechanically treated for size reduction and contaminant removal. The process is operated at thermophilic temperatures, with retention times between 15 and 20 days (Ostrem and Themelis 2004). Due to the axial mixing, reactor sizes are limited and thus where larger processing volumes are required, several reactors will be run in parallel (Arsova et al. 2010).

The Valorga process is the most popular in the world today, with more than two million tons of installed capacity (IEA 2008). It employs vertical steel tanks fitted with a large central baffle to create plug-flow conditions. Before entering digestion, waste is pretreated to separate inorganic contaminants, then the waste is mixed with water to form a thick sludge, which is fed into the bottom of the reactor. The process may be operated at either mesophilic or thermophilic temperatures (Arsova et al. 2010). A biogas mixing system is used, where recycled biogas re-enters the reactor at the bottom, which mixes the reactor's contents whilst also ensuring adequate contact between fresh feed and mature digestate. By mixing in this way, the process avoids the need to inoculate fresh feed outside the tank before digestion. Process water may be added to maintain a solids content of between 20% and 25% in the reactor (Mata-Alvarez et al. 2000). Retention times in the reactor are between 18 and 25 days, with average biogas production of 80 to 160 Nm^3/mg of waste (Ostrem and Themelis 2004). The main limitation of this process is the biogas mixing system, as the nozzles are often found to clog (Li et al. 2011).

7.4.4 Multistage Systems

In multistage systems, the first stage focuses on high-solids feed hydrolysis and the second on lower solids level methanogenesis, a scheme called a 'wet–dry configuration'. Examples include the Biotechnische

Abfallverwertung GmbH (BTA) and the STRABAG Umweltanlagen GmbH (Strabag, formerly known as the Linde-KCA-Dresden GmbH or Linde) processes.

The BTA process is a multistage low-solids process that consists of a pretreatment and separation stage before digestion. Wastes are mixed with water and fed into a hydropulper where organic and inorganic fractions are separated, then on to a hydrocyclone for grit removal before digestion (Arsova et al. 2010). The solids content of the feed is maintained at 10% and digesters are operated at mesophilic temperatures (Verma and Themelis 2002). Units are available in both single-stage and two-stage digesters, with capacities ranging between 2000 and 150,000 tons/year, average retention times of 12 to 17 days and average biogas production of 85 to 95 Nm³/tonne feed (Ostrem and Themelis 2004).

The Strabag process uses concrete horizontal, plug-flow digesters with a rectangular cross-section. Several agitators are fitted in-line along the length of the digester and a conveyor frame is fitted to the bottom to transfer solids to discharge. Pretreated waste enters the digester using a screw type feeding system. Digestion can be operated in thermophilic or mesophilic modes and with a total solids content between 15% and 45%. Biogas yields are approximately 100 m³/ton feed (Ostrem and Themelis 2004). Installed capacities vary from 1000 to 150,000 ton/year (Strabag 2012).

7.4.5 Batch Solid-State Digestion

Although continuous systems are popular with MSW, for lignocellulosic waste and energy crops, batch processing dominates. Batch reactors have the advantages of simplicity, minimal maintenance requirements, low parasitic energy losses and most importantly low capital cost. Due to their popularity, batch reactors have been the focus of much innovation and development in recent years.

A typical batch system digests organic wastes at between 30% and 40% total solids in a gastight room or vessel. Leachate or digestate from the previous batch may be added with the feed to reduce inoculum requirements. There are benefits and drawbacks to both approaches; leachate is a more concentrated form of bacteria, but results in a wetter digestate than is desired, whereas digestate does not affect dilute the solids content, it adds bulk to the incoming feed, increasing handling costs and the size of the digester required. Systems that recycle leachate are called percolation systems, an example of which is the 'garage type' reactor made by the German company Bekon.

One disadvantage of batch systems is the lack of control over the biological process, particularly due to the lack of mixing. The application of both digestate and leachate to the feed helps reduce excess variability within the digestion pile (Li et al. 2011).

Nomenclature

ACR	anaerobic contact reactor
AD	anaerobic digestion
ASBR	anaerobic sequencing batch reactor
AUF	anaerobic upflow filter
BSW	biodegradable solid waste
C/N	carbon to nitrogen ratio
COD	chemical oxygen demand
CSTR	continuously stirred reactor
DFSFF	downflow stationary fixed film
FB/EB	fixed bed/expanded bed
HRT	hydraulic residence time
MSW	municipal solid waste
SFAD	solid-feed anaerobic digester
SRT	solids (bacterial) residence time
UASB	upflow anaerobic sludge blanket
UBF	upflow sludge bed filters
VFA	volatile fatty acids
VS	volatile solids

References

Abbasi, T. and S. A. Abbasi, Biomass energy and the environmental impacts associated with its production and utilization. *Renewable and Sustainable Energy Reviews* 14 (2010) 919–937.

Abbasi, T. and S. A. Abbasi, Small hydro and the environmental implications of its extensive utilization. *Renewable and Sustainable Energy Reviews* 15 (2011) 2134–2143.

Abbasi, T., S. M. Tauseef and S. A. Abbasi, *Biogas Energy*. SpringerLink ebooks—Engineering, New York, 2012.

Al Seadi, T., D. Rutz, H. Prassl, M. Köttner, T. Finsterwalder, S. Volk and R. Janssen, *Biogas Handbook*, Ed. T. A. Seadi. University of Southern Denmark Esbjerg, Niels Bohrs Vej 9–10, DK-6700 Esbjerg, Denmark, 2008.

Amon, T., B. Amon, V. Kryvoruchko, A. Machmaller, K. Hopfner-Sixt, V. Bodiroza, R. Hrbek, J. Friedel, E. Patsch, H. Wagentristl, M. Schreiner and W. Zollitsch, Methane production through anaerobic digestion of various energy crops grown in sustainable crop rotations. *Bioresource Technology* 98 (2007) 3204–3212.

Appels, L., J. Lauwers, J. Degrève, L. Helsen, B. Lievens, K. Willems, J. Van Impe and R. Dewil, Anaerobic digestion in global bio-energy production: Potential and research challenges. *Renewable and Sustainable Energy Reviews* 15 (2011) 4295–4301.

Arsova, L., N. J. Themelis and K. Chandran, Anaerobic digestion of food waste: Current status, problems and an alternative product, M.S. Degree in Earth Resources Engineering, New York, 2010.

Austin, G. and G. Morris, Biogas Production in Africa. In *Bioenergy for Sustainable Development in Africa*; Springer Netherlands: Dordrecht, The Netherlands, 2012; 103–115.

Bajpai, P. *Microbial Degradation of Pollutants in Pulp Mill Effluents*. Academic Press, New York, 2001, pp. 79–134.

Bunger, J. Bioenergy in Denmark, *IEA Bioenergy News* 17 (2005) p. 8.

Davis, M. and D. Cornwell, *Introduction to Environmental Engineering*. WCB/McGraw-Hill, New York, 1998.

De Baere, L. Partial stream digestion of residual municipal solid waste. *Water Science and Technology* 57 (2008) 1073–1077.

Durai, G. and M. Rajasimman, Biological treatment of tannery wastewater—A review. *Journal of Environmental Science and Technology* 4 (2011) 1–17.

El-Mamouni, R., S. R. Guiot, P. Mercier, B. Safi and R. Samson, Liming impact on granules activity of the multiplate anaerobic reactor (MPAR) treating whey permeate. *Bioprocess and Biosystems Engineering* 12 (1995) 47–53.

EnviTech Biogas, *The World's Largest Biogas Park in Pekun*, EnviTec Biogas, Ed. NAWARO BioEnergie AG, Lohne, Germany, 2006.

Erkut, E., A. Karagiannidis, G. Perkoulidis and S. A. Tjandra, A Multi-Criteria Facility Location Model for Municipal Solid Waste Management in North Greece, *European Journal of Operational Research* 187 (2008) 1402–1421.

Evans, E. A., K. M. Evans, A. Ulrich and S. Ellsworth, Anaerobic processes. *Water Environment Research* 83 (2011) 1285–1332.

Hendriks A. T. W. M. and G. Zeeman, Pretreatments to enhance the digestibility of lignocellulosic biomass. *Bioresource Technology* 100 (2009) 10–18.

IEA, Energy Statistics Manual, 2005.

IEA, World Energy Outlook 2008 Edition, 2008.

Inyang, M., B. Gao, P. Pullammanappallil, W. Ding and A. R. Zimmerman, Biochar from anaerobically digested sugarcane bagasse. *Bioresource Technology* 101 (2010) 8868–8872.

Inyang, M., B. Gao, Y. Yao, Y. Xue, A. R. Zimmerman, P. Pullammanappallil and X. Cao, Removal of heavy metals from aqueous solution by biochars derived from anaerobically digested biomass. *Bioresource Technology* 110 (2012) 50–56.

Kumar, K., C. N. Dasgupta, B. Nayak, P. Lindblad and D. Das, Development of suitable photobioreactors for CO_2 sequestration addressing global warming using green algae and cyanobacteria. *Bioresource Technology* 102 (2011) 4945–4953.

Lehtomäki, A., S. Huttunen and J. A. Rintala, Laboratory investigations on co-digestion of energy crops and crop residues with cow manure for methane production: Effect of crop to manure ratio. *Resources, Conservation and Recycling* 51 (2007) 591–609.

Lettinga, G., R. Roersma, P. Grin, W. de Zeeuw, L. Hulshof Pol, L. van Velsen, S. Hovma and G. Zeeman, *Anaerobic Treatment of Sewage and Low Strength Waste Waters*. In: Proceedings of the Second International Symposium on Anaerobic Digestion, Travemünde, Germany, 1981, pp. 271–291.

Li, Y., S. Y. Park and J. Zhu, Solid-state anaerobic digestion for methane production from organic waste. *Renewable and Sustainable Energy Reviews* 15 (2011) 821–826.

Macias-Coral, M., Z. Samani, A. Hanson, G. Smith, P. Funk, H. Yu and J. Longworth, Anaerobic digestion of municipal solid waste and the effect of co-digestion with dairy cow manure. *Bioresource Technology* 99 (2008) 8288–8293.

Martin, D. J., L. G. A. Potts and V. A. Heslop, Reaction mechanisms in solid-state anaerobic digestion: II. The significance of seeding. *Process Safety and Environmental Protection* 81 (2003) 180–188.

Mata-Alvarez, J., S. Mace and P. Llabres, Anaerobic digestion of organic solid wastes. An overview of research achievements and perspectives. *Bioresource Technology* 74 (2000) 3–16.

Mosier, N., C. Wyman, B. Dale, R. Elander, Y. Y. Lee, M. Holtzapple and M. Ladisch, Features of promising technologies for pretreatment of lignocellulosic biomass. *Bioresource Technology* 96 (2005) 673–686.

Mullins P. A. and Tikalsky S. M., Centre for Climate and Energy Solutions, 2012, http://www.c2es.org/.

Murphy J. D., R. Braun, P. Weiland and A. Wellinger, Biogas from crop digestion. IEA Bioenergy, 2011, http://groengas.nl/wp-content/uploads/2013/07/2011-09-00-Biogas-from-Crop-Digestion.pdf (accessed 6 March 2014).

OECD, *Bioheat, Biopower and Biogas. Developments and Implications for Agriculture.* OECD Publishing, Paris, France, 2010.

Ostrem, K., K. Milltath and N. Themelis, *Combining Anaerobic Digestion and Waste-to-Energy.* ASME, Georgia, 2004, pp. 265–271.

Ostrem, K. and N. J. Themelis, *Greening Waste: Anaerobic Digestion for Treating the Organic Fraction of Municipal Solid Wastes.* Columbia University, New York, 2004, p. 59.

PAQUES, 2012, http://en.paques.nl/pageid=51/Anaerobic_COD_removal.html.

Qiao, W., X. Yan, J. Ye, Y. Sun, W. Wang and Z. Zhang, Evaluation of biogas production from different biomass wastes with/without hydrothermal pretreatment. *Renewable Energy* 36 (2011) 3313–3318.

Rapport J., R. Zhang, B. M. Jenkins and R. B. Williams, *Current Anaerobic Digestion Technologies Used for Treatment of Municipal Organic Solid Waste.* California Environmental Protection Agency, Sacramento, California, 2008.

Safley Jr., L. M. and P. W. Westerman, Psychrophilic anaerobic digestion of animal manure: Proposed design methodology. *Biological Wastes* 34 (1990) 133–148.

Sankar Ganesh, P., R. Sanjeevi, S. Gajalakshmi, E. V. Ramasamy and S. A. Abbasi, Recovery of methane-rich gas from solid-feed anaerobic digestion of ipomoea (*Ipomoea carnea*). *Bioresource Technology* 99 (2008) 812–818.

Schanbacher, F. *Anaerobic Digestion: Overview & Opportunities.* Ohio State University, Wooster, OH, 2009.

Strabag, Dry digestion. STRABAG Umweltanlagen GmbH, Dresden, Germany, 2012.

Tambone, F., P. Genevini, G. D'Imporzano and F. Adani, Assessing amendment properties of digestate by studying the organic matter composition and the degree of biological stability during the anaerobic digestion of the organic fraction of MSW. *Bioresource Technology* 100 (2009) 3140–3142.

Tambone, F., B. Scaglia, G. D'Imporzano, A. Schievano, V. Orzi, S. Salati and F. Adani, Assessing amendment and fertilizing properties of digestates from anaerobic digestion through a comparative study with digested sludge and compost. *Chemosphere* 81 (2010) 577–583.

UNdata, Energy statistics database. United Nations Statistical Division, 2012.

Vandevivere, P., L. De Baere and W. Verstraete, Unpublished manuscript, 1999. Found at Verma, S., 2002: Anaerobic digestion of biodegradable organics in municipal solid wastes. Department of Earth & Environmental Engineering (Henry Krumb School of Mines) Fu Foundation School of Engineering & Applied Science Columbia University.

Verma, S. and N. Themelis, Anaerobic digestion of biodegradable organics in municipal solid wastes, Master of Science Degree in Earth Resources Engineering Columbia University, New York, 2002, p. 56.

Walfer, M. Training material on anaerobic wastewater treatment. Ecosan Expert Training Course, Version 3. Seecon gmbh, Switzerland, 2008.

Walker, L., W. Charles and R. Cord-Ruwisch, Comparison of static, in-vessel composting of MSW with thermophilic anaerobic digestion and combinations of the two processes. *Bioresource Technology* 100 (2009) 3799–3807.

Ward, A. J., P. J. Hobbs, P. J. Holliman and D. L. Jones, Optimisation of the anaerobic digestion of agricultural resources. *Bioresource Technology* 99 (2008) 7928–7940.

Weiland, P. *Results and Bottle Necks of Energy Crop Digestion Plants-Required Process Technology Innovations*, Workshop: Energy Crops and Biogas, Ed. Federal Agricultural Research Centre (FAL). Utrecht, The Netherlands, 2005.

Wellinger, A. (2007) Anaerobic Digestion: Making Energy and Solving Modern Waste Problems. AD-NETT Report 2000, 195 pp. http://www.adnett.org (accessed July 2008).

Weiland, P. Biogas production: Current state and perspectives. *Applied Microbiology and Biotechnology* 85 (2010) 849–860.

Wu, X., W. Yao, J. Zhu and C. Miller, Biogas and CH_4 productivity by co-digesting swine manure with three crop residues as an external carbon source. *Bioresource Technology* 101 (2010) 4042–4047.

8

Esterification

Gary Leung and Vladimir Strezov

CONTENTS

8.1 Introduction

Esterification is a chemical reaction in which two reactants, typically alcohol and an acid, form an ester as a reaction product. Biodiesel processing usually refers to transesterification (also called alcoholysis), which involves changing one ester (oil or fat) into another (alkyl ester). Alkyl esters are also termed biodiesel. Esterification can also refer to the reaction of free fatty acids (FFAs; fatty acid chains formed by the breakdown of conventional oil triglyceride molecules) with alcohol or glycerol to form the alkyl ester biodiesel. This chapter reviews esterification as a concept for biodiesel production, including both strict esterification and the transesterification of oils and fats.

Transesterification of oils and fats is a well-developed process dating back to as early as 1853 when it was first developed by the scientists E. Duffy and J. Patrick. This was many years prior to the development of the first diesel engine. German inventor Rudolf Diesel devised the original diesel compression-ignition engine and demonstrated its performance using vegetable oil at the 1900 World Fair in Paris. At the time, he believed the utilisation of vegetable oils (such as peanut and castor oil) would be the future of his engine and that vegetable oils could one day become as important as petroleum-based fuels.

In the 1920s, technological changes were made by diesel engine manufacturers to produce smaller engines. These changes required lower viscosity of petroleum-derived diesel. The result of this and further calibration of diesel engines meant that vegetable oils no longer ran smoothly. At the same time, the petroleum industry was able to make inroads as they were able to produce much cheaper medium-weight diesel fuels from fossil resources. As a result, for many years, the development of the biomass fuel industry was virtually halted.

More recently, over the past three decades, environmental and energy security concerns have prompted extensive research and development in, and the commercialisation of, biodiesel production by esterification. Transesterification is performed to reduce the high viscosity and flashpoints of component vegetable oils and animal fats to provide fuel with properties closer to that of conventional diesel fuel. Much of the research and development has been involved in optimising esterification reaction conditions and production methods, including work to increase yields, reduce reactions times, reduce costs and simplify the production process. The high price of vegetable oils and concerns about competition with food uses causing starvation in developing countries (Pimentel et al. 2009) have also led to research and development in alternative feedstock sources including waste cooking oils, animal fats and inedible plant oils such as Jatropha and algae. Conventional transesterification involves the use of an alkali catalyst; however, research and development has gone into newer technologies, such as the use of different catalysts including lipase enzymes, noncatalytic supercritical alcohol methods and ultrasonic cavitation.

8.2 Biomass Esterification Process

Typical biodiesel production process through esterification consists of five principal steps: (1) oil production, (2) pretreatment of oils to remove components that would be detrimental to subsequent processing steps, (3) esterification whereby the pretreated oils are reacted with alcohol to form alkyl esters (biodiesel) and glycerol, (4) separation of the glycerol from the alkyl ester and (5) alkyl ester purification to remove any soaps and remaining methanol, catalyst and glycerol. Processes are generally designed to a high level of alkyl ester purity (>98%). The by-product glycerol may also be purified and sold for other applications. Figure 8.1 shows a simplified flow diagram of alkali-catalysed biodiesel processing.

8.2.1 Oils Suitable for Esterification Process

A variety of biolipids can undergo the esterification and transesterification process to produce biodiesel. Various edible and inedible vegetable oils, animal fats, waste greases and oils can be used. More than 350 oil-bearing crops have been identified (Jamieson 1932), although only a limited number of these are considered as viable potential alternative fuel sources for diesel engines. The choice of oils or fats suitable for transesterification to biodiesel is a particularly important decision because it generally has the largest influence on the total cost of producing biodiesel (Demirbas 2007).

The oils and fats used in the esterification process primarily consist of fatty acid triglycerides (also known as triacylglycerides; typically 90%–98%) and have carbon chain lengths mostly between 16 and 22 carbon atoms (Srivastava and Prasad 2000). Triglycerides are esters derived from glycerol with three fatty acids attached. Most vegetable oils are composed of 96% to 98% triglycerides. The remaining 2% to 4% consists of a range of nontriglycerides including FFAs, diglycerides, monoglycerides and phospholipids (Keshwani 2010).

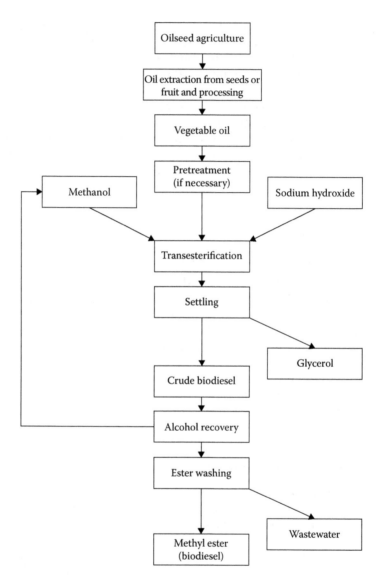

FIGURE 8.1
Simplified flow diagram of alkali-catalysed biodiesel processing.

8.2.1.1 Virgin Vegetable Feedstock Oils and Animal Fats

Rapeseed, soybean, palm and sunflower oils are the most commonly used oils for esterification and transesterification, with more limited use of mustard and hemp oil. Rapeseed is the largest source of oil for esterification globally and has long been grown in Europe due to its preference for a cool moist climate. Rapeseed (also known as rape) is a bright yellow flowering member of the family Brassicacaeae. It is grown for the production of animal feed, for vegetable oil for human consumption and for biodiesel production. Canola is a trademark variety of rapeseed species, characterised by low erucic acid and low glucosinolate contents. Rapeseeds contain approximately 38% to 50% oil on a dry basis. Rapeseed oil is similarly primarily constituted of triglycerides (91.8%–99.0%) and smaller percentages of FFAs (0.5%–1.8%) and phospholipids (up to 4.3%; Wang and Keshwani 2010).

Soybean is the second most commonly used oil for esterification and the dominant oilseed resource in the United States and Argentina. It is favoured for its high oil content for food and fuel purposes, and for its high nutritive protein content (Wang and Keshwani 2010). The oil content of soybeans is relatively low, being 15% to 23%. Soybean oil consists primarily of neutral lipids, of which triglycerides make up 95% to 97%. Phospholipids (1%–3%) and FFAs (<1%) are minor lipid components in the soybean oil.

Oil palm is a tropical plant grown in South and Central America, Africa and Asia as an important source of edible oil. Two types of oil can be extracted from the oil palm: orange red palm oil from the mesocarp and the colourless palm kernel oil from the kernel inside the nut. The oil palm grows in rainy climates and is the highest yielding oil crop. Crude palm oil feedstock can contain high FFA contents (up to 30%) and thus may require pretreatment before conventional transesterification processing.

Sunflower is the fourth largest oil source globally, following rapeseed (including soybean and palm). The annual production of sunflower oil in 2007 was around 27 million tonnes (Food and Agricultural Organisation [FAO] 2008). Major producers are Russia, Ukraine, other European countries and Argentina. Turkey, China and South Africa also produce sunflower oil (FAO 2010). Sunflower is more geographically limited due to specific climatic and soil requirements, such as long day length and fertile, moist, well-drained soil (Gupta 2002). Sunflower seeds contain 44% to 51% oil (dry basis). Other vegetable oils that have been tried for biodiesel production include linseed, cottonseed, safflower and peanut/groundnut.

Animal fats are frequently mentioned, but are rarely employed as a feedstock in industrial-scale esterification and have not been studied to the same extent as vegetable oils. Animal fats that have been investigated for esterification into biodiesel include lard (pig fat), beef tallow, chicken fat and fish oil (Lee et al. 2002; Nelson and Schrock 2006; Armenta et al. 2007; Lu et al. 2007).

8.2.1.2 Waste Oils and Fats

Waste cooking oils include yellow and brown grease (Canakci and Van Gerpen 2001; Schnepf 2003; Zhang et al. 2003a,b). The use of waste cooking oils for esterification to biodiesel is a good commercial choice due to its low cost. The waste oil can be obtained from fast food restaurants, industrial deep fryers in food processing plants, snack food factories and even household kitchens. Use of collected oils also reduces pollution as they would otherwise have been discharged to the environment (Zhang et al. 2003a). Use of waste cooking oils has some disadvantages. They contain substantially more FFAs, water and other contaminants; they are more susceptible to oxidation and are more viscous compared with fresh vegetable oils. Preliminary treatments, such as filtering, use of adsorbents and acid-catalysed pretreatment, can make waste oils and fats more suitable for conventional transesterification to biodiesel (Fortenbery 2005).

8.2.1.3 Inedible Oils

Inedible oils include Jatropha oil, neem oil, mahua oil, castor oil and tall oil (Demirbas 2009). Use of Jatropha as a feedstock for transesterification to biodiesel is a rapidly growing industry. Jatropha is lauded as it is a wild plant that can grow in dry and marginal lands without irrigation (Prueksakorn and Gheewala 2008). It is reported to have few pests and diseases, is drought-resistant and is an inedible source of oil and so does not compete with food. Extraction of Jatropha oil and transesterification to biodiesel occurs similarly to edible vegetable oils (Achten et al. 2008). The oil yield of Jatropha seed is a difficult issue as the actual mature seed yield per hectare per year is not known and systematic yield monitoring has only started recently (Achten et al. 2008). Earlier reported figures (0.4–12 t/ha annually) are not coherent as they were based on extrapolations of individual trees to hectares when planting distance greatly affects the seed yield. Adding to the issue is that Jatropha has not yet been properly domesticated and so is still considered a wild plant, with great variability in productivity between individuals. There has been a dramatic expansion in Jatropha plantations worldwide, particularly in Southeast Asia, Africa and Central and South America. Jatropha is currently grown for transesterification to biodiesel in India, the Philippines, Indonesia, Brazil, Ghana and in other developing countries.

Recent research has touted microalgal oils for esterification to biodiesel production as a potentially highly cost-efficient alternative source. Highlighted advantages include rapid growth rates and high oil yields per unit of cropland. A number of researchers have demonstrated the feasibility of biodiesel production from algal oils through various esterification techniques (Miao and Wu 2006; Xue et al. 2006; Li et al. 2007a,b).

Algae are highly robust organisms and are able to grow in a wide range of conditions. Their versatility can serve many advantages for the production of oils for biodiesel. Microalgae grow extremely rapidly, typically doubling their biomass within 24 hours. Whereas soybean and palm oil sources typically produce, approximately 446 and 5950 L/ha annually, respectively, algae has the potential to yield as much as 135,000 L/ha annually (Christi 2007). The proportion of oil content varies with the type of algae. Some types are comprised of up to 80% mass by oils, with 20% to 50% levels more common (Christi 2007). Some algae are also able to thrive in saline water, either from the sea or from underground formations bearing brackish water

(Azachi et al. 2002). Although microalgal biodiesel is technically feasible, the economics of microalgal production must substantially improve to make it a competitive fuel source (Christi 2007). Research is being performed in genetic and metabolic engineering of algal biology to reduce the costs of algal biodiesel.

8.2.2 Oil Production from Feedstock

Although high-quality biodiesel can be produced from crude vegetable oil, use of partially or fully refined oil due to their increased purity, simplifies the biodiesel production process. Because of this, some producers may select degummed or even fully refined oils, despite their higher cost. This section will discuss the practice of processing of vegetable oils, from extraction into its crude form and through subsequent processing steps of refining, bleaching and deodorisation. Rendering of animal fats is also discussed here.

8.2.2.1 Extraction of Oil

The method of oil extraction depends on the feedstock used. For oily fruits, such as palm, the extraction of oils involves mechanical pressing. For seeds, such as soybeans, rapeseed and Jatropha, extraction may be through mechanical pressing (crushing) or solvent extraction (Gunstone 2008). Solvent extraction is the most common oil extraction method due to its higher efficiency. Less commonly, small plants will use mechanical crushing as it requires a smaller investment and is considered more natural.

Before oil extraction, a general cleaning pretreatment step is performed on plants and seeds to remove foreign materials, such as stems, leaves and stones, sand and dirt. This is usually performed using screens and filters. Depending on the feedstock, pretreatment may include drying, peeling, shelling or dehulling. Seeds are often flaked, especially before solvent extraction, to increase their surface area and to increase exposure of the oil to the solvent (Wang 2002). Feedstocks may be heat-treated (cooked) to release oils out of protein–lipid interactions, rupture cell membranes, coagulate proteins and destroy enzymes that can cause problems with their use as animal feed meal.

Mechanical pressing or crushing, if performed, can be done either as a batch or continuous process. Batch processing with cold-press expeller is still used by small-scale facilities and in developing countries. Small-scale cold-press expelling technologies have recovery efficiencies of approximately 80%. Larger scale operations may use continuous screw presses with heating and under pressure to extract most of the fat (>95%; Wang 2002). Extrusion-expelling technology is becoming an increasingly popular method of processing of seeds such as soybean.

Commonly, a fat solvent, such as hexane, is used to extract oil from cracked seeds. A diffusion process is performed either by immersing seeds in solvent (for finely ground oilseeds) or by percolating the solvent through the seeds (for larger particle sizes). Typically, a seed-to-solvent ratio of 1:18 w/w% and reaction temperature of approximately 50°C is applied. The contact time depends on the processed oilseed. The solvent–oil mixture (miscella) is then filtered, whereas the solvent is recovered through vaporisation and a steam stripping process and is recycled back into the process (Wang 2002). Solvent extraction is a more efficient oil recovery method than mechanical extraction and is more effective for processing of low-oil seeds.

After extraction, the crude oil is usually approximately 95% pure. Oil-insoluble impurities such as seed fragments and meal fines, free water and waxes can be removed through filtration. Oil-soluble impurities such as FFAs, phospholipids and other gums are removed through refining.

8.2.2.2 Refining

The refining step removes undesirable components of the crude oil, namely, FFAs and phospholipids. Refining usually consist of two steps: degumming and neutralisation (Gunstone 2008).

The primary purpose of degumming is to remove phospholipids (also called gums or phosphatides), compounds in the oil that have a similar structure to triglycerides. Most crude vegetable oils typically contain 1% to 4% phospholipids. Phospholipids are removed because they are strong emulsifiers and, if present during the later alkali neutralisation step of vegetable oil production, they will inhibit the separation of soaps and lower the oil yield. Phospholipids also react with water to form insoluble sediments that are undesirable when cooking with oil.

Degumming involves mixing with water or dilute acid (phosphoric or citric) to produce a gum containing phospholipids (and trace metals). The phospholipids are recovered as crude lecithin and are separated through settling, centrifugation or filtering (Gunstone 2008). A portion of the phospholipids not easily removed by contact with water are probably calcium and magnesium salts of phosphatidic acids (Wang 2002). These can be removed through the addition or citric or phosphoric acid.

The second step of refining is neutralisation, also called caustic refining or deacidification. Because the crude oil contains FFAs, an alkaline solution, usually sodium hydroxide, is added to react with FFAs and form soaps. The soaps are removed by settling, centrifugation or filtering. The alkali solution also neutralises any acid remaining from the degumming stage (Gunstone 2008).

8.2.2.3 Bleaching

The primary purpose of bleaching is to remove colour pigments, such as chlorophyll and carotene, in the oil (Wang 2002). However, it can also simplify the biodiesel production process and increase yields by helping to remove remaining impurities, such as soaps, trace metals, residual phospholipids and sulphur compounds (Gunstone 2008). Bleaching breaks down peroxides (primary oxidation products) into lower molecular weight carbonyl products, which helps facilitate their removal through deodorisation (Wang 2002). Bleaching involves mixing the oil with absorbent bleaching clays such as bentonite and montmorillonite clays. The mixture is then heated at 80°C to 180°C (but mainly at 90°C–120°C) under a vacuum (Gunstone 2008). The amount of absorbent clay used is approximately 1%, but can vary between 0.2% and 2%, depending on the type of fat (Grün 2004). Once adsorption processes have reached equilibrium, the clay is filtered out by self-cleaning filters.

8.2.2.4 Deodorisation

Deodorisation is performed to remove trace compounds that give oils disagreeable odours or tastes. Deodorisation is a steam distillation process that occurs at high temperatures (170°C–266°C) under reduced pressure (0.25–0.92 kPa; Wang 2002). The odorous compounds are more volatile than the triglycerides, and so are evaporated by heating at low pressure. First, deaeration is performed to remove dissolved oxygen from the oil so that it does not oxidise at the high temperatures used in deodorisation. The oil is heated by injecting steam. It is held at high temperature for a sufficient time to vaporise the odorous compounds. Chelation may be performed by adding 50 to 100 mg/kg of citric acid to bind and filter off trace metals in the oil (Wei et al. 2009). Deodorisation also has the added benefit of further removing FFAs, simplifying the biodiesel esterification process.

8.2.2.5 Rendering

Rendering is the extraction of fat or oil from animal tissues using heat. Animal fats are usually rendered with dry heat, steam injection or both. (Gunstone 2008). The dry heat method involves feeding fat and bone trimmings, meat scraps and other disposed-of animal material into a cooker to be heated to 120°C to 130°C (Wei et al. 2009). Higher temperature encourages the removal of water and separates a portion of the fat from the solids. Fats are drained off from the solids in a drain pan. The solids are fed to a screw press where the remaining fat can be squeezed out (Wei et al. 2009). The fat may be centrifuged or filtered to remove particulates. It is common for the fat to then undergo steam injection to remove any remaining water.

Steam injection may be performed after dry heat rendering or as a distinct rendering process. Steam is directly injected into the animal tissue or dry heat–rendered fat under high pressure. This disintegrates the fat cells releasing the fat. The water settles to the bottom and the dry fat rises to the top of the tank and is skimmed off (Grün 2004). It may be further centrifuged to remove water.

8.2.3 Feedstock Pretreatment

If present, water may be removed from the triglyceride oils because its presence can hydrolyse the triglycerides, forming FFAs and causing the transesterification process to partially change to saponification. The formation of soap is undesirable as it can gel and bind the catalyst into a semisolid form that may prevent the reaction from continuing. Soap formation also lowers the yield of the biodiesel ester and can cause postesterification processing difficulties with glycerol separation and water washing (Van Gerpen et al. 2004). Techniques similar to those described in Section 8.2.2 to treat vegetable oil: refining, bleaching and deodorisation, may also be employed, especially degumming methods to remove phospholipids. If waste vegetable oil or animal fats are used, they may be filtered to remove dirt, charred food and other non–oil material, if found.

8.2.3.1 Determination and Treatment of FFAs

FFAs are a common contaminant found in fat and oil feedstocks. FFAs are formed when fatty acid chains split from the triglyceride molecules. The formation of FFAs usually occurs due to heat, water and the action of degrading lipase enzymes during storage of oilseeds, extraction of oil from oilseeds and storage of the crude vegetable oil. Most crude vegetable oils typically contain less than 2% FFAs and less than 1% monoglycerides and diglycerides. An exception is palm oil, which can contain up to 4% FFAs, up to 2% monoglycerides and up to 7% diglycerides (Keshwani 2010). Refined vegetable oils are highly pure with less than 0.05% FFA content. Waste cooking oils typically contain 2% to 7% FFA content, with trap grease being 40% to 100% FFAs.

High levels of FFAs (>1%) in the oil feedstock can cause problems in the transesterification process because they will react with the alkali catalyst to form soap. Soap formation may bind reactants into a semisolid mass that can impede the transesterification reaction. Soap formation also produces water, which can hydrolyse the triglycerides, further contributing to soap formation. Soap formation can cause difficulties with later separation of the glycerol from the biodiesel and with purification, and ultimately reduces the biodiesel yield (Van Gerpen et al. 2004).

Oil feedstocks containing more than 0.5% to 2.5% FFA may still be used, but may require special measures to be undertaken. The oil feedstock's FFA concentration can be determined by titration with potassium hydroxide (KOH). A number of methods exist to treat high-FFA oils. The easiest method to reduce FFAs is to mix high-FFA with low-FFA oils. This will work for the occasional high-FFA batch.

Other methods require a pretreatment process of intentionally making soap (through esterification). For FFA levels of up to 4% to 5%, and sometimes as high as 5% to 6%, depending on the water content and types of emulsifiers present, a common practice is to add extra alkali catalyst so that the FFAs can be converted to soap, which is then removed. Titration can determine the additional amount of alkali catalyst to neutralise any FFAs present and ensure complete transesterification. After removal of the soap, the remaining catalyst is then left to undergo the standard transesterification reaction. This method has the significant disadvantage of lowering yields as the oil FFA content is discarded as a soap.

If the FFA level of the feedstock is more than 5%, the amount of soap produced will inhibit glycerol separation. A number of methods for converting the FFAs to biodiesel are discussed below, with acid catalytic pretreatment being the most commonly used.

1. *Full acid catalysed esterification.* Acid-catalysed esterification has the advantage over conventional alkali-catalysed transesterification because the water and FFA contents do not cause soap formation (Van Gerpen et al. 2004). The esterification reaction of the FFAs to alcohol esters is relatively fast, typically reaching completion in 1 h at 60°C. However, the transesterification of triglycerides is generally considered too slow for industrial processing, typically taking several days to complete (Canakci and Van Gerpen 1999; Ma and Hanna 1999; Fukuda et al. 2001). Heating to 130°C can speed up the reaction to complete in 30 to 45 min (Van Gerpen et al. 2004). Water production in the reaction mixture also inhibits the reaction from reaching completion. Acid residues must be removed from the final products because these can damage engine parts (Al-Saadi and Jeffreys 1981 in de Oliveira et al. 2005).

2. *Acid catalysed pretreatment.* The most common method for treating high-FFA oils is the use of acid-catalysed esterification as a pretreatment before the conventional alkali-catalysed transesterification process (Canakci and Van Gerpen 2001). Acid catalysis pretreatment solves the reaction rate problem of full acid esterification by using both catalytic techniques. Water formation can still be a problem during acid catalysis. A number of acid pretreatment methods are used to convert the FFAs to usable biodiesel. The most commonly used method involves adding acid and a large percentage of alcohol (as high as 50:1 alcohol-to-oil molar ratio) to prevent water formation from inhibiting the reaction (Zhang et al. 2003b). An alternative method involves adding acid, heat (70°C–90°C) and a small amount of alcohol. A less energy-intensive approach involves allowing the acid-catalysed reaction to settle and removing the methanol–water mixture from the top of the biodiesel phase. Acid catalysis may be repeated until the FFA level is satisfactory (Van Gerpen et al. 2004). Typically, a 1 wt% sulphuric acid (H_2SO_4) to oil ratio is used in this process. When the FFA level is reduced to 0.5% or lower, the glycerol,

alcohol and acid catalyst are removed and conventional alkali-catalysed transesterification is performed.

3. *Glycerolysis pretreatment.* Glycerolysis involves the addition of glycerol to the feedstock and heating to high temperature (200°C), usually with a catalyst, such as zinc chloride. The glycerol reacts with the FFAs to form monoglycerides and diglycerides. Once the FFA level of the oil is reduced, conventional alkali-catalysed transesterification can be performed. The disadvantage of glycerolysis is the high temperature required and a relatively slow reaction rate.

4. *Enzymatic methods.* Transesterification using lipase enzyme catalysts is less affected by water. Although extensive research has gone into lipase enzymes, their use is not yet economically and technically competitive on an industrial scale. Section 8.3.2 has more information on these types of catalysts.

5. *Steam stripping.* For extremely high FFA levels (10%–15%), steam stripping or distillation is an effective method. Because FFAs are more volatile than triglycerides, they can be evaporated by heating with injected steam. FFAs can be held at high temperature for a sufficient time to vaporise. Steam stripping is less effective for lower FFA levels of 1% to 2%.

6. *Adsorbents.* Less commonly used are commercially available adsorbents. Adsorbents can be used when dealing with low levels of FFA, up to possibly 5%. Adsorbents extract the FFAs by chemically adsorbing them into a powder. This method can result in a fairly significant amount of waste material because the powder must be disposed of, typically into landfills (Voegele 2012).

8.2.4 Biomass Esterification

Esterification is a chemical reaction in which two reactants, typically an acid and an alcohol, form what is known as an ester as the reaction product. Transesterification involves changing one ester into another. With respect to biodiesel processing, transesterification (also called alcoholysis) involves the reaction of triglyceride oils or fats (composed of glycerol esters) with alcohol to form alkyl esters. Transesterification reactions are often catalysed by a base or acid to accelerate the adjustment of the reaction equilibrium. Glycerol is removed from the product of the reaction to leave the fatty acid esters that make up biodiesel. The transesterification reaction of a triglyceride with methanol in the presence of sodium hydroxide as a catalyst to give the methyl ester and glycerol is presented with the following expression:

$$\begin{array}{c} H_2C-OCOR \\ | \\ HC-OCOR \\ | \\ H_2C-OCOR \end{array} \ + \ 3\,CH_3OH \ \underset{\text{NaOH catalyst}}{\rightleftharpoons} \ 3\,CH_3OOCR \ + \ \begin{array}{c} H_2C-OH \\ | \\ HC-OH \\ | \\ H_2C-OH \end{array}$$

| Triglyceride | Methanol | | Methyl ester | Glycerol |

Transesterification is performed to reduce the high viscosity and flash-points of component vegetable oils or animal fats to provide a fuel with properties closer to that of conventional diesel fuel. Although vegetable oils have been used as a diesel fuel without processing in the past, extended tests showed that they caused operational problems in engines, mainly due to their high viscosity. Vegetable oils have viscosity values between 27.2 and 53.6 mm^2/s, significantly more viscous than that of conventional petroleum-derived diesel fuel (2.7 mm^2/s) at 40°C (Demirbas 2003b). Problems with using vegetable oils in conventional engines include injector coking and trumpet formation, more carbon deposits (especially on cylinders), oil ring sticking and thickening, and gelling of the engine lubricant oil due to con-tamination (Ma and Hanna 1999; Demirbas 2003a).

Viscosity is an important factor in predicting biodiesel performance because it affects the operation of fuel injection equipment, particularly at low temperatures when the increased viscosity affects the fluidity of the fuel. High viscosity leads to poorer atomisation of the fuel spray and less accurate operation of the fuel injectors. The lower viscosity of biodiesel, achieved through esterification, allows it to be easier to pump and atomise and achieve finer droplets. Transesterification of triglycerides into methyl or ethyl esters reduces the molecular weight to one-third that of triglycerides and reduces the viscosity by a factor of about 8.

Transesterification proceeds with oils or fats (commonly vegetable oils) com-bined with primary or secondary monohydric aliphatic short-chained (1–8 carbon atoms) alcohol, usually methanol or ethanol and a catalyst (usually an alkaline such as sodium hydroxide [NaOH]; Lang et al. 2001). The triglyceride oils react to form simple alkyl esters, which constitute the molecules of biodiesel fuel. Glycerol is also produced as a by-product and may be used in pharma-ceutical and cosmetic applications (Nersesian 2007). Transesterification offers a potentially cost-effective method of transforming the large, branched molecu-lar structure of bio-oils into the smaller, straight-chain molecules, of the type required by conventional diesel combustion engines (Demirbas 2009).

Transesterification is an equilibrium reaction. Because the reaction is reversible, an excess of alcohol may be used, or one of the productions removed from the reaction mixture to shift the equilibrium to the products side. Usually, the alcohol is combined with a protonated base catalyst before reacting with the glyceride. A catalyst (alkali or acid based) is required to split the oil molecules and increase solubility because the alcohol is spar-ingly soluble in the oil phase. Alkalis can catalyse the reaction by removing a proton from the alcohol, thus making it more reactive. Acids can catalyse the reaction by donating a proton to the carbonyl group, thus making it more reactive (Demirbas 2009).

The reaction mechanism for alkali-catalysed transesterification was formulated as three steps (Ma and Hanna 1999). Transesterification first reduces the triglycerides to diglycerides and subsequently to monoglycerides. The monoglycerides are finally reduced to glycerol. One mole of alkyl esters is removed during each step. This stepwise conversion of triglycerides is shown in the reactions below. The first reaction step of the methanol and triglycerides forming diglycerides and one mole of alkyl ester is rate limiting, and the other steps occur much faster (Mittelbach and Trathnigg 1990).

$$Triglyceride + alcohol(ROH) \longleftrightarrow diglyceride + (ester)RCOOR$$

$$Diglyceride + alcohol(ROH) \longleftrightarrow monoglyceride + (ester)RCOOR$$

$$Monoglyceride + alcohol(ROH) \longleftrightarrow glycerol + (ester)RCOOR$$

Reaction kinetics vary with the system temperature and pressure. For the commonly used methanol-to-triglyceride molar ratio of 6:1, transesterification kinetics are thought to be pseudo second-order for the first stages of the reaction followed by first-order or zero-order in the final stages (Darnoko and Cheryan 2000). The initial pseudo second-order rate is due to the excess methanol having low miscibility with the oil and the catalyst being in the methanol phase. The reaction speeds up as the reactants are dissolved into each other.

Alkali-catalysed transesterification is generally preferred over acid-catalysed transesterification because it is much faster and produces high levels of conversion to the desired methyl or ethyl esters (Ma et al. 1998; Canakci and Van Gerpen 1999; Ma and Hanna 1999; Fukuda et al. 2001; Zhang et al. 2003a; de Oliveira et al. 2005). Alkali catalysts include sodium hydroxide (NaOH), potassium hydroxide (KOH), carbonates and corresponding sodium and potassium alkoxides, such as sodium methoxide, sodium ethoxide, sodium propoxide, and sodium butoxide. Acid catalysts include sulphuric acid (H_2SO_4), hydrochloric acid (HCl) and sulphronic acids. Heterogeneous catalysts, such as lipases, metal oxides, and solid bases and acids (including SiO_2 and zeolites), may also be used.

Sodium hydroxide (caustic soda) is very well accepted and is widely used in industrial processing due to its low cost and high product yield (Fukuda et al. 2001; Demirbas 2003a). Other commonly used catalysts are potassium hydroxide (caustic potash) and sodium methoxide (methylate). These base catalysts are highly hygroscopic (attract and hold water molecules) and they form chemical water when dissolved in the alcohol reactant. They also absorb water from the air during storage. Care should be taken to prevent absorption of water, which will cause problems with soap formation during the transesterification reaction.

In the conventional transesterification process, the alkali catalyst is added slowly to methanol and vigorously stirred using a standard agitator or mixer until it dissolves. To ensure complete reaction of the fat or oil to its esters, excess alcohol is normally used, with the balance recovered for reuse after the reaction. The methanol and catalyst mix is then pumped into a closed biodiesel reactor and the oil or fat is added. The reaction mix is then stirred vigorously. The reaction is often conducted at 60°C to 65°C, usually just below the boiling point of methanol. This also avoids the need for pressurised reactors. The use of higher temperatures, up to just above the boiling point of alcohol, can significantly speed up the transesterification reaction (Freedman et al. 1984). Recommended reaction times vary from 1 to 8 h, although the optimal reaction time is about 2 h (Van Gerpen et al. 2004). A successful reaction produces two liquid phases, constituting the two major products of the reaction: methyl esters (biodiesel) and crude glycerol. Both products still contain a substantial amount of the methanol that was used in the reaction. The reacted mixture is sometimes neutralised at this step, if needed. The glycerol is much denser or heavier than the biodiesel so the two can be gravity separated. After several hours of settling, the glycerol segregates at the bottom and can be simply removed from the bottom of the settling vessel (Bala 2005). Phase separation can be observed within 10 min and can be complete within 2 h after stirring has stopped. Complete settling, however, can take as long as 20 h (Demirbas 2008). In some cases, a centrifuge is used to separate the two materials faster.

Alkali catalysed transesterification is extremely sensitive to water and FFA content in the oil or fat used. Water in the triglyceride and high FFA content causes the transesterification reaction to partially change to saponification, which produces soap. When water is present, particularly at high temperatures, it can hydrolyse the triglycerides to diglycerides to form FFAs. The alkali catalyst typically used to encourage the reaction reacts with the FFAs to form soap. Water in oils and fats can cause soap formation during the transesterification reaction. The soaps of saturated fatty acids tend to solidify at ambient temperatures, and thus a reaction mixture with excessive soap may gel and form a semisolid mass that is very difficult to recover. This reaction is undesirable because it binds the catalyst into a form that does not contribute to accelerating the reaction. The soap also lowers the yield of esters. Excessive soap in the products can cause difficulties in the subsequent processing of the biodiesel, including glycerol–ester separation and water washing (Van Gerpen et al. 2004).

Acid-catalysed transesterification has the advantage over alkali-catalysed transesterification because it is much more tolerant of water and FFA (>1%) in the oil feedstock. However, alkali catalysis is generally preferred over acid catalysis because the latter is considered too slow for industrial processing, typically 4000 times slower (Canakci and Van Gerpen 1999; Ma and Hanna 1999; Fukuda et al. 2001). To speed up the acid-catalysed reaction, heating may be employed to temperatures higher than 100°C, which will cause the reaction to reach completion in more than 3 h (Freedman et al. 1984). The acid in the final products must be neutralised in subsequent steps because acidic residues can damage engine parts (Al-Saadi and Jeffreys 1981 in de Oliveira et al. 2005). Commonly for high-FFA oils, acid-catalysed esterification is used as a pretreatment for the conventional alkali-catalysed transesterification procedure.

8.2.5 Parameters Affecting Esterification

Several parameters affect the transesterification of triglycerides into biodiesel, including the molar ratio of alcohol to oil, the catalyst type, reaction temperatures and FFA content and purity of the reactants (mainly water content; Demirbas 2009).

8.2.5.1 FFA and Water Content in Oils and Alcohols

FFA and water content in the reactants, namely, the oils and the alcohol, are very important factors to be considered for esterification (Meher et al. 2006a,b). The FFA content affects the type of transesterification process used as well as the yield produced from the process. FFAs are the acids in the oil that are not connected to triglyceride molecules. In conventional alkali-catalysed transesterification, the presence of FFAs and water interferes with the reaction because it causes soap formation, which consumes the catalyst and reduces the effectiveness of the catalyst (Ma et al. 1998). High water content ultimately results in lower yields, unconverted triglycerides and also potentially posttransesterification processing complications (Kusdiana and Saka 2004). Typically, when using an alkali catalyst, 3% or lower FFA content is required to carry the reaction to completion (Meher et al. 2006a,b). The FFAs and water are often removed in a refining step of vegetable oil processing or through a filtering or acid-catalysed transesterification pretreatment before performing the conventional transesterification process. Excess FFAs can also be removed as soaps in a separate transesterification step or through caustic stripping (see Section 8.2.3.1 for more information). The catalyst-free supercritical alcohol method of transesterification, by contrast, tolerates much greater percentages of water in reactants (see Section 8.3.3 for more information). Other contaminants present in the oil, such as wax, can also affect biodiesel yields. Oil feedstock pretreatment, such as settling or filtering, may be necessary prior to carrying out conventional transesterification processes.

8.2.5.2 Reaction Temperature

Generally, transesterification is carried out at temperatures close to the boiling point of methanol (60°C–70°C) at atmospheric pressures, as temperature increases the reaction time (Demirbas 2002a). However, temperatures higher than the boiling point of methanol may result in lower production yields as the oxidation of alcohol is promoted, or it can result in saponification (Ramadhas et al. 2005; Leung and Guo 2006).

8.2.5.3 Alcohol to Triglyceride Molar Ratio

The stoichiometric ratio for transesterification requires three moles of alcohol and one mole of triglyceride to yield three moles of the fatty acid ester and one mole of glycerol. However, because transesterification is an equilibrium reaction, a higher molar proportion of alcohol is typically used to shift the reaction to the product's side (Meher et al. 2006a,b). Accepted molar ratios of alcohols to triglycerides for alkali-catalysed transesterification are between 3:1 and 6:1. Increasing the molar ratio of alcohol to triglyceride increases the rate of reaction and yield to more than 98% at a 30:1 ratio (Canakci and Van Gerpen 1999). This effect, however, declines sharply beyond the 6:1 ratio, resulting in 90% conversion. Extremely high ratios of alcohol to triglyceride are avoided because the alcohol can interfere with the separation of the glycerol by increasing its solubility (Meher et al. 2006a,b). Dissolved glycerol can also cause the reaction to reverse back to the reactants, decreasing the yield of alkyl esters (Meher et al. 2006a,b). Usually, for alkali catalysed transesterification, a 100% excess of alcohol is used, with six moles of alcohol per mole of triglyceride at 60°C to 65°C. This typically yields a 98% conversion of triglyceride to methyl esters after 60 min (Freedman et al. 1986). In cases of acid-catalysed transesterification, ratios of up to 50 mol of alcohol per mole of triglyceride may be used.

8.2.5.4 Catalyst Type

Sodium hydroxide (NaOH) and potassium hydroxide (KOH) are the most commonly used catalysts for industrial biodiesel production due to their low cost and mild temperature requirements. However, the presence of water in the reactants can give rise to hydrolysis of some of the produced esters, with consequent soap formation and the associated washing and separation difficulties and reduced yield. High conversions to alkyl esters (>98%) can be achieved by using catalyst concentrations of 1 or 2 mol%. However, the biodiesel and glycerol produced must be purified to remove the alkaline catalyst and separate out any soap. Sodium hydroxide is the preferred catalyst over potassium hydroxide mainly due to its lower cost. Potassium hydroxide may give higher yields compared with sodium hydroxide (Vincente et al. 2004).

Sodium methoxide (CH_3ONa) and potassium methoxide (CH_3ONa) are more effective catalysts than sodium hydroxide and potassium hydroxide, and produce higher yields because they do not form water (Leung and Guo 2006). Reaction rates using these two catalysts are fast (30 min) and may be achieved even with low molar concentrations (0.5 mol%). Potassium methoxide is the more effective catalyst compared with sodium methoxide at equivalent molar concentrations with the same triglyceride samples. Sodium methoxide and potassium methoxide are less commonly used than sodium hydroxide and potassium hydroxide in industrial processing because they are more expensive and more sensitive to water in feedstocks (Freedman et al. 1984). Heterogeneous catalysts, such as lipases, metal oxides and solid bases and acids (including SiO_2 and zeolites) may also be used.

8.2.5.5 Nature of the Alcohol

Methanol is the most commonly used alcohol because, despite being toxic, it is generally less expensive than other alcohols. Ethanol is also used but is less reactive than methanol. Ethanol is also more sensitive to water so it must be drier than is required for methanol (Van Gerpen 2009). An advantage of ethanol is that it is considered more renewable than methanol, and because it is obtained from agricultural products, it is more environmentally friendly. Other alcohols suitable for esterification include propanol, isopropanol (Lee et al. 2004), butanol, octanol (Marchetti et al. 2007) and branched-chain alcohols (Modi et al. 2006; Kose et al. 2002).

8.2.6 Postesterification Processing

Refining is needed to ensure trouble-free operation in diesel engines and to meet biodiesel fuel quality standard requirements. For this reason, alkyl esters must be separated from the biodiesel. Steps that take place in postesterification processing include ester–glycerol separation, alcohol recovery and ester washing to purify the biodiesel and neutralise any catalysts. The order of postesterification steps for removal of glycerol and other impurities is process dependent.

8.2.6.1 Glycerol Separation for Esters (Biodiesel)

Crude glycerol is the principal by-product of the biodiesel esterification process. Glycerol is a viscous, colourless and odourless coproduct. It is usually approximately 10 wt% of the feedstock vegetable oil (Kemp 2006). For each gallon of biodiesel produced, approximately 0.3 kg of crude glycerol is also produced (Thompson and He 2006). The produced crude glycerol is of very low value due to impurities; however, further refining, dependent on economies of scale, can increase its value to food, pharmaceutical and cosmetic industries.

Glycerol–ester separation is typically the first postesterification step in most biodiesel production processes. Because the glycerol (1.05 g/cc) is much denser than the ester (biodiesel at 0.88 g/cc), this property is exploited to separate the bulk of the glycerol by-product. The product of the transesterification process is usually left for 1 to 8 h to settle to enable gravity separation. The alcohol esters are left on the top with the glycerol simply drawn off from the bottom of the settling vessel. In some cases, a centrifuge is used to accelerate separation of the two materials (Ma and Hanna 1999).

The hydrocyclone is a new device recently considered for use in biodiesel production (Van Gerpen et al. 2004). A liquid–liquid hydrocyclone has an inverted conical shape, with the liquid fed tangentially. The effect is similar to a centrifuge, with the denser material being forced toward the wall and to the bottom exit. The lighter material is forced to the centre and upward out the larger exit.

8.2.6.1.1 Glycerol Refining

The by-product crude glycerol is considered as a highly variable commodity from plant to plant (Sims 2011). This is due to the wide variability of impurities, such as residual alcohol, catalyst residue, soap, esters and carry-over oil/fat and water. Biodiesel producers have the choice of refining their crude glycerol for sale and utilisation in food, cosmetic and pharmaceutical industries (Voegele 2009), selling the crude glycerol at a very low price, or disposing of the glycerol according to regulatory requirements (Sims 2011). Generally, the purer the glycerol, the higher the market value.

Chemical or physical refining processes can be applied for further treatment of the glycerol by-product. Chemical refining uses an acid, usually sulphuric acid, to split the soap into FFAs and salts and, if not already performed, neutralise unspent catalysts. The FFAs are removed as a top layer and the salts are left in the glycerol. If the catalyst in the separated glycerol is not neutralised in earlier steps, much more acid is required because most of the catalyst and soap remains in the glycerol phase. Physical refining involves filtering or centrifugation (or both) to remove fatty, insoluble or precipitated solids, possibly pH adjustment and then water removal by evaporation. The final purification of glycerol is completed using vacuum distillation with steam stripping or an ion-exchange process, followed by activated carbon bleaching (Van Gerpen et al. 2004).

8.2.6.2 Alcohol Recovery

The residual alcohol is typically removed from the biodiesel or glycerol through conventional or vacuum distillation, or flash vaporisation. The recovered alcohol will frequently contain water which may be removed with a distillation column before the alcohol is recycled back into the process (Van Gerpen 2009). Less commonly, the alcohol may be washed out as waste during the ester washing step.

8.2.6.3 Ester Washing

The biodiesel product is often washed gently with warm (48°C–60°C) softened water to remove any residual soaps formed during transesterification. The water is also used as a medium to neutralise the remaining catalyst and remove product salts, glycerides and free glycerol. Softened water (slightly acidic) neutralises the remaining alkali catalyst and eliminates calcium and magnesium contamination. The phase separation between the ester and washwater is very clean and complete. Some processes also remove alcohol during the washing phase. The ester washing is frequently done with multiple steps in counterflow to minimise water consumption (Van Gerpen 2009). Esters are vacuum-dried through a flash process to meet stringent standards for the amount of water present in the final biodiesel product (Ma and Hanna 1999).

An alternative to water washing is to use solid adsorbents to remove the glycerol, soap, catalyst and other contaminants. One option is to add finely ground magnesium silicate (available commercially as Magnesol) to the biodiesel after the methanol has been removed. The powder attracts the polar glycerol, methanol, water and catalyst molecules and separates them from the nonpolar ester biodiesel. After filtering, the fuel is ready for use. This eliminates the need for ester washing, wastewater disposal, as well as drying of the final product. Another alternative is the use of a specialty ion exchange resin system, such as Amberlite BD10Dry, which can be used before methanol recovery. The crude biodiesel is purified from residual soap, catalyst and free glycerol by passing it through a fixed-bed column of a copolymer resin (Van Gerpen 2009).

Some systems may employ an additional step to remove small amounts of colour bodies to produce a colourless biodiesel. An activated carbon bed is an effective way to remove excessive colour (Van Gerpen et al. 2004).

8.3 Biomass Esterification Technologies

Biomass esterification plants may apply batch or continuous processing technologies or a hybrid of the two. Factors, such as feedstock availability, reaction yield and flexibility in handling multiple feedstock oils and fats such as high FFA oils, are important factors for the selection of process technologies. The following section gives an overview of the technologies available for biomass esterification.

8.3.1 Conventional Catalytic Processing Technologies

8.3.1.1 Biodiesel Production by Batch Process

The simplest method for producing biodiesel, commonly used in smaller plants (0.1–5 million gallons per year [MMgy]), is to use batch, stirred tank reactors. Batch systems usually consist of a series of tanks in which each production phase is completed before being pumped to the next phase. The reactor may be sealed or equipped with a reflux condenser. Each batch can take several days to complete.

Oils can be transesterified batch-wise with excess alcohol (commonly at 6:1 molar ratio, although 4:1 to 21:1 ratios have been reported). Operating temperatures are usually approximately 60°C to 65°C, just below the boiling point of the alcohol (methanol) used. However, temperature ranges from 25°C to 85°C have also been reported (Ma and Hanna 1999; Demirbas 2002b; Bala 2005). The most commonly used catalyst in the batch process is sodium hydroxide, followed by potassium hydroxide. Typical catalyst loadings range from 0.3% to approximately 1.5%. Typical reaction times range from 20 min to more than 1 h (Van Gerpen et al. 2004).

Figure 8.2 shows the process flow for a typical two-step batch system with a separate settling tank (Van Gerpen et al. 2004). The oil is first charged into the system, followed by the precombined catalyst and methanol. Thorough mixing is necessary at the beginning of the reaction to bring the reactants into intimate contact (Van Gerpen et al. 2004). Toward the end of the reaction, less mixing can help increase the extent of reaction by allowing the inhibitory product, glycerol, to phase separate from the ester–oil phase. Most small plants (<5 MMgy), are built as a two-step batch system; with separate steps consisting of a reactor vessel and a settling tank. Alternatively, the product esters and glycerol may also allowe to settle and separate in the reactor. Some processes may also separate using a centrifuge (Van Gerpen et al. 2004).

Alcohol is removed from both the glycerol and ester stream using an evaporator or a flash unit (Van Gerpen et al. 2004). The esters are washed gently using warm, slightly acidic water to neutralise the catalyst and remove residual methanol and salts. After drying, the product biodiesel is transferred to storage. The glycerol may be neutralised through washing and either sold as crude glycerol or sent to a glycerol refining unit.

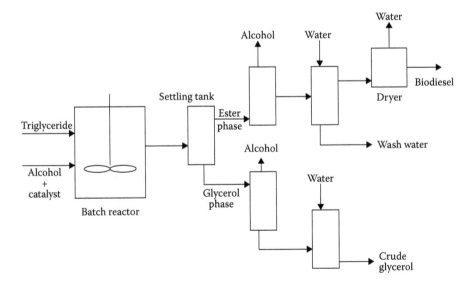

FIGURE 8.2
Batch reaction process for biodiesel production.

High FFA feedstocks (>1%–2%) are commonly pretreated through acid-catalysed esterification. Acid-catalysed esterification requires a slightly modified system with the addition of an acid esterification vessel and storage for the acid catalyst (Van Gerpen et al. 2004). The feedstock is sometimes dried (down to 0.4% water) and filtered before being charged into the acid esterification tank. Premixed sulphuric acid and methanol are added to the oil and the system is agitated. Temperatures similar to those used in transesterification are used and sometimes the system is pressurised (Van Gerpen et al. 2004). The mixture is neutralised with excesses base catalysts. The process then continues through the transesterification batch processes described above, in which any remaining FFAs are converted into soaps.

Batch plants require lower overall investment than continuous plants. They offer higher flexibility because the feedstock source can be varied and the reaction conditions for each batch can be altered depending on the FFA level and other impurities. The trend, however, is toward continuous production plants due to their higher production rates and lower operating costs.

8.3.1.2 Biodiesel Production with Continuous Flow Processing

Larger plants (> 10 MMgy) typically use more efficient continuous flow processes involving continuous stirred-tank reactors (CSTRs) in series or plug-flow reactors (PFRs). Continuous flow processing is suited to large-capacity facilities, where economies of scale can begin to take effect (Bart et al. 2010). Continuous systems operate 24 h/day and are highly automated with excellent quality control. One type of PFR system is schematically shown in Figure 8.3 (Van Gerpen et al. 2004).

The CSTRs can be varied in volume to allow for a longer residence time in the first CSTR to achieve a greater extent of reaction. Alcohol is introduced into the process in fractions. For example, approximately 80% of the alcohol and catalyst may be added to the oil in the first CSTR. After the initial reaction, glycerol is removed through decanting, and the remaining 20% of the alcohol and catalyst can be added to react in the second CSTR. The reaction in the second CSTR is rather rapid, with 98% or greater completion rates. This technique allows for complete reaction to be achieved, whilst potentially using less alcohol than single-step systems.

Intense mixing, using pumps or motionless mixers in the reactors, initiates the esterification reaction and ensures that the composition throughout the reactor is essentially constant. This has the effect of increasing the dispersion of the glycerol in the ester phase (Van Gerpen et al. 2004) but requires longer times for phase separation.

8.3.2 Lipase Enzyme–Catalysed Transesterification

Although conventional alkali-catalysed transesterification gives high conversion levels of oil feedstocks to alkyl esters in short times, the process has

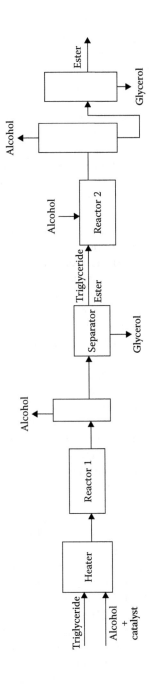

FIGURE 8.3
PFR system.

several drawbacks: FFAs and water interfere with the reaction by causing soap formation, glycerol recovery is difficult, the catalyst must be removed from the product, and it can be energy intensive (Meher et al. 2006a,b). In recent years, significant research has gone into lipase enzyme–catalysed transesterification due to its many touted advantages over conventional transesterification processes. A major advantage is that lipase enzymes or whole cells can be immobilised to mitigate posttransesterification processing issues involved with catalyst removal, product separation and purification. Other advantages of lipase enzyme–catalysed transesterification include mild reaction conditions and lower energy requirements, high selectivity, regeneration and reuse of enzymes genetic engineering can improve their efficiency, they can accept new substrates, they have enhanced thermostability and they may also be considered as natural and produce less side effects and waste, especially wastewater, and so are more environmentally favourable.

Lipases are water-soluble proteins widely distributed amongst animals, plants and microorganisms. Lipases are enzymes that catalyse the hydrolysis of the glycerol ester of triglyceride bonds, and therefore, also the synthesis of glycerol esters (esterification and transesterification; Wei et al. 2009). Lipases can be produced in high yields from microorganisms, such as bacteria and fungi. There are at least 35 lipases available commercially, but only a few can be obtained in industrial quantities. Some of the more promising commercially available microbial lipases are derived from *Chromobacterium viscosum*, *Candida rugosa*, *Rhizomucor miehei*, *Pseudomona fluorescens* and *Apergillus niger* (Wu et al. 1996).

Much of the recent research has involved determining the best enzyme source (type of microorganism that generates the enzyme) and optimising the reaction conditions (FFA level, water content, temperature, time, solvent or no solvent, pH, etc.) to establish suitable characteristics for scaling-up to industrial applications. Specific enzyme catalysts require different reaction and residence times. A number of studies deal with the use of enzymes with differing characteristics, different alcohols, oils and fats, and under varied reaction conditions (Ranganathan et al. 2008; Fjerbaek et al. 2009).

Although lipase enzyme technologies have been successfully applied in the laboratory, technical issues exist with implementing them on an industrial scale, related to slow reactions, constrained chemical equilibriums and low yields (Voegele 2012). Their high costs are also an obstacle to commercialisation (Iso et al. 2001). Although enzymes are commercially available, their incorporation into biodiesel esterification production systems had only reached the pilot stage from 2010 (Biofuels International 2010).

Despite this, researcher efforts and biotechnology companies remain optimistic about the potential use of lipase enzymes as catalysts for industrial esterification of biodiesel. Research and development is expected to increase the economic and technical competitiveness of lipase enzymatic approaches compared with chemical transesterification. Enzyme technologies offer the prospect of significantly increasing the cost-effectiveness of industrial biodiesel production, especially through the use of crude, waste and other low-quality high-FFA oils. Genetic engineering, the production of intracellular (whole cell immobilised) rather than extracellular immobilised lipases and reuse are some of the major efforts to improve cost-effectiveness of enzymatic system technologies (Ranganathan et al. 2008; Nagao et al. 1996).

8.3.3 Noncatalytic Supercritical Alcohol Transesterification

In conventional alkali-catalytic transesterification, FFAs and water in the feedstock react with the alkali catalyst to form soap, inhibiting catalyst effectiveness and reducing yields. Noncatalytic supercritical alcohol transesterification avoids these problems by using supercritical temperatures and pressures to increase alcohol and oil miscibility. The supercritical method handles the high-FFA feedstocks well (up to 36 wt%; Kusdiana and Saka 2004). Supercritical alcohol transesterification also avoids problems related to time-consuming and complicated removal of the catalyst and washing out of soaps from the biodiesel product, which add to production costs and energy consumption.

In conventional transesterification, a catalyst is used to split oil molecules to increase the solubility of the two-phase nature of normal oil/methanol mixtures. Supercritical alcohol transesterification solves this problem by forming a single phase as a result of the lower value of the dielectric constant of methanol in the supercritical state (Saka and Kusdiana 2001; Demirbas 2003). Methanol has a critical temperature of 239.45°C and critical pressure of 8.09 MPa; however, higher temperatures (250°C–400°C) and pressures (20–65 MPa) have been investigated. The result has been that reactions are completed in a much shorter time compared with catalytic processing.

Noncatalytic supercritical methanol transesterification can be performed in a high-pressure stainless steel cylindrical reactor (autoclave; Demirbas 2006). Heat may be supplied from an external heater. In a typical run, the autoclave is charged with excess methanol and vegetable oil (up to 40:1 molar ratio). After each run, the gas is vented, and the autoclave is poured into a collecting vessel. The remaining contents are removed from the autoclave by washing with methanol (Demirbas 2006). The supercritical alcohol transesterification method achieves very fast reaction rates. Using methanol at 300°C, the yield of conversion increases to 95% during the first 10 min. Table 8.1 compares the supercritical methanol and the conventional catalytic methanol transesterification methods, showing the benefits of this developing technology (Saka and Kusdiana 2001).

Compared with conventional catalytic transesterification, noncatalytic supercritical alcohol transesterification has a shorter reaction time and allows for much simpler processing and purification of the methyl esters (biodiesel). Although noncatalytic supercritical alcohol transesterification techniques are potentially low cost with a simpler technology, as of 2012, it was still at the pilot or very early commercial stage, largely due to process safety concerns and associated capital costs (Geiver 2011a).

TABLE 8.1

Comparison between the Conventional Catalytic Methanol Method and the Supercritical Methanol Method

	Conventional Catalytic Methanol Transesterification	Supercritical Methanol Transesterification
Catalyst	Alkali (NaOH or KOH)	None
Reaction temperature (°C)	35–65	>239.45
Reaction pressure (MPa)	0.1	>8.09
Reaction time	1–8 h	2–15 min
FFAs	Saponified products	Methyl esters, water
Removal for purification	Methanol, catalyst, glycerol, soaps	Methanol
Process	Complicated	Simple

8.3.4 Ultrasonic and Shockwave Cavitation

Ultrasonic irradiation causes the cavitation of bubbles near the phase boundary between the immiscible oil and alcohol. The formation and collapse of bubbles vastly enlarge the surface area between the two phases for which the esterification reaction can take place (Leung et al. 2010). Cavitation causes localised heating at the phase boundary, leading to intensive mixing and enhancing the reaction (Stavarache et al. 2005; Santos et al. 2009; Thanh et al. 2009). Because of this, the esterification reaction can be performed without external thermal heating or at lower process temperatures.

Ultrasound reactors can achieve high yields (>99%) whilst reducing batch processing times from 1 to 4 h to less than 30 s (Kotrba 2010). Separation times can be reduced from up to 10 h, down to 1 h. Ultrasound is also employed in commercial continuous flow processing plants. Sonification is most commonly performed at increased pressures of 0.1 to 0.3 MPa (Kotrba 2010). Use of ultrasound reactors reduces the required amounts of excess methanol by up to 50% (Hielscher Ultrasonics 2011a). Molar ratios between 1:4 and 1:4.5 (oil/methanol) are sufficient for most feedstocks. The amount of catalyst required is also decreased by up to 50% compared with conventional continuous flow processing (Hielscher Ultrasonics 2011a). Ultrasound technology is also more energy efficient compared with conventional mechanical mixing (Hielscher Ultrasonics 2011a). Intensified mixing also allows for the use of waste cooking oils and animal fats. Major costs of ultrasonic processing are the cost of devices, maintenance and utility costs.

The ShockWave Power Reactor (SPR) employs similar cavitation principles to achieve higher yields and reduce reaction times (Geiver 2011b). Rather than using ultrasound, SPR employs 'controlled' cavitation using a spinning rotor with depressions (Hydro Dynamics, n.d.; Geiver 2011b). As the device spins, microscopic bubbles are formed and collapse in the depressions, giving off shockwaves into the liquid. This increases the surface area at the phase boundary between the reactants to enhance the esterification reaction. SPR is already used in at least eight biodiesel plants (Geiver 2011b).

8.3.5 BIOX Cosolvent Process

The BIOX production process applies an inert cosolvent in an oil-rich single phase continuous process esterification system. The system has attracted considerable attention because it is able to achieve conversion yields of more than 99% at near-ambient temperatures in less than 90 min, compared with previous processes that required several hours (BIOX Corporation 2010). The BIOX process, shown in Figure 8.4, uses a cosolvent, tetrahydrofuran (THF), in a two-step, single phase, continuous process at atmospheric pressures and near-ambient temperatures. Acid-catalysed esterification pretreatment is first performed on high FFA-content (up to 10%) oil feedstocks, followed by conversion of triglycerides by way of alkali-catalysed transesterification. The cosolvent THF is used to dissolve the two phases of the methanol/oil system into a single phase (Boocock et al. 1998). Use of a cosolvent allows the process to overcome slow reaction times caused by the extremely low solubility of the methanol in the oil phase. THF was selected for its low boiling point of 67.8°C, which is only 2°C higher than methanol. Other cosolvents have also been investigated, such as methyl tertiary butyl ether, oxolane and dimethyl sulphoxide (Mahajan et al. 2006; Zhou et al. 2003). No separate pretreatment step is needed, as is the case with conventional transesterification processes. Separation of the glycerol and biodiesel is clean and the final products contain no catalyst or water residues. The cosolvent must also be removed from the biodiesel and glycerine. The THF cosolvent and the unreacted methanol are codistilled and recycled back into the process (Boocock et al. 1996). The BIOX process is not feedstock-specific and is able to achieve conversion yields higher than 99% when using up to 10% FFA feedstocks (Van Gerpen et al. 2004).

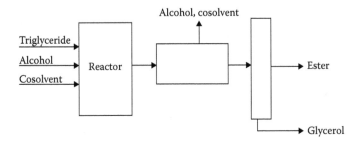

FIGURE 8.4
BIOX cosolvent process.

8.3.6 Microwave-Enhanced Transesterification

Microwave irradiation and RF energy can also be used to provide potentially more energy-efficient heating to significantly expedite esterification reactions (Shahid and Jamal 2011). Microwaves are able to transfer energy directly into the sample, unlike conventional thermal heating, which relies on conduction currents. With homogenous catalysts, similar to supercritical alcohol techniques, heating results in enhanced diffusion of the alcohol–catalyst mixture with the oil.

The microwave-enhanced transesterification process is still at the research and development phase. Microwave technology suffers from a scale-up problem as microwaves have limited penetration depth and are absorbed after passing through just a few centimetres of liquid (Bart et al. 2010). To overcome this problem, microwaves with ultrasonification have been employed at one early pilot 110 L/h process (Kotrba 2011).

8.3.7 *In situ* Transesterification

In the *in situ* transesterification process, alcohol contacts the triglycerides still resident in oilseeds, instead of reacting with pre-extracted oil (Georgogianni et al. 2008). By combining oil extraction and transesterification into one step, the alcohol acts as both an extraction solvent and the esterification reagent. This method potentially reduces or eliminates the expenses associated with solvent or mechanical extraction and refining of oil, and simplifies the steps in biodiesel production.

Although still not commercially developed, *in situ* transesterification has been investigated using catalysed methanol and ethanol transesterification with a variety of different oilseeds (Carapiso and Garcia 2000). *In situ* transesterification has been demonstrated as an effective method for biodiesel production using a number of different lipid-bearing materials, including soy flakes, distillers dried grains with solubles and meat and bone meal (Haas et al. 2007). When the appropriate catalysis is selected, *in situ* transesterification can produce yields comparable or even greater than those obtained from conventional transesterification with pre-extracted vegetable oil (Harrington and D'Arcy-Evans 1985; Kildiran et al. 1996; Carapiso and Garcia 2000). The yield of *in situ* transesterification; however, may be more sensitive to water and FFA content of the oilseed feedstock.

8.4 Current Status of Biomass Esterification Activities

Most of the biodiesel on the market today is produced through the esterification process. A majority of the plants use alkali-catalysed transesterification techniques due to their high conversion yields, relatively short reaction times and the low temperature requirements. Oils with higher FFA content, such as palm oil and waste cooking oils, are commonly pretreated with acid-catalysed esterification before undergoing the conventional alkali-catalysed transesterification technique (Voegele 2012). Some producers use steam stripping (10%–15% FFA content) and glycerolysis (up to 5% FFA content) to deal with FFAs in oils, although these techniques are generally less popular than acid-catalysed pretreatment (Mosali and Bobbili 2011).

Although noncatalytic supercritical alcohol transesterification techniques are potentially low-cost simple technologies, as of 2011, they were still at the pilot or very early commercial stage, largely due to process safety concerns and associated capital costs (Geiver 2011a). Shockwave cavitation was being used in eight different biodiesel plants as of 2011, with one described as one of the largest production facilities in the United States (Geiver 2011b). Ultrasound cavitation technology is employed in a number of commercial-scale plants (Kotrba 2010); however, its prevalence in the industry could not be determined. Users of ultrasound technology would, however, seem to be very pleased with their results (Kotrba 2010; Hielscher Ultrasonics 2011a,b). Hielscher Ultrasonics (2011b) offers small-scale and medium-scale biodiesel reactors for production of up to 10 kl/h and full-scale industrial biodiesel reactors for up to 100 kl/h production.

Significant research has gone into lipase enzyme catalysts for the treatment of FFAs. Various biotechnology companies market proprietary enzyme systems for oil processing, either for food and cooking use or for biodiesel production (Novozymes 2010; Verenium 2010). Enzymatic systems may be built into new plants being constructed or retrofitted to existing plants. Despite intensive research and commercial availability, the use of enzyme catalysts on industrial scales is limited. Biodiesel producers cite the high costs of enzyme systems and technical issues, such as slow reaction rates and low yields, as reasons for preference for other techniques usually consisting of acid catalysis pretreatment (Voegele 2012; Iso et al. 2001).

Business models for biodiesel production plants typically follow two scales that allow them to ride out market fluctuations. Large-scale biodiesel companies (10 MMgy and larger) either own large corporate farms to supply sufficient oil to achieve a profitable economy of scale, or use their large size to negotiate on all levels of operation including long-term feedstock supply and off-take agreements. A drawback can be the cost of transporting large quantities of feedstock to the plant. Larger plants mostly use continuous-flow processes involving CSTRs or PFRs (Bart et al. 2010). Large-scale operations make up approximately 29% of plants in the United States (Seybold 2008) and are favoured in Argentina and Europe. Small-scale operations (0.1–9 MMgy) are common in the United States (approximately 38%; Seybold 2008). Small-scale plants have lower running costs and usually have access to local vegetable oil and waste oil feedstocks. Smaller plants often use batch reactors (Bart et al. 2010). The current trend is toward larger plants.

World biodiesel production by region and production of selected countries is shown in Table 8.2. The data are derived from the U.S. Energy Information

TABLE 8.2

World Biodiesel Production by Region and Selected Countries (million litres per year)

Region/Country	2000	2001	2002	2003	2004	2005	2006	2007	2008	2009	2010
North America	0	32	40	54	106	355	994	1953	2664	2044	1316
Canada	0	0	0	0	0	12	46	93	99	122	139
United States	—	32	40	54	106	344	948	1854	2560	1916	1171
Central and South America	6	12	23	23	29	32	131	653	2,079	3304	4952
Argentina	6	12	12	12	12	12	35	209	807	1341	2089
Brazil	0	0	0	0	0	1	69	404	1164	1608	2397
Columbia	0	0	0	0	0	0	0	6	81	331	418
Peru	0	0	12	12	17	17	23	23	12	12	29
Europe	876	1088	1410	1894	2385	3601	5601	7102	8745	10,090	10,626
Belgium	0	0	0	0	0	1	28	186	313	470	493
France	342	342	371	424	447	487	673	1085	1996	2379	2147
Germany	250	313	511	812	1161	1915	3018	3308	3192	2611	2843
Italy	93	162	238	308	360	447	673	534	760	905	841
Spain	93	93	87	116	128	186	70	203	250	812	928

Region											
Eurasia	0	0	0	0	6	17	19	42	145	221	189
Lithuania	0	0	0	0	6	6	12	29	75	110	99
Middle East	0	0	0	0	0	0	0	0	0	0	6
Israel	0	0	0	0	0	0	0	0	0	0	6
Africa	0	0	0	0	0	0	0	0	3	5	10
South Africa	0	0	0	0	0	0	0	0	0	1	2
Asia and Oceania	0	6	7	8	17	129	487	628	1574	2236	2381
Australia	0	0	0	0	6	12	23	41	52	99	81
China	0	6	6	6	6	46	232	116	290	348	348
India	0	0	0	0	0	12	23	12	12	58	116
Indonesia	0	0	0	0	0	12	23	58	116	348	464
Korea, South	0	0	1	2	6	12	52	99	186	290	377
Malaysia	0	0	0	0	0	0	64	145	261	261	116
Philippines	0	0	0	0	0	12	23	35	64	116	139
Thailand	0	0	0	0	0	23	23	70	447	609	638
World	882	1138	1480	1979	2543	4134	7232	10,378	15,210	17,900	19,480

Source: U.S. Department of Energy. International Energy Statistics, 2012. Available at http://www.eia.gov/cfapps/ipdbproject/IEDIndex3.cfm?tid=79&pid=79&aid=1 (accessed February 2012).

Administration (U.S. Department of Energy 2012). Global biodiesel production increased rapidly from 2004 to 2007, with slower growth beyond 2008. In 2010, estimated biodiesel production reached 19.5 billion litres, increasing by 9% from 2009. Europe remains at the centre of global biodiesel production, with the region accounting for approximately 55% of the global production in 2010. The dominance of the region, however, has waned in recent years as other regions have ramped up production. In 2004, Europe accounted for 94% of the global biodiesel production. Growth in the region slowed in recent years, increasing only 5.3% between 2009 and 2010, compared with 15.3% between 2008 and 2009 (peak growth was 55.5% between 2004 and 2005).

The top biodiesel-producing countries in 2010 are shown in Figure 8.5, as is production by the rest of the world. Germany is the world's largest biodiesel-producing country with 2.8 billion litres, growing by 8.9% in 2010. Brazil is the second largest producing country with production up 49.7% in 2010, to 2.4 billion litres. France is the third highest producing country with 2.1 billion litres, but with production decreasing by 9.8% compared with the previous year. Production in Argentina grew by 55.8% to 2.1 billion litres to make it the fourth largest biodiesel-producing country. The United States was the fifth with 1.2 billion litres; however, production decreased by 38.9%, which was its second year in decline.

Biodiesel production across the world is largely facilitated by national governmental agricultural subsidies and favourable tax policies and regulations. Initial government subsidies are especially necessary due to the high start-up costs of industrial biodiesel production. Biodiesel producers often depend on national governmental agricultural subsidies of feedstock crops, such as

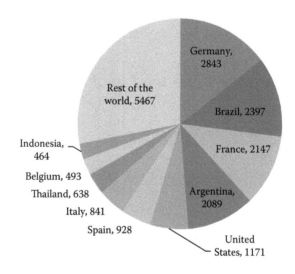

FIGURE 8.5
Biodiesel production in million litres for top countries in 2010.

rapeseed and soy because the raw cost of vegetable oils for esterification to biodiesel is often already higher than the final cost of petroleum-derived diesel fuel (Organisation for Economic Co-operation and Development [OECD] 2004). Biodiesel producers are also very sensitive to commodity price fluctuations of feedstock crops.

Biodiesel production in Europe and the United States experienced rapid growth from 2004 up until 2007. This was largely driven by detailed political directives to achieve biodiesel substitution in petrodiesel fuel blends. Producers in the United States also benefit from subsidised methyl ester (B99) exports to the European Union (EU). In Europe, a favourable taxation system allowed biodiesel to achieve approximate cost parity with conventional petroleum-derived diesel.

Since 2008, high feedstock prices for soybean oil in the United States have, in part, contributed to a slowdown of biodiesel production. As a result, most operations have operated below capacity, with many closing or being placed on standby. The fortunes of many biodiesel producers in the United States are particularly connected to a $1/gal federal tax credit for blending biodiesel in petrodiesel. When the tax credit first expired on 1 January 2010, 40 to 50 plants were left to idle, of which 20% to 25% closed permanently (Milne 2010). The tax credit was retroactively reinstated for the year in December 2010 and renewed for 2011. The biodiesel tax credit had not been reinstated for 2012 as of February, despite lobbying by producers (Kotrba 2012).

Similar to the United States, high rapeseed oil prices have contributed to the slowdown in European biodiesel production since 2007, with many operations running at a loss. European producers have also faced increased competition from relatively cheap imports from outside the EU (including from Argentina, Canada and increasingly Indonesia; REN21 Secretariat 2011). German producers have been dealing with the phaseout of a tax system (from 2007 to 2012) that favours rapeseed biodiesel. As a result, some German producers have been directed toward lower-priced raw materials such as soybean or palm oil (in summer blends; Bart et al. 2010). A legally specified overall blend quota (B7) for biofuels, introduced in January 2009, has since aided German producers. EU biodiesel production capacity was only utilised 44% for the first two quarters of 2011 (European Biodiesel Board 2011). In 2010, biodiesel production declined in some of the EU countries including France, Italy and Austria. A number of production facilities in Germany and Southern Europe have ceased operation. For example, one of Germany's leading biodiesel producers, Campa AG, stopped production at its 45 MMgy plant in Ochsenfurt and put the construction of a 60 MMgy plant in Straubling on hold. The slowdown in the biodiesel industry has been exacerbated by weak economic conditions in the United States and Europe, difficulties obtaining finance, thin capitalisation of projects and increasing construction costs with consequent slowdown in construction and production.

Argentina, Brazil, India, China and southeast Asian countries are building up biodiesel capacities at a strong pace. Production in Argentina and Brazil is largely soybean-based and the crop is cheap and available locally with sufficient milling facilities. In Argentina, more than 53% of the entire agricultural land surface is utilised for soybean production (6 Mt/year soybean oil on 15 Mha; Bart et al. 2010). A principal criticism is related to deforestation (on 600 kha) associated with soy cultivation in forested areas, such as the Humid Chaco. In Argentina, producers benefit from a differential export tax structure that favours export of biodiesel over soybean oil and soybeans. The export tax for biodiesel is approximately 12% lower than for vegetable oil. That investment incentive is driving the huge expansion of biodiesel production in Argentina, much of it aimed for export to Europe. Argentina favours large-scale plants for processing soybean oil, which are able to achieve significant economies of scale and global cost competiveness.

In Asia, where palm oil is the primary feedstock, production in Indonesia grew by 33% to 0.5 billion litres in 2010. Thailand remains the largest producer in Asia with 0.6 billion litres. Australian biodiesel production is small. Table 8.3 presents the biodiesel production facilities in Australia (Biofuels Association of Australia 2010). Only 81 ML was produced in 2010 out of 350 ML capacity due to an unfavourable tax regime and increasing feedstock prices. Predominant feedstocks are used cooking oil and tallow. This capacity is provided by five biodiesel producers with seven plants. However, only five of these plants were operating as of January 2012 (Biofuels Association of Australia 2010). The largest Australian producer of biodiesel is Australian Renewable Fuels, which now operates three plants nationally after the acquisition of the Biodiesel Producers plant at Barnawatha, Victoria (Australian Competition and Consumer Commission [ACCC] 2011). Australian biodiesel producers face challenges concerning the availability and the high price of feedstocks. As a result, new biodiesel projects have faced repeated deferrals and ongoing uncertainty. For example, National Biodiesel's plans to build what would have been Australia's largest capacity facility at 300 ML in New South Wales are in their third year of deferral and therefore its future is uncertain (APAC Biofuels Consultants 2011 as cited in ACCC 2011).

Edible vegetable oils still account for approximately 90% of feedstock for biodiesel production (OECD/FAO 2011). Their high cost has motivated a general shift to the use of waste oils and inedible vegetable oils for biodiesel production. In established biodiesel-producing countries, such as Germany and the United States, growth in the use of virgin vegetable oil feedstock is limited, with markets shifting to non-food stocks and large-scale and more technologically advanced plants. India, China, Brazil and other developing countries are particularly supportive of the use of inedible feedstocks for biodiesel production.

Waste cooking oils and inedible plant oils offer a means of reducing the cost of producing biodiesel. The waste oil can be obtained from fast-food restaurants, industrial deep-fryers in food processing plants, snack food factories,

TABLE 8.3

Biodiesel Plants in Australia

Biodiesel Plant	Location	Owner	Total Installed Capacity (ML; as of 1 January, 2012)	Feedstocks	Status (as of 1 January, 2012)
ARF Largs Bay	Adelaide, South Australia	Australian Renewable Fuels	45	Tallow, used cooking oil	In production
ARF Picton Plant	Picton, West Australia	Australian Renewable Fuels	45	Tallow, used cooking oil	In production
BPL Biodiesel Plant	Wodonga, Victoria	Australian Renewable Fuels	60	Tallow, used cooking oil	In production
BIA Biodiesel Plant	Maitland, New South Wales	Biodiesel Industries Australia	20	Used cooking oil, vegetable oil	In production
Smorgon Fuels—BioMax Plant	Melbourne, Victoria	Smorgon Fuels Pty. Ltd.	15–100	Tallow, canola oil and juncea oil	In production, possible expansion
N/A	Darwin, Northern Territory	Vopak	130	Palm oil	Not in production
Eco Tech Biodiesel Plant	Narangba, Queensland	Gull Group	30	Tallow, used cooking oil	Not in production
Total capacity (ML)			350		
National Biodiesel Plant	Port Kembla, New South Wales	National Biofuels Group	300	Soya	Not yet constructed

Source: Biofuels Association of Australia. Biodiesel production facilities in Australia, 2010. Available at http://www.biofuelsassociation.com.au/index.php?option=com_content&view=article&id=59&Itemid=67 (accessed February 2012).

TABLE 8.4

Quantity of Waste Edible Oil in Various
Counties Worldwide

Country	Quantity (million tons/year)
China	4.5
Malaysia	0.5
United States	10
Taiwan	0.07
European	0.7–1.0
Canada	0.12
Japan	0.45–0.57

Source: Gui, M.M. et al., *Energy* 33:1646, 2008.

and even household kitchens. Waste cooking oils contain substantially more
FFAs and water than fresh vegetable oils and so the biodiesel production
process is usually adapted, often involving an acid-catalysed pretreatment.
Estimates suggest that more than 15 million tonnes of waste edible oil is generated annually worldwide. The United States generates approximately 10
million tonnes and China generates about 4.5 million tonnes of waste edible
oil (Gui et al. 2008). Table 8.4 shows the quantity of waste edible oils in various countries worldwide (Gui et al. 2008).

Use of the inedible oil from Jatropha as a feedstock for transesterification to
biodiesel is a rapidly growing industry. Jatropha can be grown in marginal,
nonagricultural lands; requires little water; and does not compete with food
and so is not affected by increasing food prices. There has been a dramatic
expansion in Jatropha plantations worldwide, particularly in Southeast Asia,
Africa and Central and South America. Jatropha is currently grown for
transesterification to biodiesel in India, the Philippines, Indonesia, Brazil,
Ghana and in other developing countries. Jatropha cultivation in most cases
is still on a project or small-scale level, and so does not yet allow for large-
scale biodiesel production. As of 2010, Jatropha still accounted for less than
2% of the feedstock used for biodiesel production (OECD/FAO 2011).

8.5 Conclusion

The majority of biodiesel is produced using conventional alkali-catalysed
transesterification techniques using batch or continuous processes. There
is an ongoing shift to more efficient large-scale continuous process facilities. Much of the research and development has been involved in optimising esterification reaction conditions and production methods, including

work to increase yields, reduce reaction time and reduce costs and simplify the production process. Key technologies have also emerged including lipase enzyme catalysts, noncatalytic supercritical alcohol techniques and ultrasonic cavitation. Although these technologies have experienced mostly limited commercial implementation, they offer promising prospects to increase the economic and technical competitiveness of esterified biodiesel.

Commercial production of biodiesel through esterification has developed rapidly over the past decade. Biodiesel production reached nearly 20 billion litres globally by 2010. Yet, it still only makes up a minor fraction (<1%) of the overall world consumption of diesel fuel. Commercial esterification to convert vegetable oils and animal fats to biodiesel is not, for the most part, competitive with petroleum-derived diesel production methods, except with favourable fiscal policies and tax incentives. Currently, biodiesel production is made up of esterification of mainly vegetable oil feedstocks: rapeseed, soybean, sunflower and palm oils. The high cost of these vegetable oil feedstocks is a significant economic problem for biodiesel producers. Due to limited arable land, use of vegetable oils is unlikely to ever significantly displace petroleum diesel as a source of diesel fuel. The increasing use of waste cooking oils and the development of inedible plant oils, such as Jatropha and algae for esterification to biodiesel, will reduce the cost of biodiesel production through esterification. Combined with advancing technologies, which offer greater capability to deal with the high FFAs and other impurities in lower cost fuels, esterification has the potential to form part of the solution to the energy and greenhouse gas crisis.

References

Achten, W.M.J.; Verchot, L.; Franken, Y.J.; Mathijs, E.; Singh, V.P.; Aerts, R.; Muys, B. (2008). *Jatropha* Bio-diesel Production and Use. *Biomass and Bioenergy* 32: 1063–1084.

Armenta, R.E.; Vinatoru, M.; Burja, A.M.; Kralovec, J.A.; Barow, C.J. (2007). Transesterification of Fish Oil to Produce Fatty Acid Ethyl Esters Using Ultrasonic Energy. *Journal of American Oil Chemists' Society* 84: 1045–1052.

Australian Competition and Consumer Commission (ACCC) (2011). *Monitoring of the Australian Petroleum Industry-Report of the ACCC into the Prices, Costs and Profits of Unleaded Petrol in Australia 2011*. Commonwealth of Australia. http://www.accc.gov.au/content/index.phtml/itemId/1020827 (Accessed February 2012).

Azachi, M.; Sadka, A.; Fisher, M.; Goldshlag, P.; Gokhman, I.; Zamir, A. (2002). Salt Induction of Fatty Acid Elongase and Membrane Lipid Modifications in the Extreme Halotolerant Alga *Dunaliella Salina*. *Plant Physiology* 129: 1320–1329.

Bala, B.K. (2005). Studies on Biodiesels from Transformation of Vegetable Oils for Diesel Engines. *Energy Education Science and Technology* 16: 45–52.

Bart, J.C.J.; Palmeri, N.; Cavallaro, S. (2010). *Biodiesel Science and Technology: From Soil to Oil*. CRC Press; Cambridge, UK.

Biofuels Association of Australia (2010). Biodiesel Production Facilities in Australia. http://www.biofuelsassociation.com.au/index.php?option=com_content& view=article&id=59&Itemid=67 (Accessed February 2012).

Biofuels International (2010). Novozymes and Piedmont Launch Enzymatic Biodiesel Plant. *Biofuels International* 4(7): 16, September 2011.

BIOX Corporation (2010). BIOX Corporation >> Production Processes. http://www. bioxcorp.com/production-process (Accessed February 2012).

Boocock, D.G.B.; Konar, S.K.; Mao, V.; Sidi, H. (1996). Fast One-Phase Oil-Rich Processes for the Preparation of Vegetable Oil Methyl Esters. *Biomass and Bioenergy* 11: 43–50.

Boocock, D.G.B.; Konar, S.K.; Mao, V.; Lee, C. (1998). Fast Formation of High-Purity Methyl Esters from Vegetable Oils. *Journal of American Oil Chemists' Society* 75: 1167–1172.

Canakci, M.; Van Gerpen, J. (1999). Biodiesel Production via Acid Catalysis. *Transactions of the American Society of Agricultural Engineers* 42: 1203–1210.

Canakci, M.; Van Gerpen, J. (2001). Biodiesel Production from Oils and Fats with High Free Fatty Acids. *Transactions of the American Society of Agricultural Engineers* 44: 1429–1436.

Carapiso, A.I.; Garcia, C. (2000). Development in Lipid Analysis: Some New Extraction Techniques and in situ Transesterification. *Lipids* 35: 1167–1177.

Christi, Y. (2007). Biodiesel from Microalgae. *Biotechnology Advances* 25: 294–306.

Darnoko, D.; Cheryan, M. (2000). Kinetics of Palm Oil Transesterification in a Batch Reactor. *Journal of American Oil Chemists' Society* 77: 563–567.

de Oliveira, D.; Di Luccio, M.D.; Faccio, C.; Rosa, C.D.; Bender, J.P.; Lipek, N.; Amroginski, C.; Dariva, C.; de Oliveira, J.V. (2005). Optimization of Alkaline Transesterification of Soybean Oil and Castor Oil for Biodiesel Production. *Applied Biochemistry and Biotechnology* 121–124: 553–560.

Demirbas, A. (2002a). Biodiesel from Vegetable Oils via Transesterification in Super-critical Methanol. *Energy Conversion and Management* 24: 835–841.

Demirbas, A. (2002b). Diesel Fuel from Vegetable Oil via Transesterification and Soap Pyrolysis. *Energy Sources* 24: 835–841.

Demirbas, A. (2003a). Biodiesel Fuels from Vegetable Oils via Catalytic and Non-catalytic Supercritical Alcohol Transesterification and Other Methods: A Survey. *Energy Conversion and Management* 44: 2093–2109.

Demirbas, A. (2003b). Fuel Conversional Aspects of Palm Oil and Sunflower Oil. *Energy Sources* 25: 457–466.

Demirbas, A. (2006). Biodiesel Production via Non-catalytic SCF Method and Biodiesel Fuel Characteristics. *Energy Conversion and Management* 47: 2271–2282.

Demirbas, A. (2007). Importance of Biodiesel as Transportation Fuel. *Energy Policy* 35: 4661–4670.

Demirbas, A. (2008). Comparison of Transesterification Methods for Production of Biodiesel from Vegetable Oils and Fats. *Energy Conversion and Management* 49: 125–130.

Demirbas, A. (2009). Progress and Recent Trends in Biodiesel Fuels. *Energy Conversion and Management* 50: 14–34.

European Biodiesel Board (2011). *PRESS RELEASE: 2010–2011: EU Biodiesel Industry Production Forecasts Show First Decrease in 2011 Since Data is Gathered.* http:// www.ebb-eu.org/EBBpressreleases/EBB%20press%20release%202010%20 prod%202011_capacity%20FINAL.pdf (Accessed February 2012).

Fjerbaek, L.; Christensen, K.V.; Norddahl, B. (2009). A Review of the Current State of Biodiesel Production Using Enzymatic Transesterification. *Biotechnology and Bioengineering* 102: 1298–1315.

Food and Agricultural Organisation (FAO) (2008). FAOSTAT. http://faostat.fao.org/ (Accessed January 2012).

Food and Agricultural Organisation (FAO) (2010). *Sunflower Crude and Refined Oils Agribusiness Handbook.* http://www.fao.org/docrep/012/al375e/al375e.pdf (Accessed February 2012).

Fortenbery, T.R. (2005). Biodiesel Feasibility Study: An Evaluation of Biodiesel Feasibility in Wisconsin. Staff Paper Series, Agricultural & Applied Economics; University of Wisconsin-Madison.

Freedman, B.; Pryde, E.H.; Mounts, T.L. (1984). Variables Affecting the Yields of Fatty Esters from Transesterified Vegetable Oils. *Journal of the American Oil Chemists' Society* 61: 1638–1643.

Freedman, B.; Butterfield, R.O.; Pryde, E.H. (1986). Transesterification Kinetics of Soybean Oil. *Journal of American Oil Chemists' Society* 63: 1375–1380.

Fukuda, H.; Kondo, A.; Noda, H. (2001). Biodiesel Fuel Production by Trans-esterification of Oils. *Journal of Bioscience and Bioengineering* 92: 405–416.

Geiver, L. (2011a). Proving Out the Supercritical Processing. *Biodiesel Magazine.* http://www.biodieselmagazine.com/articles/7791/proving-out-supercritical-processing (Accessed February 2012).

Geiver, L. (2011b). Ready to Burst. *Biodiesel Magazine.* http://www.biodieselmagazine. com/articles/7598/ready-to-burst (Accessed February 2012).

Georgogianni, K.G.; Kontominas, M.G.; Pomonis, P.J.; Avlonitis, D.; Gergis, V. (2008). Conventional and in situ Transesterification of Sunflower Seed Oil for the Production of Biodiesel. *Fuel Processing Technology* 89: 503–509.

Grün, I.U. (2004). Fats: Edible Fat and Oil Processing. In J.S. Smith and Y.H. Hui (eds.), *Food Processing: Principles and Applications.* Blackwell; IA; pp. 353–360.

Gui, M.M.; Lee, K.T.; Bhatia, S. (2008). Feasibility of Edible Oil vs. Non-edible Oil vs. Waste Edible Oil as Biodiesel Feedstock. *Energy* 33: 1646.

Gunstone, F. (2008). *Oils and Fats in the Food Industry.* Blackwell; Oxford.

Gupta, M.J. (2002). Sunflower Oil. In F.D. Gunstone (ed.), *Vegetable Oils in Food Technology: Composition, Properties and Uses.* CRC Press; Boca Raton, FL; pp. 128–156.

Haas, M.J.; Scott, K.M.; Foglia, T.A.; Marmer, W.N. (2007). The General Applicability of in situ Transesterification for the Production of Fatty Acid Esters from a Variety of Feedstocks. *Journal of the American Oil Chemists' Society* 84: 963–970.

Harrington, K.J.; D'Arcy-Evans, C.A. (1985). Comparison of Conventional and in situ Methods of Transesterification of Seed Oil from a Series of Sunflower Cultivar. *Journal of the American Oil Chemists' Society* 62: 1009–1013.

Hielscher Ultrasonics (2011a). Ultrasonics Improve Biodiesel Process Efficiency. http://www.hielscher.com/ultrasonics/biodiesel_processing_efficiency.htm (Accessed February 2011).

Hielscher Ultrasonics (2011b). Ultrasonics Improve Biodiesel Process Efficiency. http://www.hielscher.com/ultrasonics/biodiesel_ultrasonic_mixing_reactors. htm (Accessed February 2011).

Hydro Dynamics (n.d.). Technology—Hydro Dynamics Inc. Cavitation Reactors. http://www.hydrodynamics.com/technology (Accessed February 2011).

Iso, M.; Chen, B.; Eguchi, M.; Kudo, T.; Shrestha, S. (2001). Production of Biodiesel Fuel from Triglycerides and Alcohol Using Immobilized Lipase. *Journal of Molecular Catalysis B: Enzymatic* 16: 53–58.

Jamieson, G.S. (1932). *Vegetable Fats and Oils, the Chemistry, Production and Utilization of Vegetable Fats and Oils for Edible, Medicinal and Technical Purpose.* Chemical Catalog Co.; New York.

Kemp, W.H. (2006). *An Introduction to Biodiesel. Biodiesel Basics and Beyond: A Comprehensive Guide to Production and Use for the Home and Farm.* Aztec Press; Ontario, Canada.

Keshwani, D.R. (2010). Biomass Chemistry. In J. Cheng (ed.), *Biomass to Renewable Energy Processes.* CRC Press; Boca Raton, FL; pp. 7–40.

Kildiran, G.; Yücel, S.O.; Türkay, S. (1996). In-situ Alcoholysis of Soybean Oil. *Journal of the American Oil Chemists' Society* 73: 225–228.

Kose, O.; Tuter, M.; Aksoy, H.A. (2002). Immobilized *Candida Antarctica* Lipase-catalysed Alcoholysis of Cottonseed Oil in a Solvent-free Medium. *Bioresource Technology* 83: 125–129.

Kotrba, R. (2010). Ultrasonic Biodiesel Processing. *Biodiesel Magazine.* http://www.biodieselmagazine.com/articles/4202/ultrasonic-biodiesel-processing (Accessed February 2012).

Kotrba, R. (2011). New Technologies Continue to Develop. *Biodiesel Magazine.* http://www.biodieselmagazine.com/articles/8123/new-technologies-continue-to-develop (Accessed February 2012).

Kotrba, R. (2012). Northwest Producers Unite, Tell Congress to Reinstate Tax Credit. *Biodiesel Magazine.* http://www.biodieselmagazine.com/articles/8335/northwest-producers-unite-tell-congress-to-reinstate-tax-credit (Accessed February 2012).

Kusdiana, D.; Saka, S. (2004). Effects of Water on Biodiesel Fuel Production by Supercritical Methanol Treatment. *Bioresource Technology* 91: 289–295.

Lang, X.; Dalai, A.K.; Bakhshi, N.N.; Reany, M.J.; Hertz, P.B. (2001). Preparation and Characterization of Bio-diesels from Various Bio-oils. *Bioresource Technology* 80: 53–62.

Lee, K.T.; Foglia, T.A.; Chang, K.S. (2002). Production of Alkyl Ester as Biodiesel from Fractionated Lard and Restaurant Grease. *Journal of American Oil Chemists' Society* 79: 191–195.

Lee, G.C.; Wang, D.L.; Ho, Y.F.; Shaw, J.F. (2004). Lipase-Catalysed Alcoholysis of Triglyceride for Short-Chain Monoglyceride Production. *Journal of American Oil Chemists' Society* 84: 533–536.

Leung, D.Y.C.; Guo, Y. (2006). Transesterification of Neat and used Frying Oil: Optimization for Biodiesel Production. *Fuel Processing Technology* 87: 883–890.

Leung, D.Y.C.; Wu, X.; Leung, M.K.H. (2010). A Review on Biodiesel Production Using Catalyzed Transesterification. *Applied Energy* 87: 1083–1095.

Li, N.W.; Wu, H.; Zong, M.H.; Lou, W.Y. (2007a). Lipase-Catalysed Transesterification of Rapeseed Oils for Biodiesel Production with a Novel Organic Solvent as the Reaction Medium. *Journal of Molecular Catalysis* 28: 333–338.

Li, X.; Xu, H.; Wu, Q. (2007b). Large-Scale Biodiesel Production from Microalga Chlorella Protethacoids through Heterotrophic Cultivation in Bioreactors. *Biotechnology and Bioengineering* 98: 764–771.

Lu, J.K.; Nie, K.L.; Xie, F.; Wang, Y.J.; Zhu, S.L. (2007). Enzymatic Synthesis of Fatty Acid Methyl Esters from Lard with Immobilized *Candida sp. Process Biochemistry* 42: 1367–1370.

Ma, F.; Clements, L.D.; Hanna, M. (1998). The Effects of Catalyst, Free Fatty Acids, and Water on Transesterification of Beef Tallow. *Transactions of the American Society of Agricultural Engineers* 41: 1261–1264.

Ma, F.M.; Hanna, M.A. (1999). Biodiesel Production: A Review. *Bioresource Technology* 70: 1–15.

Mahajan, S.; Konar, S.K.; Boocock, D.G.B. (2006). Standard Biodiesel from Soybean Oil by a Single Chemical Reaction. *Journal of the American Oil Chemists' Society* 7: 641–644.

Marchetti, J.M.; Miguel, V.U.; Errazu, A.F. (2007). Possible Methods for Biodiesel Production. *Renewable and Sustainable Energy Reviews* 11: 1300–1311.

Meher, L.C.; Dharmagadda, V.S.S.; Naik, S.N. (2006a). Optimization of Alkali-Catalysed Transesterification of *Pongamia pinnata* Oil for Production of Biodiesel. *Bioresource Technology* 97: 1392–1397.

Meher, L.; Sagar, D.; Naik, S. (2006b). Technical Aspects of Biodiesel Production by Transesterification—A Review. *Renewable and Sustainable Energy Reviews* 10: 248–268.

Miao, X.; Wu, Q. (2006). Biodiesel Production from Heterotrophic Microalgal Oil. *Bioresource Technology* 97: 841–846.

Milne, B. (2010). US Biodiesel Industry Struggles to Catch a Tax Break. *Biofuels International* 4(7): 38–39, September 2011.

Mittelbach, M.; Trathnigg, B. (1990). Kinetics of Alkaline Catalyzed Methanolysis of Sunflower Oil. 92: 145–148.

Modi, M.K.; Reddy, J.R.C.; Rao, V.V.S.K.; Prasad, R.B.N. (2006). Lipase-Mediated Transformation of Vegetable Oils into Biodiesel Using Propan-2-ol as Acyl Accepter. *Biotechnology Letters* 28: 637–640.

Mosali, R.; Bobbili, S. (2011). Homogenous Catalyst and Effects on Multifeedstock Processing. *Biodiesel Magazine*. http://www.biodieselmagazine.com/articles/ 7793/homogenous-catalyst-and-effects-on-multifeedstock-processing (Accessed February 2012).

Nagao, T.; Shimada, Y.; Sugihara, A.; Tominaga, Y. (1996). Expression of Lipase cDNA from *Fusarium Heterosporum* by *Saccharomyces cerevisiae*: High-Level Production and Purification. *Journal of Fermentation and Bioengineering* 81: 488–492.

Nelson, R.G.; Schrock, M.D. (2006). Energetic and Economic Feasibility Associated with the Production, Processing, and Conversion of Beef Tallow to a Substitute Diesel Fuel. *Biomass and Bioenergy* 30: 584–591.

Nersesian, R.L. (2007). Energy for the 21st Century: A Comprehensive Guide to Conventional and Alternative Sources. In M.E. Sharpe (ed.), *Bioenergy and Biofuel from Biowastes and Biomass*. American Society of Civil Engineers; Reston, VA; pp. 389–410.

Novozymes (2010). Oils & Fats. http://www.novozymes.com/en/solutions/food-and-beverages/oils-fats/Pages/default.aspx (Accessed February 2012).

OECD/FAO (2011). *OECD-FAO Agricultural Outlook 2011–2020*. OECD Publishing and FAO. http://dx.doi.org/10.1787/agr_outlook-2011-en (Accessed February 2012).

Organisation for Economic Co-operation and Development (OECD) (2004). *Biomass and Agriculture: Sustainability, Markets and Policies*. OECD Publishing; Paris.

Pimentel, D.; Marklein, A.; Toth, M.A.; Karpoff, M.N.; Paul, G.S.; McCormack, R.; Kyriazi, J.; Krueger, T. (2009). Food versus Biofuels: Environmental and Economic Costs. *Human Ecology* 37: 1–12.

Prueksakorn, K.; Gheewala, S.H. (2008). Full Chain Energy Analysis of Biodiesel from *Jatropha curcas* L. in Thailand. *Environmental Science and Technology* 42: 3388–3393.

Ramadhas, A.S.; Jayaraj, S.; Muraleedharan, C. (2005). Biodiesel Production from High FFA Rubber Seed Oil. *Fuel* 84: 336–340.

Ranganathan, S.V.; Narasimhan, S.L.; Muthukumar, K. (2008). An Overview of Enzymatic Production of Biodiesel. *Bioresource Technology* 99: 3978–3981.

REN21 Secretariat (2011). *Renewables 2011 Global Status Report.* Paris. http://www.ren21. net/Portals/97/documents/GSR/REN21_GSR2011.pdf (Accessed February 2012).

Saka, S.; Kusdiana, D. (2001). Biodiesel Fuel from Rapeseed Oil as Prepared in Supercritical Methanol. *Fuel* 80: 225–231.

Santos, F.P.P.; Rodrigues, S.; Fernandes, F.A.N. (2009). Optimization of the Production of Biodiesel from Soybean Oil by Ultrasound Assisted Methanolysis. *Fuel Processing Technology* 90: 312–319.

Schnepf, R. (2003). Biodiesel Fuel and U.S. Agriculture. http://www.biodiesel. org/resources/reportsdatabase/reports/gen/20030707_gen-379.pdf (Accessed January 2012).

Seybold, J. (2008). Taking the Pulse of the Biodiesel Industry. *Biodiesel Magazine.* http://biodieselmagazine.com/articles/2060/taking-the-pulse-of-the-biodiesel-industry (Accessed February 2012).

Shahid, E.M.; Jamal, Y. (2011). Production of Biodiesel: A Technical Review. *Renewable and Sustainable Energy Reviews* 15: 4732–4745.

Sims, B. (2011). Clearing the Way for Byproduct Quality. *Biodiesel Magazine.* http:// www.biodieselmagazine.com/articles/8137/clearing-the-way-for-byproduct-quality (Accessed February 2012).

Srivastava, A.; Prasad, R. (2000). Triglycerides-based Diesel Fuels. *Renewable and Sustainable Energy Reviews* 4: 111–133.

Stavarache, C.; Vinatoru, M.; Nishimura, R.; Maeda, Y. (2005). Fatty Acid Methyl Esters from Vegetable Oils by Means of Ultrasonic Energy. *Ultrasonics Sonochemistry* 12: 367–372.

Thanh, L.T.; Okitsu, K.; Sadanga, Y.; Takenaka, N.; Maeda, Y.; Bandow, H. (2009). Ultrasound-Assisted Production of Biodiesel Fuel from Vegetable Oils in a Small Scale Circulation Process. *Bioresource Technology* 101: 639–645.

Thompson, J.C.; He, B.B. (2006). Characterization of Crude Glycerol from Biodiesel Production from Multiple Feedstocks. *Applied Engineering in Agriculture* 22: 261–265.

U.S. Department of Energy (2012). International Energy Statistics. http://www.eia.gov/ cfapps/ipdbproject/IEDIndex3.cfm?tid=79&pid=79&aid=1 (Accessed February 2012).

Van Gerpen, J.H.; Shanks, B.; Pruszko, R.; Clements, D.; Knothe, G. (2004). *Biodiesel Production Technology.* Report from Iowa State University for the National Renewable Energy Laboratory, NREL/SR-510-36244.

Van Gerpen, J. (2009). Biodiesel: Small Scale Production and Quality Requirement. In J. R. Mielenz (ed.), *Biofuels: Methods and Protocols.* Humana Press; New York; pp. 281–290.

Verenium (2010). Verenium-Purifine® Phospholipase C (PLC). http://www.verenium. com/prod_purifine.html (Accessed February 2012).

Vincente, G.; Martinez, M.; Aracil, J. (2004). Integrated Biodiesel Production: A Comparison of Different Homogenous Catalysts Systems. *Bioresource Technology* 92: 297–305.

Voegele, E. (2009). Glycerin: Research Turns UP New Uses. *Biodiesel Magazine.* http://www.biodieselmagazine.com/articles/3237/glycerin-research-turns-up-new-uses (Accessed January 2012).

Voegele, E. (2012). A Critical Component. *Biodiesel Magazine.* http://www.biodiesel magazine.com/articles/8295/a-critical-component (Accessed February 2012).

Wang, T. (2002). Soybean Oil. In F.D. Gunstone (ed.), *Vegetable Oils in Food Technology: Composition, Properties and Uses.* Blackwell; Oxford; pp. 18–58.

Wang, Z.; Keshwani, D.R. (2010). Biomass Resources. In J. Cheng (ed.), *Biomass to Renewable Energy Processes.* CRC Press; Boca Raton, FL; pp. 41–70.

Wei, D.-Z.; Yang, F.; Su, E. (2009). Chemical Conversion Process for Biodiesel Production. In J. Cheng (ed.), *Biomass to Renewable Energy Processes.* CRC Press; Boca Raton, FL; pp. 337–435.

Wu, X.Y.; Jääaskeläinen, S.; Linko, Y. (1996). An Investigation of Crude Lipases for Hydrolysis, Esterification, and Transesterification. *Enzyme and Microbial Technology* 19: 226–231.

Xue, F.; Zhang, X.; Luo, H.; Tan, T. (2006). A New Method for Preparing Raw Material for Biodiesel Production. *Process Biochemistry* 41: 1699–1702.

Zhang, Y.; Dube, M.A.; McLean, D.D.; Kates, M. (2003a). Biodiesel Production from Waste Cooking Oil: 2. Economic Assessment and Sensitivity Analysis. *Bioresource Technology* 90: 229–240.

Zhang, Y.; Dube, M.A.; Mclean, D.D.; Kates, M. (2003b). Biodiesel Production from Waste Cooking Oil: 1. Process Design and Technological Assessment. *Bioresource Technology* 89: 1–16.

Zhou, W.; Konar, S.K.; Boocock, D.G.B. (2003). Ethyl Esters from the Single-Phase Base-Catalyzed Ethanolysis of Vegetable Oils. *Journal of the American Oil Chemists' Society* 80: 367–371.

9

Fermentation of Biomass

Katrin Thommes and Vladimir Strezov

CONTENTS

9.1 Introduction

A major challenge to reducing our dependence on fossil fuel resources is the production of sustainable liquid fuels. Ethanol is amongst the most well-known liquid fuels and has been used for car engines since the late 1800s (Rothmann et al. 1983). Ethyl alcohol, or chemically, C_2H_5OH or EtOH, can be produced from renewable biomass materials and is therefore considered a 'green' fuel. Its utilisation as a transportation fuel can help reduce both the consumption of crude oil and the associated production of greenhouse gases.

Although alcohols have been known as fuels for combustion engines for more than a century, ethanol was only established as an alternative fuel during the oil crisis in the 1970s. Today, it accounts for the majority of the biofuel production worldwide (Walter et al. 2008). Ethanol can be used as liquid biofuel or as a gasoline 'antiknock' additive to increase the octane number. The oxygen it contains also helps reduce the emissions of carbon monoxide and particulate matter during the combustion process. Disadvantages of ethanol as gasoline substitute include a lower energy density, higher corrosiveness and comparatively high production costs (Balat et al. 2008).

Because many countries have implemented programmes to support alternative fuels and reduce dependence on oil imports, global fuel ethanol production has increased significantly over the last decade. The percentage of ethanol used in petrol ranges from 5% (Sweden) to 85% or more (Brazil), depending on the country and subsidies (Balat 2005). Ethanol can be produced synthetically or biologically. Bioethanol fuel is obtained through the fermentation of biomass materials including energy crops (such as corn, wheat and sugarcane) and lignocellulosic biomass (such as agricultural wastes and forest residues). On a commercial scale, nearly all of the biologically produced ethyl alcohol is obtained from corn or sugarcane, with the United States and Brazil being the main producers (Walter et al. 2008).

The cost and complexity of the bioethanol production process greatly depends on the type of feedstock used. Overall, these feedstocks can be divided into three categories: (a) sugar-containing feedstocks (e.g. sugarcane, sugar beet and sorghum), (b) starch-based feedstocks (e.g. corn, wheat and barley) and (c) lignocellulosic materials (e.g. agricultural wastes such as wheat straw, corn stover, grass and forest residuals). Based on the substrates used in the production process, ethanol is often grouped into first (crops, sugar), second (lignocellulose) or third (algae, seaweed) generation bioethanol (Nigam and Singh 2011). Given that second and third generation feedstocks are obtained from nonfood crop sources and are present in significant quantities, their use has been of increasing interest to develop. Although the potential production of bioethanol could replace a large amount of gasoline, the commercial scale is still limited by its economic and technical feasibility.

The fermentation process to convert sugars to ethanol is well established. Production cost, however, is a limiting factor in bioethanol production, and competitiveness with fossil fuels can only be reached through the optimisation of process designs and the development of suitable technologies.

9.2 Fermentation Process

9.2.1 General Concept of Fermentation

The process of fermentation has been known for centuries and generally refers to the conversion of simple sugars to ethanol and carbon dioxide in the presence of microorganisms such as yeasts (Figure 9.1). This process usually takes place under anaerobic conditions.

The most widely used microorganism for the production of ethanol is *Saccharomyces cerevisiae*, also known as 'Baker's yeast'. The yeast cells produce ethanol to provide energy for cell growth. There are several metabolic

$$\text{Sugar} \xrightarrow{\text{Microorganisms}} \text{Ethanol} (+ CO_2 + \text{by-products})$$

$$\underset{100\,g}{C_6H_{12}O_6\ (\text{Hexoses})} \longrightarrow \underset{51.14\,g}{2\,C_2H_5OH} + \underset{48.86\,g}{2\,CO_2}$$

$$\underset{100\,g}{3\,C_5H_{10}O_5\ (\text{Pentoses})} \longrightarrow \underset{51.14\,g}{5\,C_2H_5OH} + \underset{48.86\,g}{5\,CO_2}$$

FIGURE 9.1
Chemical reaction for fermentation.

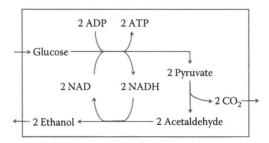

FIGURE 9.2
Simplified Embden–Meyerhof pathway of alcohol fermentation in a yeast cell (*S. cerevisiae*).

pathways that control the conversion of sugars to EtOH, with glycolysis or the Emdben–Meyerhof–Parnas (EMP) pathway being the central one for hexose sugars such as glucose (Taherzadeh and Karimi 2008). In the yeast cell, the latter is converted to pyruvate and then to ethanol in a sequence of reactions involving adenosine triphosphate (ATP), nicotinamide adenine dinucleotide (NADH) and enzymes (Figure 9.2). The major product, ethanol, is accompanied by several by-products such as biomass, glycerol and carboxylic acid. This biological reaction takes place at ambient temperature and under atmospheric pressure.

Stoichiometrically, 1 mol of glucose would be converted into 2 mol of ethanol. As outlined in the chemical reaction in Figure 9.1, the theoretical yield in this case would be 0.51 g of ethanol starting from 1 g of glucose. Due to the formation of by-products, however, the yields obtained during a fermentation process are usually in the range of 90% to 95% (Scragg 2009).

Pentose sugars (five-carbon chain) can also be converted to ethanol under anaerobic conditions through a pentose phosphate pathway (PPP) and glycolysis. The general overall reaction equation is displayed in Figure 9.1. The reactions involved in pentose sugar conversion are significantly slower than those for hexoses (six-carbon chain) and only a few microorganisms have been found to be able to produce ethanol from pentose sugars (Chandel et al. 2011). Industrial applications have thus far been limited.

9.2.2 Feedstock for Bioethanol Production

The three main types of feedstock (sugar, starch and lignocellulosic materials) contain different types of sugars and other substrates resulting in significant structural differences. Table 9.1 provides an overview of the components and structures of the different feedstocks that influence the number and complexity of process steps prior to fermentation. A breakdown of the worldwide commercial bioethanol production quantities (by country and region) is listed in Table 9.2.

TABLE 9.1

Components and Structure of the Three Different Feedstocks Used for Bioethanol Production

Feedstock	Materials	Components	Structure	Resulting Sugars for Fermentation
Sugar-based	Sugarcane, sugar beet, sorghum	Sucrose	Disaccharide	Glucose (C6)
Starch	Corn, wheat, barley, potato, cassava	Starch	Polymer of α-glucose subunits linked via α-1,4 and α-1,6-glycosidic bonds	Glucose
Lignocellulose	Forest residuals (hardwood, softwood, grasses), agricultural wastes (straw, bagasse, leaves), cardboard and paper	Cellulose	Linear polymer of glucose linked via β-1,4-glycosodic bonds	Glucose
		Hemicellulose	Branched polymer of pentoses (xylose, arabinose) and hexoses (mannose, glucose, galactose) and glucuronic acids	Xylose (mainly), arabinose, mannose, glucose, galactose
		Lignin	Branched, substituted, aromatic polymers	Separated, not used for fermentation

TABLE 9.2

Commercial Bioethanol Production in 2011

Region	Country	Predominant Feedstocks	2011 Production (ML)	Worldwide (%)
North and Central America		Corn	54,760	65
	United States	Corn	52,620	62
	Canada	Corn, wheat	1750	2
South America		Sugarcane	21,640	26
	Brazil	Sugarcane	21,100	25
Europe		Wheat (and other grains), sugar beet	4430	5
Asia/Pacific		Sugarcane, cassava	3520	4
	China	Corn, wheat, cassava, sweet sorghum	2100	2
	Australia	Sugarcane	330	<1
Africa		Sugarcane	150	<1
World			84,500	

9.2.2.1 Sugar-Containing Feedstocks

The most common sugar containing feedstocks include sugarcane and sugar beet. Sugarcane is grown in tropical and subtropical regions, including Australia, Brazil and India. Sugar beet is the main fermentation material used in temperate climate zones, such as Europe.

Sugar-based crops contain sucrose, a disaccharide composed of 12 carbon atoms. Sucrose can be used for fermentation by microorganisms, such as *S. cerevisiae*, because enzymes catalyse the conversion (hydrolysis) of sucrose to glucose and fructose, which are sugar monomers with six carbon atoms. The glucose and fructose can then be fermented to obtain ethanol (Balat et al. 2008).

9.2.2.2 Starch-Based Feedstocks

Worldwide, corn is the most used starch-based feedstock, with the majority of corn-based bioethanol production located in North America. In Europe, wheat is the most common starch-based feedstock for ethanol production (Balat et al. 2008).

Starch contains glucose sugars in the form of polymers (amylose and amylopectin). These carbohydrate chains (composed of D-glucose monomers) cannot be directly utilised by microorganisms (e.g. yeasts) but have to be broken down into glucose monomers prior to fermentation. This conversion is achieved by a hydrolysis step (enzymatic or acid) that yields the desired C6 sugar (Taherzadeh and Karimi 2008).

9.2.2.3 Lignocellulosic Biomass

Lignocellulosic biomass, such as agricultural waste or forest residues, are an abundant source of carbohydrates that do not directly compete with food crops for land use. Biomass materials, such as grass and straw, display a more complex structure than sugar-based or starch-based feedstocks. They mainly consist of three polymers (in varying ratios): cellulose, hemicellulose and lignin. Cellulose and hemicellulose are carbohydrates that can be converted to fermentable sugars. Lignin is a cross-linked polymer in the cell wall that is often bound to the cellulose fibres. It interferes with the hydrolysis of cellulose and hemicellulose and therefore should be removed prior to fermentation through pretreatment. The pretreatment of lignocellulosic materials to access molecules that can be converted into fermentable sugars is one of the major challenges in bioethanol production (Taherzadeh and Karimi 2008; Menon and Rao 2012). Cellulose is a linear polymer composed of glucose subunits that are linked together by β-1,4-glycosidic bonds. Its poor accessibility and low solubility in most solvents complicates the hydrolysis to glucose. Hemicellulose is a branched, heterogeneous polymer that contains pentoses (C5 sugars: D-xylose, L-arabinose) and hexoses (C6 sugars: D-mannose, D-glucose and D-galactose). The polymer chains are generally shorter than those in cellulose and are more easily hydrolysed due to their higher solubility (Jordan et al. 2012).

9.2.3 Process Steps

The type of raw material used for the fermentation process plays an important role in bioethanol production design. Generally, there are four steps involved: (a) pretreatment, (b) hydrolysis and saccharification, (c) fermentation of monomeric sugars to ethanol and (d) separation and purification. An overview of the processing steps can be found in Table 9.3 and Figure 9.3.

9.2.3.1 Pretreatment

The main purpose of pretreatment is to alter the crop or biomass material structure to improve the rate and yields of the downstream production process (hydrolysis or fermentation). Depending on the feedstock type, the pretreatment step can range from a simple procedure (such as milling or heating) to being the most challenging step in the entire bioethanol production process (e.g. for lignocellulosic material).

For sugar-based substances, the only pretreatment required is the extraction of the sugar juice. Starchy materials mostly require milling and liquefaction to break down the polymers into oligomers. For the pretreatment of lignocellulosic materials, a range of processes has been developed to prepare the biomass for fermentation. They include physical treatment methods

TABLE 9.3

Overview of Processing Steps for Different Feedstock Materials

Feedstock	Preparation/ Pretreatment	Hydrolysis/ Saccharification	Fermentation	Ethanol Recovery/ Purification
Sugar based	Extraction of sugar juice/ molasses	Disaccharide to monomer by yeast	Glucose using yeast	Distillation, dehydration
Starch	Milling, cooking, extraction of starch	Liquefaction, enzymatic or acid hydrolysis, saccharification of oligomers (from hydrolysis) to monomers	Glucose using mainly yeast	Distillation, dehydration
Lignocellulosic material	Physical: chipping, grinding, milling Physical–chemical: steam explosion, ammonia fibre explosion, CO_2 explosion Chemical: alkaline, acid, ozonolysis, organosolv Biological: fungal	Acid hydrolysis (dilute or concentrate) Enzymatic hydrolysis	(Detoxification) hexoses, pentoses using yeasts, fungi, bacteria	Distillation, dehydration, lignin removal

(e.g. extrusion, mechanical treatment), biological treatment (e.g. fungi), chemical treatments (e.g. acid, lime, ozonolysis, organosolv) and physicochemical methods (e.g. steam explosion, ammonia fibre explosion, ammonia recycled percolation, wet oxidation, CO_2 explosion, microwave and ultrasound; Balat et al. 2008, Sánchez and Cardona 2008; Limayem and Ricke 2012).

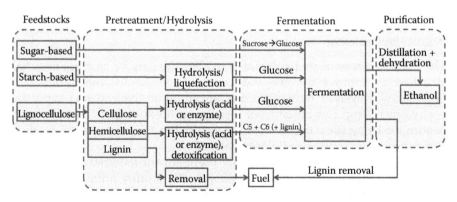

FIGURE 9.3
Simplified diagram of processing steps for different feedstock materials.

9.2.3.2 Hydrolysis/Saccharification

Following pretreatment, it may be necessary to hydrolyse the resulting substances (starch/oligomers, cellulose, hemicellulose) to obtain fermentable sugar monomers. The hydrolysis step (reaction with water) can be catalysed by acid or by enzymes.

Acid hydrolysis can be performed using concentrated or diluted acid. Sulphuric acid is the most widely used catalyst for this purpose. Enzyme hydrolysis breaks down the bonds in polymeric sugars using a suitable enzyme complex. Starchy materials and oligomers can be treated with the enzyme amylase to yield glucose monomers. For the treatment of cellulose, the enzyme cellulase is suitable to break down the polymers into fermentable C6 sugars. Significant improvements in enzyme cost and efficiency over the last few decades have made this method a viable alternative to acid treatments (Taherzadeh and Karimi 2008).

9.2.3.3 Fermentation

After hydrolysis, the fermentable sugars are converted to alcohols by microorganisms. Various fermentation processes and microorganisms can be used to optimise the design. Industrial fermentation processes that utilise sugar-based or starchy materials as feedstocks can generally be classified as batch, fed-batch or continuous operations with the former two being the most widely used modes of operation (Inui et al. 2009). For lignocellulosic materials, the fermentation step may be integrated with the hydrolysis step to increase yields and decrease cost (Section 9.3; Cardona and Sánchez 2007; Chandel et al. 2007).

9.2.3.3.1 Microorganisms

Microorganisms play a central role in the conversion of sugars to ethanol. The ideal strain should produce high ethanol yields by having high fermentation reaction and growth rates. It should also operate at a low pH (to reduce contamination), but at a high temperature (to reduce the need for cooling), and it should be robust and tolerate the presence of potential inhibitors (Taherzadeh and Karimi 2008). In addition, the suitable microbe should be capable of fermenting hexose and pentose sugars to be used in ethanol production from lignocellulosic materials.

The microorganisms used for fermentation can be classified as yeasts, bacteria and fungi. There are several different microbes that are capable of producing high ethanol concentrations from varying substrates (sugars). The type of fermentable sugars (oligomers, hexoses or pentoses) in the substrates as well as the ideal type of microorganism depends on the feedstock used. An overview of selected microorganisms and their characteristics can be found in Table 9.4.

Yeasts have been the most widely used microbes in ethanol production, with *S. cerevisiae* (Baker's yeast) being the most popular organism for

TABLE 9.4

Overview of the Characteristics of Selected Microorganisms for Bioethanol Production

Microbe	Strain/Species	T (°C)	pH Range	Carbon Source (Sugar)	EtOH Yield (%)	Literature	Application and Status
Yeasts	*S. cerevisiae*	28–32	3–5	Glucose, fructose, sucrose, galactose, mannose, maltose	73–94	Lin and Tanaka 2006; Mousdale 2008; Sánchez and Cardona 2008	Industrial scale: sugarcane, corn, wheat
	P. stipitis			Glucose, mannose, galactose xylose, arabinose	73–83	Limayem and Ricke 2012; Hahn-Hägerdal 2007; Chandel et al. 2011	Research scale: lignocellulose
Bacteria	*Z. mobilis*	30–35	6–8	Glucose, fructose, arabinose xylose	85–97	Dien et al. 2003, Limayem and Ricke 2012	Pilot/demonstration scale: lignocellulose
	E. coli	35		Glucose, galactose, mannose, arabinose xylose	88–90	Dien et al. 2003	Pilot/demonstration scale: lignocellulose
Fungi	*Mucor indicus*	30–37	3.5–5	Glucose, xylose, hydro-lysate	35–85	Binot et al. 2010; Taherzadeh and Karimi 2008	Research scale: lignocellulose
	Fusarium oxysporum	28–32		Glucose, xylose, cellulose	40–75	Singh and Kumar 1991; Ruiz et al. 2007	Research scale: lignocellulose

fermentation. A pH between 4.5 and 5 and a temperature of approximately 30°C are ideal conditions for cell growth. The yeast is inhibited by its fermentation product (ethanol) resulting in a maximum ethanol concentration that can be reached in the solution (up to 20%; Lin and Tanaka 2006, Rao et al. 2011). *S. cerevisiae* can metabolise C6 sugars such as glucose, fructose, mannose, galactose and C12 disaccharides, such as sucrose and maltose. Like most yeast strains, however, *S. cerevisiae* cannot be used for the fermentation of pentoses, such as xylose and arabinose, which are found in substrates coming from lignocellulosic feedstocks. The yeast *Pichia stipitis* is amongst the few microorganisms that naturally ferment pentose sugars. The yeast strain has shown potential for industrial application but displays low alcohol and acid tolerance. Recent research activities have been directed toward genetically modifying *S. cerevisiae* to be able to ferment pentose sugars (Hahn-Hägerdal et al. 2007; Young et al. 2010; Madhavan et al. 2012).

Yeasts are not the only ethanol-producing organisms. Many bacteria are able to ferment sugars and have received increasing consideration for larger scale applications within the last two decades (Dien et al. 2003). Amongst the most promising strains are *Zymomonas mobilis* and *Escherichia coli*.

Z. mobilis has a higher specific ethanol productivity than Baker's yeast, leading to higher ethanol yields. Fermentation takes place via a different pathway (Entner–Doudoroff) in which more glucose is used for ethanol production than for cell growth (Lin and Tanaka 2006). Despite its advantages in converting hexose sugars, *Z. mobilis* displays the drawback of not being able to efficiently convert sucrose, which has limited its industrial application in ethanol production from sugarcane and sugar beet substrates. It also has low tolerance to inhibiting substances and low pH values (which are positive for limiting unwanted bacteria growth; Taherzadeh and Karimi 2008).

E. coli is also amongst the promising bacteria for fermentation due to its ability to utilise a variety of sugars, including hexoses as well as pentoses such as xylose. It can also be relatively easily genetically engineered. The main disadvantage of *E. coli* organisms is their narrow pH range (between 6.0 and 8.0), which increases the cost for sterilisation of the process reactor. They also display low ethanol tolerance (Dien et al. 2003).

A number of fungi are also able to produce ethanol from sugars. The species *Fusarium* and *Mucor* are amongst the pentose fermenting microbes and display a high optimum temperature, which helps decrease the cost for cooling in industrial processes. However, most fungi generally display low ethanol productivity and long fermentation periods (Kuhad et al. 2011). Problems can also arise due to growth on reactor walls and fermentation equipment, which can lead to difficulties in measurements and cleaning, and may limit its industrial application (Taherzadeh and Karimi 2008).

9.2.3.3.2 Fermentation Process Types

In addition to the ethanol-producing microorganisms, the configuration of the fermentation process is important for the feasibility of the ethanol production. Ideal parameters should lead to high productivity (ethanol yield through high conversion of sugars) with low capital and operating costs. The choice of the operating mode depends on a number of factors, including the substrate, the microorganism and the presence of inhibiting substances (from previous process steps such as hydrolysis). Controlling parameters, such as pH and temperature, play an important role in optimising process conditions. An overview of the characteristics of the three main types of process modes can be found in Table 9.5 and Figure 9.4.

In batch processes, the required materials for fermentation (substrates, yeast cells, nutrients) are introduced into the bioreactor together. During the ethanol forming process, no materials are added or removed except gas and pH control solutions. The fermenter is usually equipped with a mixing system to keep conditions uniform throughout the medium. At the end of the process, the fermented materials are removed and further processed. The fermenter is cleaned and sterilised before being charged with a new batch. The conversion efficiency is usually good (90%–95% of theoretical yield) with a final ethanol concentration of 10% to 16% (Lin and Tanaka 2006). Batch operations have the advantage of low investment costs, uncomplicated management of feedstocks and sterilisation. The process is robust and does not require highly trained labour to be maintained (Inui et al. 2009).

TABLE 9.5

Overview of the Characteristics of the Main Fermentation Process Types

Process	Conversion Efficiency	Productivity	Capital Cost	Operating Cost	Comment
Batch (traditional)	High	Low due to long downtimes	Low	High	Can be improved by cell recycling and multiple fermenters in series (Melle–Boinot), large capacity
Fed-batch	High	Determined by feed rate	Moderate	High	*In situ* detoxification of hydrolysates, high flexibility
Continuous	Moderate	High	Moderate	Low	Good for large-scale production, interruptions (due to contamination or mutation) can be costly

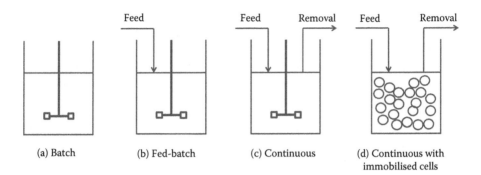

FIGURE 9.4
Schematic diagram of fermentation systems.

A major drawback of this mode of operation is its long 'downtime' between fermentation processes, which results in low overall productivity. To overcome this disadvantage, processes have been improved by operating several fermenters in parallel and by recycling yeast cells to reduce the initial lag period. The Melle–Boinot fermentation process is one of the most applied industrial batch processes (especially for sugarcane in Brazil) and uses several fermenters and yeast recycled (up to 80%) by centrifugation from previous batches (Sánchez and Cardona 2008).

If inhibiting substances are present in the batch material (such as in lignocellulosic hydrosylates) in low concentrations, they can undergo detoxification in the batch fermenter, resulting in longer lag phases (whilst inhibitors are converted). Higher concentrations, however, can lead to complete deactivation of the fermentation process (Taherzadeh and Karimi 2008).

The fed-batch process is similar to the batch process, with medium and cells present in the reactor at the commencement of each batch. The substrate concentration, however, is held constant during the fermentation process through the continuous addition of sugars and nutrients. The feed flows must be the same as the rate of substrate consumption to achieve this. The substrate levels are usually kept at a concentration that is low but still sufficient to provide for high ethanol productivity. Online instrumentation facilitates the adjustment of concentrations during fermentation. The process batch is completed when the ethanol concentration becomes high enough to inhibit the fermentation metabolism.

Due to the constantly low substrate concentration in the reactor, fed-batch processes have been useful to avoid substrate inhibition or catabolic repression (Çaylak 1998). They also do not have the problem of cell washout, and mutation or plasmid instability of cultures as is often found in continuous processes. Fed-batch processes, however, require advanced control systems and skilled labour to successfully carry out flow control operations. Similar to batch processes, fed-batch operations also have 'downtimes' due to the required emptying, cleaning and sterilisation between batches (Inui et al. 2009).

Fed-batch operations can be divided into two models: operations with feedback control (indirect control and direct control) and operations without feedback control (intermittent, constant rate, exponentially and optimised; Harada et al. 1996). The possibility of *in situ* detoxification of inhibiting substances (when kept at low concentrations) has made fed-batch processes popular in bioethanol production from lignocellulosic materials.

In continuous processes, the substrates, the culture medium and the required nutrients are added to the agitated bioreactor (containing the microorganisms) in a continuous flow. From the top of the reactor, the product (ethanol), cells and residual sugars are collected throughout the process. The mixture is usually aerated to ensure the optimal growth of the cells (through sufficient oxygenation). This helps maintain the high consumption rates of sugars and high production rates of ethanol and cells. Ideally, the flows are regulated in a way that the composition of the solution in the reactor remains constant throughout the process.

A major advantage of continuous processes is the higher productivity because the 'downtime' is significantly shorter than in batch or fed-batch processes. They also require smaller reactor volumes and operations can be automated, which is important for large-scale processes. Due to the high productivity and throughput rates, however, continuous operation modes only display little flexibility and can tolerate only minor fluctuations in substrate quality or temperature. This requires technology (automation and continuous sterilisation) that can be expensive. Another disadvantage is the high risk of cell washout and cell mutation (Inui et al. 2009).

Continuous operations can be classified into operations with feedback control (turbidostats, cell concentration at constant level; phauxostats, pH at constant level; nutristats, nutrient concentration at constant level) and operations without feedback control (chemostat; Harada et al. 1996).

To increase productivity through higher ethanol concentration and complete conversion of sugars, continuous systems can be operated using several fermenters in series. A different strategy to enhance productivity in continuous processes has been the application of immobilised cells. In this method, the yeast cells are not freely suspended in the bioreactor medium, but are attached to a support or bound to one location. This ensures that the cells stay in the reactor and allows for high cell densities and high flow rates without cell washout (Verbelen et al. 2006; Inui et al. 2009). The immobilisation of yeast cells can be realised through: (a) attachment to the surface, (b) use of porous matrix, (c) containment behind a barrier or (d) flocculation of the cells (Verbelen et al. 2006; Sivakumar et al. 2010). The success of an immobilised cell process depends on the stability of the immobilised cells and the exchange rates between substrate and the cell on the support system (biocatalyst; Cardona et al. 2009). The complexity of immobilised processes has limited their industrial application, and most systems remain untested for large-scale continuous bioethanol productions (Walker 2010).

9.2.3.4 Purification

After fermentation, the reactor product contains approximately 2 to 12 wt% ethanol. Solids can be separated from the liquid by centrifugation or by settling. Distillation of the liquids is used to concentrate the ethanol. A simple distillation, however, can yield no more than 95.67 wt% of ethanol in the mixture because it forms an azeotrope with water. For the purification of ethanol to the desired grade, a number of industrial distillation systems have been developed. These include two-column and multicolumn systems, vacuum rectification and vapour decompression, amongst others (Madson and Monceaux 1995; Huang et al. 2008). Due to the high energy demand of these processes, several other techniques have been developed but have not been widely implemented yet (Taherzadeh and Karimi 2008). The ethanol content after industrial distillation is usually approximately 95 wt%. Dehydration (drying) of the produced ethanol to concentrate it beyond this percentage is performed using molecular sieves or membrane technologies (Madson and Monceaux 1995; Balat et al. 2008; Huang et al. 2008).

9.2.3.5 Existing Process Designs for Bioethanol Production

Most of the world's bioethanol is produced by either the United States or Brazil. The industrial technologies for sugarcane and corn processing have matured over many years, although efforts to improve productivity and reduce costs are ongoing. The fermentation technologies to convert lignocellulosic materials into ethanol have yet to reach the commercial scale. However, research and development of various integrated process designs and engineering of microorganisms have made significant progress over the last decade (Cardona and Sánchez 2007; Chandel et al. 2011; Limayem and Ricke 2012). Parameters important for the performance of a process include (volumetric) productivity (in grams of EtOH per litre and hour), the ethanol yield (grams of EtOH per gram of substrate, or as a percentage), the pH and temperature range and the alcohol and inhibitor tolerance.

9.2.4 Fermentation Process Designs for Sugar-Containing Materials

Sucrose-containing feedstocks are composed of mainly sugarcane juice and molasses, and sugar beet molasses. Fermentation of these materials can be performed using batch, fed-batch or continuous processes (Figure 9.4). Because sugarcane is the dominant feedstock amongst the sugar-containing materials, the main industrial process designs used in the sugarcane bioethanol industry (mainly Brazil) are presented as examples in the following. Approximately 70% to 85% of Brazil's ethanol production processes are batch or fed-batch, and between 15% and 30% of the facilities employ continuous fermentation processes (Sánchez and Cardona 2008; Amorim et al. 2011). Before the fermentation step, the sugarcane is washed, crushed and milled to extract the juice and molasses. The bagasse, the solid residue from the extraction, is often processed further to generate energy. Research efforts have also been made toward using bagasse as lignocellulosic feedstock for further bioethanol production (Cardona et al. 2010).

9.2.4.1 Batch and Fed-Batch Fermentation (Melle–Boinot)

The simple traditional batch process has mainly been replaced by batch operation modes that include cell recycling or a series of fermenters. A widely used batch fermentation process in Brazil is the Melle–Boinot process, which was invented in the 1930s. In many cases, this method has been modified to a fed-batch process with cell recycling (Basso et al. 2011; Soccol et al. 2005). Fed-batch processes are similar to the batch operation mode and are currently the most employed processes in Brazil's bioethanol industry (Amorim et al. 2011). A semicontinuous process with cell recycling usually achieves higher productivities compared with batch fermentation. Furthermore, inhibition due to high substrate or product concentration can be decreased by controlling the feed rate and maintaining low substrate levels (Cardona et al. 2009).

A simplified schematic diagram of a typical Melle–Boinot process is shown in Figure 9.5. The sugar solution from the extraction step is purified, pasteurised, and the pH and sugar content (Brix) are adjusted before entering the fermenter. *S. cerevisiae* is the dominant microorganism used for the fermentation process. The sugars are converted to ethanol and the resulting wort undergoes decanting and centrifuging. Yeast cells are recycled to the fermenter and the ethanol solution is distilled and further dehydrated to obtain the fuel ethanol. A list of selected typical parameters for a Melle–Boinot

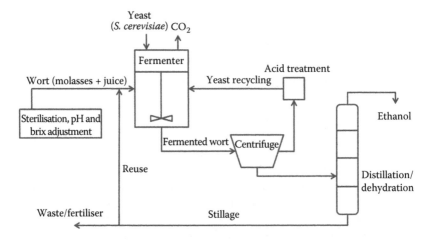

FIGURE 9.5
Schematic diagram of a typical Melle–Boinot process with cell recycling.

TABLE 9.6

Selected Typical Parameters for Batch, Fed-Batch and Continuous Processes Used in Ethanol Production from Sugarcane Feedstocks

Parameter	Batch (Traditional)	Fed-Batch	Continuous
Temperature (°C)	32–35	32–35	32–36
pH	4–5	4–5	4–5
Productivity (g/L h)	1–7	9–31	5–26
Ethanol yield (%)	85–92	73–89	84–95
Ethanol concentration (in broth) (% v/v)	7–11	6–11	7–12
Fermentation time (h)	6–12	~9	4–7

batch and fed-batch fermentation process is presented in Table 9.6. A variation to this process employs the recirculation of stillage, which can reduce water consumption and stillage volume (Cardona et al. 2009).

9.2.4.2 Continuous Fermentation

Since the 1980s, continuous fermentation processes have been implemented in a number of facilities in Brazil and other countries. Continuous stirred tank reactors (CSTR) ensure a homogeneous distribution of substrates in the reactor content during the constant fermentation process. Very high productivity (due to long running times), and easier maintenance and operation control are some of the advantages of this method (Sánchez and Cardona 2008; Cardona et al. 2009). Some typical parameters for continuous fermentation processes can be found in Table 9.6. As in batch and fed-batch processes, *S. cerevisiae* is mainly used as the fermenting microorganism. Efforts to improve continuous processes have been directed toward increased productivity through decreasing ethanol inhibition effects and optimising yeast recovery and production. Only a limited number of these advanced continuous processes have reached the commercial level. Amongst them are series-arranged continuous flow systems and processes with recirculation of yeast and wastewater.

Alfa Laval commercialised a continuous process in Brazil that uses one fermenter but operates with yeast recirculation. The process is known as Biostil technology. In the Biostil process, the yeast is cultivated in the fermentation vessel and a continuous stream is constantly removed to a centrifuge. The recycled yeast cells are sent back to the fermenter and the yeast-free fermented wort is processed in a distillation unit. From here, the concentrated ethanol is removed and the stillage is recycled back to the fermenter (blackset; Kosaric and Velikonja 1995; Ingledew 2003). Fermenters arranged in a cascade (multistage) have also been found to enhance yields (Cardona et al. 2009). The ethanol produced in the first fermenter is transported to the next and hence inhibition effects are reduced (Figure 9.6). The configuration can also be chosen in a way that the sugar is only partially converted in the first reactor allowing the second reactor to be of lower productivity (Taherzadeh and Karimi 2008).

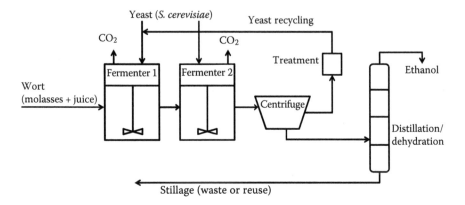

FIGURE 9.6
Simplified schematic diagram of a two-stage continuous fermentation.

Aeration also plays an important role in continuous processes because it controls cell growth, productivity and density (Sánchez and Cardona 2008). The use of immobilised cells can improve continuous fermentation processes by reducing cell washout and facilitating the recovery step. Due to the complexity of the systems, however, this technology has not yet been widely implemented in industrial ethanol production (Cardona et al. 2009).

9.2.5 Fermentation Process Designs for Starchy Materials

Amongst the starchy feedstocks, corn is the most widely used material, especially in the United States. Processing of other starchy substrates, such as wheat or barley, requires similar technologies to those that utilise corn. Because yeasts are not able to convert starch to ethanol, these materials need to be hydrolysed before fermentation to obtain fermentable sugars. There are two main processes for converting corn to fuel ethanol—the dry milling process and the wet milling process. Between 75% and 90% of the corn processing facilities in the United States employ the dry milling process (O'Brien 2010; Gosh and Prelas 2011). An overview of the processing steps of both processes can be found in Figure 9.7. Both approaches produce side products, such as dried distiller's grain and solubles (DDGS), corn oil and corn meal, which can be used for other purposes (e.g. animal feed; U.S. Department of Energy 2010).

9.2.5.1 Wet Milling Process

The wet milling process was developed approximately 150 years ago, before the dry milling process. The corn kernels are first processed to separate corn into the starch, fibre, gluten and germ components. This involves a number

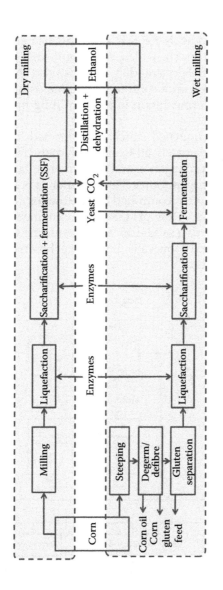

FIGURE 9.7
Simplified overview of steps for dry and wet milling processes converting corn to ethanol.

of steps including soaking/steeping to soften the kernels, followed by grinding, removal of starch and gluten from the germs, removal of fibre from the starch and gluten slurry, separation of starch from gluten, followed by washing and purification to obtain the starch suitable for further processing. This starch product is then liquefied at elevated temperatures (90°C–110°C). Due to milder reaction conditions and fewer side reactions, enzymes (amylases) are generally preferred to acids for this step (Sánchez and Cardona 2008). The product is liquefied starch, which contains dextrines (low molecular weight glucose polymers). Fermentation systems used in wet milling processes are mainly operated on a continuous regime using cascade fermentations. Typical cascade fermentation in a wet milling process is shown in Figure 9.8.

Saccharification of the liquefied starch is performed in an external step at temperatures of approximately 60°C using glycoamylase as the enzyme. This is followed by yeast propagation and prefermentation using *S. cerevisiae* with the addition of a nitrogen source. Fermentation is performed at 30°C to 32°C. The temperature is often controlled by continuous circulation through an external heat exchanger. A low pH (~3.5) is maintained to reduce the risk of infection (especially during saccharification) requiring the use of stainless steel reactors (Madson and Monceaux 1995; Drapcho et al. 2008; Inui et al. 2009; Gosh and Prelas 2011).

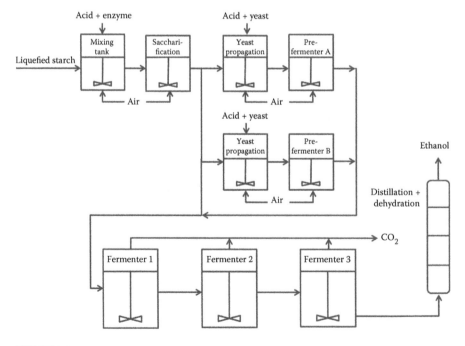

FIGURE 9.8
Simplified diagram of a continuous cascade fermentation (wet milling process).

Due to the number and requirements of the processing steps, wet milling processes are generally found to have a higher capital investment and energy demands than dry milling processes.

9.2.5.2 Dry Milling Process

Most of the newer fuel ethanol plants use the dry milling process. The main difference from the wet milling process is that the whole corn kernel is ground and processed in the fermentation step without separation of other components (germ, fibre, etc.). The ground corn is mixed with water to form a mash. Similar to the wet milling process, the mash undergoes liquefaction at higher temperatures (90°C–110°C) using amylases and a pH of around 6. After cooling down to a temperature of approximately 60°C, the saccharification is carried out using glycoamylases. The fermentation step can be performed using batch or continuous operations. For dry milling processes, batch fermentation is common with fermentation times of approximately 48 h. The milling, liquefaction, saccharification and distillation, however, are carried out in a continuous operation mode. Three or more fermenters are used in the batch mode to ensure a constant supply of fermented broth (Madson and Manceaux 1995; Gosh and Prelas 2011).

In the 1970s, simultaneous saccharification and fermentation (SSF) was developed, which decreased the risk of contamination and increased the yield. Most dry milling plants now utilise the SSF technology. In this configuration, the liquefied mash is cooled down to 32°C, the pH is adjusted to between 4.5 and 5, glycosamylase is added and the mixture is sent into the fermenter where the yeast (*S. cerevisiae*) is added. The dextrins in the liquefied starch are metabolised by the glycoamylases and the resulting glucose is directly fermented by the yeast. Fermentation times are between 48 and 72 h. Elimination of the external saccharification step reduces the risk of bacterial contamination, and the higher pH of 4.5 to 5 allows the use of carbon steel reactors instead of stainless steel resulting in reduced costs (Bothast and Schlicher 2005; Drapcho et al. 2008; Inui et al. 2009; Gosh and Prelas 2011). A typical dry milling SSF process is shown in Figure 9.9.

9.2.5.3 Very High Gravity Fermentation

Very high gravity (VHG) fermentations aim to reduce costs of bioethanol productions by minimising the water requirements of the process and therefore reducing energy and distillation costs. In this method, high or very high gravity mashes are fermented with concentrations in the reactor, which usually exceed 200 g/L. The high substrate concentration results in high ethanol concentrations at the end of the fermentation process (>15% v/v; Cardona et al. 2009; Puligundla et al. 2011). This, however, can lead to inhibition effects and slow or incomplete fermentations may be observed. Research has been undertaken to find more resistant yeast strains that can tolerate higher

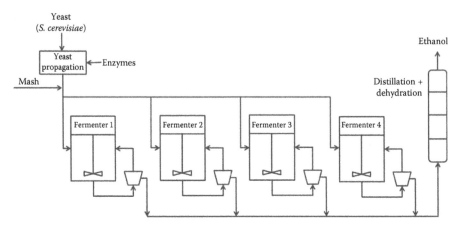

FIGURE 9.9
Simplified diagram of a wet milling batch process using SSF.

ethanol concentrations and ideally can be recycled several times (Mussatto et al. 2010). The implementation of VHG fermentations has been proposed as one of the methods with the most potential to improve continuous bioethanol production from wheat starches. It can decrease energy and water costs without additional investment for infrastructure and equipment (Bai et al. 2008).

9.2.6 Process Design for Fermentation of Lignocellulosic Biomass

The process to convert lignocellulosic materials into bioethanol is more complex than those employed in existing corn or sugarcane treatment facilities (see Section 9.3). Lignocellulosic biomass includes many types of feedstock materials (straw, bagasse, soft woody, grass, etc.) that may require different preparation and pretreatment methods. There are two pathways for ethanol production from biomass material (Figure 9.10). The syngas pathway involves the gasification of biomass followed by fermentation or catalytic conversion of the syngas (not described in more detail here). The biochemical pathway involves traditional fermentation using microorganisms. The lignocellulosic structure has to be broken down to separate the cellulose, hemicellulose and lignin components. A number of pretreatment methods have been developed and are described (Mosier et al. 2005; Sánchez and Cardona 2008; Alvira et al. 2010). Depending on the pretreatment method, the hemicellulose is either solubilised or hydrolysed, and is found in the liquid process stream, whereas the cellulose and the lignin usually remain in the solid state. The cellulose (and hemicellulose) then have to be hydrolysed (with acid or enzymes) to obtain sugars (hexoses and pentoses) suitable for the fermentation process. The general steps of ethanol production from lignocellulose are shown in Figure 9.10.

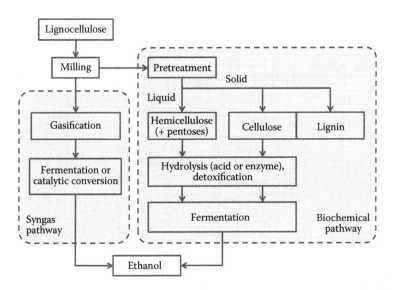

FIGURE 9.10
Overview of pathways and steps for bioethanol production from lignocellulosic feedstocks.

The required technologies and microorganisms are still under development, with a number of plants that have reached pilot or demonstration scale. The fermentable sugars (hexoses and pentoses) obtained from plant biomass are metabolised in different ways, and efforts to optimise the fermentation process and sugar conversion have been ongoing in recent years. In particular, the fermentation of pentose sugars remains a major challenge (Young et al. 2010; Kuhad et al. 2011). The integration of several process steps has been a promising approach to reduce cost and increase economic feasibility (Cardona and Sánchez 2007; Gosh and Prelas 2011). In these cases, hydrolysis is usually performed using enzymes. A number of integration schemes for lignocellulose-based ethanol plants are presented in the following subsections.

9.2.6.1 Separate or Sequential Hydrolysis and Fermentation

In this traditional method, the hydrolysis and fermentation are two distinct process steps and the fermentation of hexoses and pentoses is carried out in separate reactors. In a common configuration A, the pretreated biomass is hydrolysed and then introduced into the first fermenter where the glucose is metabolised by yeasts (or other microorganisms). After fermentation, the mixture is distilled to remove the produced ethanol. The remaining pentoses (mainly xylose) are then processed in a second reactor, which utilises microorganisms suitable for the conversion of pentoses to ethanol. This is followed by a second distillation (Figure 9.11; Hamelink et al. 2005; Gosh and Prelas 2011).

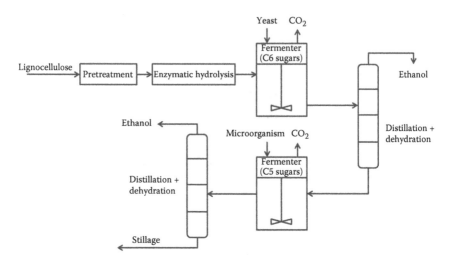

FIGURE 9.11
Process flow diagram of a configuration A of SHF.

In another method, the solids (which contain the cellulose) are separated after the first hydrolysis step. The sugars in the liquid (mainly pentoses) from the hemicellulose are fermented in one reactor. The cellulose is hydrolysed and the resulting glucose is fermented in another reactor. The product recovery of both fermenters is combined (Cardona et al. 2009). The second configuration B of separate or sequential hydrolysis and fermentation (SHF) is shown in Figure 9.12. SHF may require higher capital costs but an advantage of this method is that each step can be performed at its ideal conditions

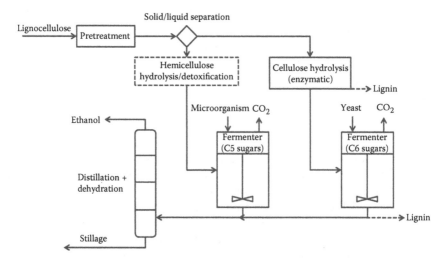

FIGURE 9.12
Process flow diagram of a configuration B of SHF.

(temperature, pH) and different microorganism can be used for the fermentations. SHF processes can be performed in batch, fed-batch or continuous regimes (Hamelinck et al. 2005; Scragg 2009).

Examples of bioethanol plants that utilise SHF process are the Canadian company, Iogen Corporation (Iogen 2012) and the Spanish company, Abengoa (Abengoa 2012), which both use straw as the biomass feedstock.

9.2.6.2 Simultaneous Saccharification and Fermentation

Similar to the SSF process in corn-processing plants, in this process configuration, the cellulose hydrolysis step and the glucose fermentation step are combined. The glucose that is produced through enzymatic hydrolysis is directly converted to ethanol in the same reactor vessel. This also helps avoid reaction inhibition caused by the substrate glucose. SSF requires lower capital cost and was found to give a higher ethanol yield (Hamelinck et al. 2005; Lin and Tanaka 2006). The process rate, however, is reduced by the different optimal conditions between enzyme hydrolysis and fermentation. The optimal temperature for yeasts is usually around 30°C, but can be increased by using thermotolerant yeasts (Hasunuma and Kondo 2012). The hydrolysis optimum is found between 45 and 50°C and most often a compromise of approximately 38°C is used in the SSF process (Scragg 2009; Zhao et al. 2012). The cost of cellulase, the enzyme to hydrolyse cellulose, also plays an important role. Short hydrolysis times mean higher cellulase costs but decrease the overall fermentation times and hence costs. The optimum compromise is usually found between 3 and 4 days (Hamelinck et al. 2005). A typical SSF process is shown in Figure 9.13.

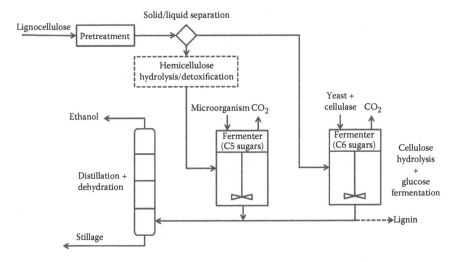

FIGURE 9.13
Simplified flow diagram of a fermentation process using SSF.

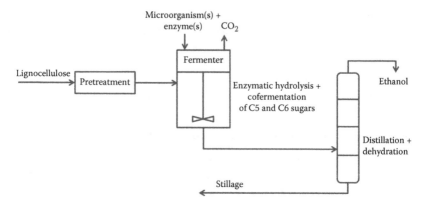

FIGURE 9.14
Simplified flow diagram of a fermentation process using SSCF.

9.2.6.3 Simultaneous Saccharification and Cofermentation

Simultaneous saccharification and cofermentation (SSCF) is similar to SSF but whereas the liquid stream containing the pentoses is usually processed separately in the SSF process, the processing of hexoses and pentoses is combined in SSCF. The solid cellulose is not separated after the pretreatment, but both the hemicellulose sugars as well as cellulose are processed (hydrolysis and fermentation) in one reactor vessel (Drapcho et al. 2008). SSCF displays the same advantages as SSF over SHF including higher ethanol yields and productivity, as well as overcoming the product's inhibition effects. In addition, it requires even less fermentation equipment (Ojeda et al. 2011). Figure 9.14 shows a typical SSCF process.

After pretreatment, the product stream undergoes enzymatic hydrolysis, and the fermentation of the resulting pentose and hexose sugars is carried out by using suitable microorganisms (yeasts, fungi or bacteria). Two organisms can be used in combination for the fermentation but ideally a single organism would be used for the fermentation of all sugars. This remains a major challenge in the research and development of lignocellulosic ethanol production. However, progress has been made in the area of metabolically engineered microorganisms (Olofsson et al. 2008).

9.2.6.4 Consolidated Bioprocessing

In consolidated bioprocessing (CBP), the hydrolysis and fermentation steps and the enzyme production are carried out in a single reactor vessel. One microorganism or a combination of microorganisms that is able to produce the required enzymes for hydrolysis and convert the fermentable sugars into ethanol is used. No organism has been found in nature that displays all the desirable features for this processing scheme. Biological engineering of fungi

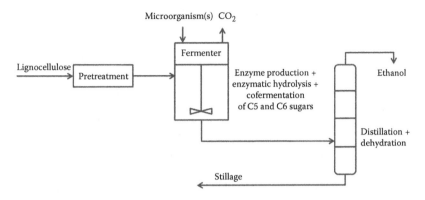

FIGURE 9.15
Simplified flow diagram of a fermentation process using CBP.

and bacteria is therefore required to further develop this technology (Elkins et al. 2010).

CBP has been recognised as a potential method for economic bioethanol production from biomass, and intensive research has been undertaken in this area (Xu et al. 2009; Olson et al. 2012). Fewer processing steps and integrated enzyme production would lower capital and operating costs. The concept of CBP is illustrated in Figure 9.15.

9.2.7 Current State of Biomass Fermentation Processes

Worldwide ethanol production has significantly increased over the last 10 years. Although the amount of bioethanol produced in 2001 was approximately 20,000 ML, this number more than tripled by 2011 (>80,000 ML; Scragg 2009; Renewable Fuel Association [RFA] 2012). In the two main producer countries, the United States and Brazil, large-scale production started in the 1970s. Improvements in bioethanol production technologies, which use starch-based or sugar-based feedstocks, have been ongoing since then. The United States has more than 200 bioethanol production facilities, including some large commercial facilities with capacities of more than 0.5 BL/year. Brazil has more than 400 bioethanol production facilities, with predominantly smaller-scale commercial plants (~100–200 ML/year) located in areas where the sugarcane is grown (RFA 2012; UNICA 2012).

Both the feedstocks (starch and sugar) currently used for commercial ethanol production are also food crops. Increases in bioethanol production therefore consume a portion of the world's food crop production (Rajagopal et al. 2007). Growing concern has led to an interest in lignocellulosic materials as a source of fermentable sugars, and research efforts have been directed toward commercialising suitable technologies and processes.

9.2.7.1 Starch-Based and Sugar-Based Facilities

9.2.7.1.1 Brazil

As a result of the oil crisis and the low sugar prices in the 1970s, the Brazilian government set up the National Alcohol Program, ProAlcool, with the goal of substituting petrol with bioethanol. Under the plan, the production of bioethanol from sugarcane and molasses was highly subsidised and purchase of produced ethanol by the state-owned company PETROBAS was guaranteed (Soccol et al. 2005; Goldemberg 2008). The ethanol industry and its usage has grown significantly since then. As of 2011, less than half of the sugarcane grown in Brazil is used for sugar production whereas approximately 55% is converted into ethanol (Valdes 2011). In Brazil, ethanol accounts for approximately 50% of the transportation fuel used in vehicles. Two types of ethanol are produced and used: anhydrous and hydrous EtOH. Anhydrous ethanol is used in unmodified engines and is blended with gasoline (10%), whereas hydrous ethanol can be utilised in modified engines as the only fuel or mixed with gasoline. Approximately two-thirds of Brazilian ethanol is hydrous and one third is anhydrous.

There are more than 430 bioethanol plants located in Brazil, producing more than 21,000 ML in 2011 (RFA 2012). Approximately two-thirds of these can be found in the State of São Paolo, where most of the sugarcane is grown (Goldemberg 2008). Larger plants (>200 ML/year of ethanol) account for approximately 10% to 20% and medium sized plants (<200 ML/year of ethanol) account for approximately 70% to 80%. The rest are smaller facilities that produce less than 50 ML/year (UNICA 2012). The yeast *S. cerevisiae* is used as the ethanol-producing microorganism in almost all industrial-scale plants in Brazil. Some of the largest plants operating in Brazil are listed in Table 9.7.

The ethanol and sugar industry in Brazil is controlled by a relatively small number of companies, which results in a linked network of sugar mills, holding groups and cooperatives (Schurig 2008). The influence of foreign investors has grown steadily in recent years. Many of the sugar mills produce both sugar and ethanol. Cosan is one of the largest sugar groups (composed of five companies) in Brazil and is a leader in bioethanol production, operating more than 20 sugar mills with an overall production of 1.8 BL in 2011/2012 (Cosan 2012). Sao Martinho is also one of the largest sugar companies in the country that produces sugar, ethanol and other sugar-based products. The yearly production of its three mills, Sao Martinho, Iracema and Boa Vista, is between 400 and 500 ML (Sao Martinho 2012). Copersucar is the largest private cooperative in Brazil composed of more than 30 producers with a total ethanol production of more than 3.5 BL in 2010/11 (Copersucar 2012).

9.2.7.1.2 North America

Although commercial plants started to appear in the 1970s, the ethanol industry in the United States remained small in the 1980s. After the use of

TABLE 9.7

Large Commercial Sugar and Ethanol Facilities in Brazil

Plant/Mill (Company/ Corporation)	Location	Ethanol Production/ Capacity (ML/year per harvest)	References
Sao Martinho (Sao Martinho)	Pradópolis, São Paolo	400	UNICA 2012; Sao Martinho 2012
Da Barra (Cosan)	Barra Bonita, São Paolo	300–400 (1800 m³/day)	Cosan 2012; UNICA 2012
Madhu (previously Equipav; Renuka do Brazil/Shree Renuka)	Promissao, São Paolo	300–400 (1600 m³/day)	Renuka do Brasil 2012; UNICA 2012
Vale do Rosario/Biosev (Luis Dreyfus Commodities Bioenergia and Santelisa Vale)	Morro Agudo, São Paolo	200–250	Luis Dreyfus Commodities 2012; UNICA 2012
Colorado (Group Colorado)	Guaira, São Paolo	250–300	Colorado 2012; UNICA 2012
Sao Jose–Macatuba (Zilor/Copersucar)	Macatuba, São Paolo	200–250	Zilor 2012; UNICA 2012
Barra Grande (Zilor/Copersucar)	Lençóis Paulista, São Paolo	200–250	Zilor 2012; UNICA 2012
Itamarati/Usinas Itamarati (autonomous)	Nova Olympia, Mato Grasso	200–300	Itamarati 2012

leaded compounds as fuel additives was banned in the 1980s, the interest in ethanol as a fuel additive grew. Despite governmental subsidies, low gasoline prices, together with fluctuating corn prices, kept the bioethanol industry from growing significantly (Solomon et al. 2010). During the last decade, however, the ethanol industry grew rapidly due to the restriction placed on methyl tert-butyl ether (used as oxygenating fuel additive) and due to the Renewable Fuel Standards programme, which requires a certain amount of renewable fuel to be blended into transportation fuel (EPA Renewable Fuel Standard 2012). More than 200 biorefineries could be found in the United States. Most of the plants are located in the Midwest and are attached to or close to large corn farms and processing facilities (Solomon et al. 2010). The three largest companies (Table 9.8) account for more than 30% of the ethanol production; however, less than 50% of the total ethanol amount is produced by the 10 biggest companies.

E10, a mixture of 10% anhydrous ethanol and 90% gasoline is widely used in the United States. In Canada, the Federal Renewable Fuel Regulations (Environment Canada Renewable Fuel Regulations 2012) require the addition of 5% (average) to gasoline. The main feedstock in North America is corn, which is processed in wet or dry milling facilities, with the yeast *S. cerevisiae* being the widely applied microorganism for fermentation.

TABLE 9.8

Largest Ethanol Producers in North America

Country	Company	Overall Capacity (ML/year)	Number of Plants
United States of America	POET	6420	27
	Archer Daniels Midland	6130	9
	Valero Renewable Fuels	4200	10
	Green Plains Renewables	2800	9
Canada	GreenField Ethanol	610	4
	Suncor St. Clair	400	1

One of the main fuel ethanol producers in the United States is Archer Daniels Midland (see Table 9.9). The company owns some of the largest corn processing facilities including both dry and wet mills. The plants, which are located in Iowa, Illinois and Nebraska, also produce other products (24 in total) from corn (Archer Daniels Midland 2012).

The company POET operates the largest number of plants in the United States, with an average production per facility of approximately 15 ML/year. POET facilities mainly use the dry milling process with SSF (POET 2012).

TABLE 9.9

Largest Commercial Ethanol Production Facilities in the United States

Company	Location	Process	Capacity (ML/year)	References
Archer Daniels Midland	Columbus, NE	Dry milling, continuous fermentation	1140	ADM 2012; RFA 2012; Ethanol Producer Magazine 2012
	Decatur, IL	Wet mill	1100	
	Cedar Rapids, IA	Dry mill	1040	
	Cedar Rapids, IA	Wet mill	910	
	Clinton, IA	Wet Mill	890	
Cargill Inc.	Blair, NE	Wet Mill	740	Cargill 2012; RFA 2012; Ethanol Producer Magazine 2012
Aventine Renewable Energy	Pekin, IL	Wet mill and dry mill	600	Aventine 2012; RFA 2012; Ethanol Producer Magazine 2012
Tharaldson Ethanol LLC	Casselton, ND	Dry milling	580	Tharaldson 2012; RFA 2012; Ethanol Producer Magazine 2012
Marquis Energy LLC	Hennepin, IL	Dry mill	530	Marquis Energy 2012; RFA 2012; Ethanol Producer Magazine 2012

TABLE 9.10

Main Producers of Ethanol in Europe

Member State	Number of Plants	Overall Capacity (ML/year)	Production 2010 (ML/year)
France	14	1855	1050
Germany	10	1155	760
Poland	9	680	200
Belgium	3	650	315
Spain	5	554	470
United Kingdom	2	470	320
Sweden	2	300	205

TABLE 9.11

Largest Ethanol-Producing Facilities in Europe

Company	Location	Predominant Feedstock	Capacity (ML/year)	References
Abengoa Bioenergy	Rotterdam, Netherlands	Wheat (or corn)	480	Abengoa 2012
Ensus	Teesside/Wilton, UK	Wheat	400	Ensus 2012
CropEnergies AG	Zeitz, Germany	Wheat	360	CropEnergies 2012
Tereos	Origny, France	Wheat	300	Tereos 2012
BioWanze	Wanze, Belgium	Wheat and sugar beet	300	BioWanze 2012
Abengoa Bioenergy and Oceol	Lacq, France	Corn	250	Abengoa 2012

9.2.7.1.3 Europe

Europe is only a minor producer of bioethanol when compared with Brazil or the United States, but production has steadily increased in recent years. There are approximately 70 commercial biorefineries with a combined capacity of more than 7.5 BL, which produced more than 4 BL of fuel ethanol in 2010 (Flach et al. 2011; EPure Statistics 2012). The main producers are listed in Table 9.10. The underutilisation mainly occurred due to high wheat prices and competitive imports. France, Germany, Spain and the Benelux Countries are amongst the main producers and wheat or sugar beet is predominantly used as the feedstock (Table 9.11).

9.2.7.2 Lignocellulose-Based Bioethanol Facilities

Lignocellulosic materials are an abundant biomass source for fermentation, with the potential to reduce the demand for food crop feedstocks used for ethanol production. Commercialisation of lignocellulosic ethanol production, however, has been difficult due to various factors including the costs

of enzymes as well as technical challenges in certain production steps
(e.g. pretreatment). Many countries support lignocellulose research and
development, but the progression from laboratory to commercial scale
remains a challenge (Banerjee et al. 2010). Prices for cellulose enzymes to
hydrolyse cellulosic feedstocks have dropped in recent years and lignocellulose feedstocks are only now beginning to be considered an alternative
to sugar-based and starch-based materials. Several countries have pilot or
demonstration plants in operation, and several commercial-scale facilities
are planned or under construction. Selected plants and projects are listed
in Tables 9.12 and 9.13.

Several plants located in the United States are supported by federal
funding from the 'Biofuel Initiative', which aims to make lignocellulosic ethanol cost-competitive by 2012 (U.S. Department of Energy 2012;
Menon and Rao 2012). Biorefineries processing lignocellulosic biomass
have also been built in Canada, Europe, Brazil and Japan (Solomon et
al. 2010). Despite these facilities and projects, there remains scepticism
as to whether lignocellulosic ethanol will become economically feasible
enough to be a large-scale product.

9.2.7.2.1 United States and Canada

Several pilot and demonstration facilities have been constructed in the
United States and Canada, supported by government funding. Various feedstocks and technologies have been used with the goal of finding a way of
making lignocellulosic-based ethanol cost-competitive and therefore suitable for commercial-scale plants.

The Spanish company Abengoa, which has been operating a successful
pilot plant in Babilafuente (Spain), is building a commercial cellulosic ethanol plant in Hugoton, Kansas. Crop residues (wheat and corn), grasses and
wood wastes will be used as feedstocks, and the process will include steam
explosion pretreatment followed by enzymatic hydrolysis and fermentation
of both C5 and C6 sugars (SSF process; Bacovsky et al. 2010; Abengoa 2012).

One of the world's first demonstration facilities to produce cellulosic ethanol is owned by the Canadian company Iogen. The plant in Ottawa, operating
since 2004, converts agricultural residues (straw) into ethanol using a steam
explosion pretreatment method and an SHF process (multistage hydrolysis
process) with C5 and C6 fermentation. The lignin that is separated during
the process is used for energy generation (Iogen 2012).

Since 2009, Blue Sugars' (formerly KL Energy Corporation) demonstration
plant has been operating in Upton, Wyoming. Their continuous process technology includes a thermal–mechanical pretreatment followed by SHF with
onsite enzyme production and cofermentation of pentose and hexose sugars.
Various feedstocks are used including agricultural, forestry and industrial
residues (wood waste, paper, grasses, etc.; Blue Sugars 2012).

POET-DSM Advanced Biofuels LLC, a joint venture between the ethanol
producer POET and the global health and nutrition company, Royal DSM,

TABLE 9.12

Selected Lignocellulosic-Based Ethanol Facilities in North America, South America and Asia

Country	Company	Location	Feedstock	Process Technology	Output (ML/year)	Status (Startup Date)	References
United States	Abengoa Bioenergy	Hugoton, Kansas	Corn stover, agricultural waste	Enzymatic hydrolysis, SSF, C5 and C6 fermentation	95	Commercial, under construction (2014)	Bacovsky et al. 2010; Abengoa 2012
	Blue Sugars (KL Energy Corporation)	Upton, Wyoming	Wood waste, cardboard, paper	Thermomechanical pretreatment, SHF, enzymatic hydrolysis, C5 and C6 cofermentation	5.8	Demo (2007)	Bacovsky et al. 2010; Blue Sugars 2012
	DuPont Danisco (DDCE)	Vonore, Tennessee	Corn stover, cobs, switchgrass	Ammonia pretreatment, SHF, fermentation with *Z. mobilis*	1	Pilot (2010)	DDCE 2012
	Mascoma (Frontier Renewable Resources)	Rome, New York	Multiple feedstocks (incl. hardwood)	CBP, enzyme production, hydrolysis and fermentation in one step	0.8	Demo (2008)	Mascoma 2012
	POET DSM	Emmetsburg, Iowa	Corn cobs, agricultural residues	Enzymatic hydrolysis, genetically modified strains of yeast, C6 and C5 fermentation	95	Commercial (planned for 2014)	POET-DSM 2012
	Verenium	Jennings, Louisiana	Sugarcane bagasse, wood products, switch grass	Dilute acid steam explosion, separate C5 and C6 fermentation (SSF)	5.3	Demo (2009)	Verenium 2012
Canada	Iogen Corporation	Ottawa, Ontario	Wheat, barley and oat straw	SHF, Enzymatic hydrolysis, C5 and C6 fermentation	2	Demo (2004)	Iogen 2012
Brazil	GraalBio	Alagaos, São Paulo	Straw and sugarcane bagasse	Steam explosion, SSF, modified yeasts for C6 and C5 fermentation	82	Commercial (planned for 2014)	GraalBio 2012
Japan	DINS Sakai (Bioethanol Japan Kansai)	Sakai, Osaka	Construction wood residues, paper and food waste	Genetically engineered *E. coli* KO11, mainly fermentation of C5 but also C6, acid hydrolysis, SHF	1.4–4	Demo (2007)	Biofuel Database 2012

TABLE 9.13

Lignocellulosic-Based Ethanol Facilities in Europe

Country	Company	Location	Feedstock	Process Technology	Output (ML/year)	Status (Startup Date)	References
Denmark	BioGasol/ Technical University of Denmark	Bornholm	Various (grasses, garden waste, straw)	Four-step SSF, Carbofrac pretreatment, Pentoferm C5 fermentation technology (bacteria)	5.1	Demo (2009)	Gnansounou 2010; BioGasol 2012
	Inbicon (DONG Energy)	Kalundborg	Wheat straw	Hydrothermal pretreatment, SSF, C6 fermentation, C5 molasses production	5.4	Demo (2009)	Larsen et al. 2008; Gnansounou 2010; Inbicon 2012
Norway	Borregaard Industries Ltd.	Sarpsborg	SSL from spruce wood pulping	From SSL, enzymatic hydrolysis, SHF, C6 fermentation, C5 testing	20	Commercial (1930)	Borregaard 2012
Spain	Abengoa Bioenergy	Babilafuente	Wheat straw, corn stover	Steam explosion pretreatment, enzymatic hydrolysis, SSF, C6 fermentation	5.1	Demo (2010)	Gnansounou 2010
Sweden	SEKAB	Örnsköldsvik	Wood chips, sugarcane bagasse	Dilute acid pretreatment, SSF or SHF, modified yeast strains	5.7	Demo (2011)	Gnansounou 2010; SEKAB 2012

is planning to build a commercial cellulosic ethanol plant (Project Liberty) adjacent to POET's existing ethanol refinery in Emmentsburg, Iowa. In this plant ethanol will be produced from corncobs, leaves and other residues. A coproduct from the process will be biogas, which will be used to generate energy for the plants (POET-DSM 2012).

DuPont Danisco Cellulosic Ethanol (DDCE), a joint venture between DuPont and Danisco, has been operating a demonstration plant in Vonore, Tennessee, since 2008 and is planning to construct a commercial-scale facility in Nevada, Iowa (beginning 2012), with a capacity of around 27 million gallons (100 ML) per year. Genetically modified microorganisms based on the bacterium *Z. mobilis* are part of the technology allowing fermentation of both C6 and C5 sugars (Bacovsky et al. 2010; DDCE 2012).

Verenium's demonstration plant in Jennings, Louisiana, which was acquired by BP in 2010, uses dilute acid steam explosion pretreatment followed by separate C5 and C6 fermentation. The hydrolysis/saccharification (resulting in C6) and fermentation of cellulose is performed simultaneously (SSF). BP was planning to build a commercial-scale plant in Florida (Highlands), which uses energy grass and cane as feedstocks to produce approximately 36 million gallons (135 ML) of cellulosic ethanol, but these plans were cancelled in 2012 (Bacovsky et al. 2010; BP 2012).

Mascoma operates a demonstration facility in Rome, New York, which uses engineered microorganisms to combine enzyme production, hydrolysis and fermentation in one step (CBP). The first commercial facility using this technology was planned for construction in Kinross, Michigan, through the joint venture Frontier Renewable Resources LLC (Mascoma 2012).

9.2.7.2.2 Europe

The European Union target of replacing 10% of the fuel with renewables by 2020 and the funding that has been given to development projects have resulted in the construction of several demonstration facilities in Europe (Gnansounou 2010; Table 9.13).

BioGasol's demonstration facility in Ballerup, Denmark, was started in 2008 as the BornBioFuel Project, and the company has been working on the second phase of the project (BornBioFuel2) with operations on a semi-industrial scale. A combination of steam explosion and wet oxidation is used as pretreatment. This is followed by enzymatic hydrolysis and glucose fermentation with yeast. After the removal of lignin, the remaining pentose sugars are processed in the next step using an engineered bacterium (derived from bacterium found in hot springs in Iceland) under anaerobic conditions (BioGasol 2012).

Another Danish company, Inbicon (DONG Energy), has been exploring the concept of Industrial Symbiosis with nine companies working together in Kalundborg to utilise each other's residues and by-products. The fermentation technology includes a hydrothermal pretreatment followed by (high gravity) hydrolysis and SSF of glucose using yeasts. Other products of the process are lignin pellets and C5 molasses which can be used for biogas generation or animal feed (Inbicon 2012).

Borregard in Norway uses wood materials to produce a range of products including ethanol. In the pulp mill facility in Sarpsborg, spruce wood chips are cooked (to produce pulp for the paper mill). This process hydrolyses the hemicellulose, and the resulting sugars in the sulfite-spent liquor (SSL) are used for fermentation (Borregaard 2012).

In Sweden, SEKAB operates a demonstration facility in Örnsköldsvik, which was started in 2005. The plant uses wood (from conifers) as feedstock; however, the process also works with other agricultural materials such as straw or bagasse. Their 'e-technology' uses an acid and steam pretreatment, followed by either SSF or SHF. A special yeast strain allows the fermentation of both hexose and pentose sugars. Lignin and biogas are coproducts of the process, which can be used for energy generation. The company is planning to gradually scale up the process to commercial scale (Gnansounou 2010; SEKAB 2012).

9.2.7.2.3 South America and Asia

Asian countries such as Japan, India and China are also in the processes of developing and constructing facilities for cellulosic ethanol production which can use wood waste and agricultural residues as feedstocks (Menon and Rao 2012; Table 9.13).

The Japanese corporation DINS Sakai/Osaka (formerly Bioethanol Japan) operates a wood waste to ethanol facility in Osaka with a capacity of 1.4 ML/year, which is expected to be expanded to 4 ML/year (Table 9.13). The pretreatment stage involves dilute acid and, for the fermentation step, engineered *E. coli* is used to convert pentose and hexose sugars (Biofuel Database 2012).

The research focus in South America and especially in Brazil has been on developing processes for the conversion of sugarcane bagasse to ethanol. The Brazilian company Dedini has developed the Dedini hydrolysis rapida (DHR) process, which uses an organosolv pretreatment followed by acid hydrolysis and cofermentation with sugarcane juice (Dedini 2012).

GraalBio (Graal Group) has announced the construction of a cellulosic ethanol plant in Alagaos (Brazil) with a capacity of 82 ML/year. Sugarcane straw and bagasse will be used as feedstock and the technology includes a steam explosion pretreatment followed by enzymatic hydrolysis and fermentation (PROSEA technology by Chemtex; GraalBio 2012; Chemtex 2012).

Several other companies, which are not mentioned here, are in the process of planning commercial lignocellulosic ethanol facilities, often supported by federal projects and funding. Further developments and the constructions of new facilities are expected worldwide in the coming years.

9.3 Comparison of Existing Fermentation Processes and Challenges for Future Operations

Most of the fermentation process designs used in sugar-based or starch-based plants have been proven on the commercial scale with capacities reaching more than 0.5 BL/year. The technology of choice depends on many factors including the feedstock, infrastructure and local environmental factors. The cost of the raw material is often the main cost factor followed by energy consumption.

Lignocellulosic-based facilities have still not reached commercial scale although many pilot and demonstration plants are in operation using various technologies. In most cases, the feedstocks are abundant but production costs are still high because many processes are not energy efficient enough to be cost-competitive. The necessary pretreatment to break up the lignocellulosic structure is energy-intensive and in most cases, the production or purchase of enzymes is costly.

The technologies used for the fermentation of biomass have various advantages and limitations. The main process designs for first generation fuel ethanol feedstocks are listed and compared in Table 9.14. An overview of processes using second generation feedstocks can be found in Table 9.15.

9.3.1 Limiting Factors

9.3.1.1 Sugar-Based and Starch-Based Facilities

Large corn and sugarcane processing facilities operate at commercial scales with advanced technologies that have been continually improved for decades. Although no major breakthroughs are expected in this area, pertinent issues such as cost and efficiency of enzymes, stability and contamination of yeast cultures and wastewater treatment present opportunities for improvement. Overall, however, the success and feasibility of first generation ethanol are mainly influenced by factors that are not directly related to process technologies.

To be competitive with fossil fuels, bioethanol production costs have to be below a certain amount. Production and development are supported by increasing oil prices but the main costs of ethanol production from sugar and grain arises from the feedstock itself. Although improvements in production technologies have steadily reduced the cost of the processes, the price of the material inputs, especially corn and wheat, has fluctuated over recent years and has influenced overall ethanol production costs significantly. Feedstock commodity prices for corn in the United States have also been affected by the demand for food crops and change in crop yields (International Energy Agency [IEA] 2008).

TABLE 9.14

Overview of Bioethanol Production Processes Using First Generation Feedstocks

Main Feedstock	Design	Capital Cost	Status	Advantages/Strengths	Disadvantages/Challenges
Sugar based: sugarcane, sugar beet, molasses	Melle–Boinot (batch and fed-batch)	Capital and operation cost low	Commercial, used in many sugar facilities in Brazil	Usually complete conversion of substrate, efficient through yeast recycling and reuse of stillage, baker's yeast not expensive, no hydrolysis needed. High sugar energy to fuel conversion	Downtimes due to cleaning of reactors between batches, can be labour intensive
	Continuous	Can be higher capital cost but labour and operation costs usually low	Commercial, used in approximately 30% of facilities in Brazil	Continuous process, no downtimes, higher efficiency and productivity, bakers's yeast not expensive, no hydrolysis needed	Mutation and contamination of yeast strains may occur, leading to costly interruptions
Starch based: corn, wheat	Wet milling	More capital- and energy-intensive than dry milling, important input cost: cost of corn	Commercial, used in 10% to 25% of ethanol facilities in the United States	Separation of other components before fermentation and production of valuable by-products (energy efficient)	High capital costs, more steps, water intensive process
	Dry milling	Lower capital cost per gallon, important input cost: cost of corn	Commercial, most employed process in the United States	Fewer steps than wet milling, maximised capital return per gallon	Fewer side products that can be used
	Dry milling with SSF	Lower than non-SSF, fewer reactors needed	Commercial, employed mainly with dry milling processes in the United States	Fewer steps than regular wet and dry milling processes	Optimum conditions between hydrolysis and fermentation different—compromise, longer hydrolysis times
	VHG fermentation	Moderate, no extra installations needed	Demonstration scale, employed with wheat as feedstock	Significant energy and waste savings, increases throughput rate without increasing plant capacity	Increased yeast stress (increased osmotic pressure and ethanol concentration)

TABLE 9.15

Overview of Bioethanol Production Processes Using Second Generation Feedstocks

Main Feedstock	Design	Capital Cost	Status	Advantages/Strengths	Disadvantages/Challenges
Lignocellulosic based: straw, wood, bagasse, corn cobs, forestry, and agricultural residues	Separate hydrolysis and fermentation (SHF)	High capital costs due to separate cellulase production for hydrolysis	Demonstration scale, planned for commercial plants	Steps can be carried out at optimum conditions using different microorganisms for C5 and C6, separated lignin can be used for energy generation	More steps leading to greater energy consumption, pretreatment energy intensive
	SSF	Cost due to separate cellulose production for hydrolysis	Demonstration scale	Simple design, easy to operate, reduced end product inhibition of enzymatic hydrolysis, water and energy savings through fewer steps and reactors	Optimum conditions between hydrolysis and fermentation different— compromise necessary, longer hydrolysis times
	SSCF	Lower capital cost	Pilot/demonstration scale	Fewer vessels, fewer steps, more efficient fermentation through use of pentose and hexose sugars	Lignin cannot be separated before fermentation, which leads to very viscous broth, engineered microorganism needed that can ferment both C6 and C5
	CBP	Lower capital cost, cost reduced due to minimum number of steps	Pilot/demonstration scale	Process combined in one step, no separate enzyme production needed	No large-scale operation, still in the research phase, coordination of cellulolytic enzymes, hydrolysis of cellulose and hemicelluloses, and fermentation necessary

Energy cost is another key factor in bioethanol production, together with water and wastewater management. Corn processing facilities with steps such as hydrolysis (especially in wet milling processes), as well as sugarcane distilleries, require large amounts of water/steam and energy (Amorim et al. 2011). Many facilities have started using process residues for energy production to partially cover their demands.

The sugarcane industry has received public criticism for agricultural practices related to the harvest and transportation of sugarcane as well as the burning of the fields (Amorim et al. 2011). The sustainability of corn and wheat production has also come under scrutiny. High nutrient inputs together with soil erosion and a large water footprint are associated with bioenergy crops (Solomon et al. 2010; Bonin and Lal 2012). These factors have adversely influenced calculations of overall net energy balances and greenhouse gas (GHG) emissions of fuel ethanol (Amorim et al. 2011; Larsen 2008).

Another limiting factor for sugarcane-based ethanol plants is the several months–long idle period associated with crop harvesting. Although starch processing facilities operate throughout the whole year, the production time of Brazilian sugarcane distilleries is limited to 4 to 6 months per year. This is due to the length of the harvesting period (up to 8 months a year) and the fact that the harvested sugarcane cannot be stored or transported over long distances (Amorim et al. 2011).

A challenge for both sugar-based and starch-based ethanol production is the stability and potential microbial contamination of the fermenting microorganisms. Bacterial contaminants can lead to loss of efficiency and costly cleaning and sterilisation operations (Beckner et al. 2011). Yeast strains (*S. cerevisiae*) are commonly used in fermentation operations for first generation feedstocks. They have to be able to survive stressing industrial conditions and multiple recycle operations to minimise bacterial contaminations (Amorim et al. 2011).

One of the most important limiting factors for the extent of ethanol production from starch and sugars, however, will most likely be the availability of the biomass materials. Geography and agricultural factors limit the scale of crop production and the available resources are likely to be insufficient to cover the growing demand for biofuels, and to eventually replace gasoline as transportation fuel on a global scale (Bonin and Lal 2012).

9.3.1.2 Lignocellulosic-Based Facilities

Although no major cost-reducing process design breakthroughs are expected for starch-based and sugar-based technologies, second generation bioethanol is still in the research and development stage, and the optimisation of process technologies and related issues are likely to lead to more efficient production setups. There are a number of limitations and challenges relating to the key process steps (pretreatment, hydrolysis and fermentation; Table 9.16), and research activities have been ongoing in these areas.

TABLE 9.16

Overview of Bioethanol Challenges and Developments

Feedstock	Challenges/Limitations		Research and Developments
	Technological	Others	
First generation: sugar (sucrose)	Fermentation: yeast stability, contamination, ethanol tolerance, water/steam consumption	Feedstock: cost, yields, agricultural and geographical limitations Environment: controversial views on agricultural practices (transport, harvesting, fertilisers, burning of fields), net energy balance	Environment: steam and bioenergy production from bagasse, or second generation biofuel Fermentation: selection of new, more resistant yeast strains to reduce contamination and competing wild yeast strains
First generation: starch	Hydrolysis: high energy input, high temperatures, enzyme cost Fermentation: ethanol productivity, tolerance	Feedstock: cost, yields, agricultural and geographical limitations, competition with food supply Environment: controversial views on GHGs, net energy balance, water/steam consumption	Feedstock: development of corn hybrids 'self-processing grain' Hydrolysis: development of new enzymes (that can operate at lower temperatures) Fermentation: modification of yeast strains (recombinant strains) to increase resistance, ethanol tolerance and productivity High gravity fermentations
Second generation: lignocellulose	Pretreatment: high capital cost, energy and water intensive Hydrolysis: high enzyme cost, low temperature tolerance Fermentation: pentose and hexose fermentation, productivity, ethanol tolerance, stability	Feedstock: logistics of supply, infrastructure, storage, public acceptance and support Environment: still too energy intensive (and energy from nonrenewable sources)	Feedstock: integrated biorefineries Pretreatment: optimisation of existing processes (steam explosion, acid treatment), recycling of acids, minimise formation of inhibitors Hydrolysis: reduction in cost of cellulases (*T. reesel*), recycling of cellulase Fermentation: characterisation of fermenting organisms, genetic engineering, recombinant strains, more tolerance to inhibitors

The cost and scalability of cellulosic ethanol production are major limitations on the way to its commercial availability. The pretreatment step is often considered the most cost-intensive and is therefore a limiting factor for low-cost productions (Limayem and Ricke 2012). Many pretreatment methods consume large amounts of energy, chemicals and water. In addition, the cost for enzymes to break down cellulose and hemicellulose is high (Wyman 2007). Lignocellulosic hydrolysis requires up to 100 times more enzymes than needed in the processing of starch (Merino and Cherry 2007).

Another major current challenge is the limited availability and discovery of microorganisms that can efficiently ferment both pentose and hexose sugars (Sims et al. 2010; Weber et al. 2010). The integration approaches described in Section 9.3 and listed in Table 9.15 can only be optimised if suitable yeasts, bacteria or fungi are employed. Many discoveries and developments that are achieved on a laboratory scale fail to reach the industrial scale. Fermentation of a variety of sugars (pentose and hexoses), high ethanol yields, good ethanol tolerance and robustness (against contamination) are crucial for suitable microorganisms in the further development and commercialisation of lignocellulosic ethanol (Limayem and Ricke 2012).

Similar to first generation feedstocks, overall energy and water consumption is also an important factor for lignocellulosic-based ethanol productions. Although biomass may be abundant, the infrastructure and storage facilities needed for efficient processing may not be in place (IEA 2008). The concept of integrated biorefineries (refer to Section 9.3.2.2) and the production of valuable coproducts (heat, energy and other chemicals) has therefore become more and more interesting in recent years (Sims et al. 2010).

Although first and second generation feedstocks are considered renewable, public acceptance for fuel ethanol remains limited. Although corn and sugar feedstocks are subject to the food versus fuel debate, lignocellulosic ethanol has mainly been criticised for unproven and cost-intensive technologies. Further research and development funding is likely to be necessary to overcome economic and technological hurdles (Sims et al. 2010).

9.3.2 Developments and Directions for the Future

9.3.2.1 Bioethanol Production from First Generation Feedstocks

Although no major breakthroughs are expected in the sugar and starch processing industry, improvements in fermentation technologies and process designs can help increase productivity and decrease production costs (Table 9.16; Singh et al. 2010).

Corn hybrids could improve the overall process and ethanol yield. In a conventional corn dry-grind process, the enzyme α-amylase is added in the liquefaction step to break down the starch. The following step is saccharification or, in most cases, SSF. In amylase corn, a corn hybrid, the amylase is produced and stored in the kernel (Singh 2008). The presence of water and high temperatures activate the amylase contained within the corn. If a small amount (3%) of the processed corn is replaced with amylase corn, no additional amylase is needed, which reduces the overall cost (Singh 2008).

Another option to reduce costs in dry grind corn processes is the use of raw starch hydrolysing enzymes (granular starch hydrolysing enzymes). These enzymes are able to convert starch into dextrins (liquefaction) at low temperatures, but can also convert dextrins into fermentable sugars (glucose). This makes it possible to combine all three steps into one step (simultaneous liquefaction, saccharification and fermentation; Wang et al. 2007; Singh et al. 2010).

Fermentation efficiencies could also be improved with new or modified yeast strains that are more resistant against stresses from industrial processes (temperature, pH, osmotic pressure and ethanol). In the Brazilian sugar industry, the search for an improved strain of *S. cerevisiae* has been ongoing. The sugarcane fermentation process includes intensive yeast cell recycling and a suitable yeast strain could therefore increase ethanol productivity and reduce production costs (Basso et al. 2008). Successful implementation of new yeast strains in industrial processes is challenging and significant funding has gone into research to understand the genetics and select improved *S. cerevisiae* strains that are suitable for industrial fermentations (Amorim et al. 2011).

The challenge of reducing energy and water usage in starch-based and sugar-based facilities has also been the focus of research and development activities. Cogeneration of electricity from by-products such as sugarcane bagasse has been introduced in many distilleries in Brazil (Amorim et al. 2011). In the corn processing industry, the production of valuable by-products (such as DDGS and corn oil) has improved the overall performance and economics of corn ethanol (Gibbons and Hughes 2011). VHG fermentations have been amongst the promising technological improvements that could offer water and energy savings. Higher concentrations of substrate lead to higher concentrations of ethanol, and efforts have been directed toward applying VGH fermentations to industrial processes (Bai et al. 2008; Puligundla et al. 2011).

A major trend in sustainable fuel production has been process integration and the development of integrated biorefineries. Coproduction and the combination of first and second generation feedstock processes offer the potential for improved efficiency and reduction of water usage and wastewater streams (Cardona and Sánchez 2007; Gibbons and Hughes 2011).

9.3.2.2 Bioethanol Production from Second Generation Feedstocks

Ethanol production from second generation feedstocks still shows significant potential for technical improvements and research efforts have been focussed on increasing process efficiencies and reducing costs, as well as water and energy consumption. To reach an economically viable ethanol production using lignocellulosic feedstocks, each step (pretreatment, hydro-lysis and fermentation) has to be optimised so that high ethanol yields can be obtained with the lowest possible cost.

The pretreatment of the substrates plays an important role because it is costly and affects all downstream operations. The selection and optimisation of pretreatment methods has been the focus of many research efforts (Young et al. 2010; Menon and Rao 2012). The choice of the pretreatment method largely depends on the type of feedstock, which determines the structure of the lignocellulose material. Several chemical, physical–chemical, physi-cal and biological pretreatment approaches have been proposed and tested, but only very few achieve considerable sugar yields with low enough costs (Sánchez and Cardona 2008; Young et al. 2010; Hu and Ragauskas 2012). The optimisation and integration of pretreatment methods has remained a chal-lenge and an opportunity to reduce the cost of cellulosic ethanol.

Another key research area is the enzymatic saccharification and hydro-lysis of lignocellulose substrates. The enzymes used in this step determine the amount of fermentable sugars that can be obtained from the biomass and hence influence the overall ethanol yield. Research goals include the reduction of production costs and the improvement of enzyme properties. Most enzymes used for bioethanol production are derived from fungi, with the fungus *Trichoderma reesei* being the most employed. An efficient way to reduce costs is to reduce the amount of enzyme needed or to increase productivity of the fungal strains to decrease enzyme production costs. Significant results have been achieved in these research areas, especially in cellulase production, engineering and biotechnology (Merino and Cherry 2007; Chandel et al. 2012).

In the fermentation step, microorganisms that can metabolise the sugars obtained from the lignocellulosic biomass are required. These sugars include a range of pentoses and hexoses. Most of the commercially used microorgan-isms such as *S. cerevisiae* are only able to efficiently ferment a limited number of sugars. Several approaches to improving fermentation operations have been explored and the metabolic engineering of bacteria and yeasts strains has been the focus of research efforts (Chandel et al. 2011; Jang et al. 2012).

E. coli can metabolise a wide range of sugars but with relatively low etha-nol yields. To improve its performance, *E. coli* strains have been engineered by introducing genes, blocking unfavourable pathways and influencing by-product formation. Several strains of *E. coli* (including KO11 and SZ110), which achieve improved ethanol yields of up to 95%, have been developed (Jang et al. 2012).

Because yeasts are the most suitable microorganisms for fermentation, they have been the focus of many research activities. Different engineering approaches have been used to enable pentose fermentation (Jeffries 2006). Progress has been made in the optimisation of pathways and in pentose transport, but challenges remain in the development of a robust industrial yeast strain that is able to ferment a wide range of sugars with high efficien-cies (Laluce et al. 2012). Efforts have also been directed toward increasing tolerance to toxic fermentation inhibitors, which may be present from the pretreatment step (Madhavan et al. 2012).

Despite advances in the area of pentose-fermenting organisms, the development and application of industrially engineered microorganisms that display sufficient fermentation performance and inhibitor tolerance remains a challenge (Hahn-Hägerdal et al. 2007; Young et al. 2010). Another key area of interest has been the development of suitable systems for CBP. The one-step process with a microorganism that produces cellulases and ethanol, could significantly lower the cost of bioethanol production (Lynd et al. 2005; van Zyl et al. 2007; Olson et al. 2012).

For both first and second generation feedstocks, the concept of process integration plays an important role. The advantages of advanced combined biorefineries include reductions in energy costs, improved waste management and water usage, smaller operation units and combined downstream steps (Cardona and Sánchez 2007). An advanced biorefinery could, for example, combine the use of corn and lignocellulose materials such as corncobs. It would also produce valuable by-products and could use lignin as an energy source (Gibbons and Hughes 2011; Jenkins and Alles 2011). For the integrated biorefinery concept to be realised, technological improvements in the pretreatment, hydrolysis and fermentation steps are necessary.

Alternative feedstocks other than sugar, starch or lignocellulosic materials have also attracted research interest. Microalgae are amongst the potential third generation feedstocks. Advantages include their high rate of productivity with high starch and cellulose and low lignin contents (Singh and Dhar 2011). Research activities have explored both microalgae and macroalgae as renewable sources for bioethanol, and progress has been made in extraction and conversion processes including dark fermentations (under anaerobic conditions) and engineered microalgae producing ethanol within the microalgal cell. Several technological hurdles have to be overcome before bioethanol from algae feedstocks can become economically viable, and interdisciplinary research and collaborations will be necessary to realise production on a larger industrial scale (John et al. 2011; Jones and Mayfield 2012).

References

Abengoa, http://www.abengoabioenergy.com/ (Accessed October, 2012).

Alvira, P.; Tomás-Pejó, E.; Ballesteros, M.; Negro, M.J. (2010). "Pretreatment technologies for an efficient bioethanol production process based on enzymatic hydrolysis: A review." *Bioresource Technology* **101**: 4851–4861.

Amorim, H.V.; Lopez, M.L.; de Castro Oliveira, J.V.; Buckeridge, M.S.; Goldman, G.H. (2011). "Scientific challenges of bioethanol production in Brasil." *Applied Microbiology and Biotechnology* **91**: 1267–1275.

Archer Daniels Midland, http://www.adm.com/ (Accessed October 2012).

Aventine Renewable Energies, http://www.aventinerei.com/ (Accessed October 2012).

Bacovsky, D.; Dallos, M.; Woergetter, M. (2010). "Status of 2nd generation biofuels demonstration facilities in June 2010." International Energy Agency (IEA) Bioenergy Task 39, Commercializing 1st and 2nd Generation Liquid Biofuels from Biomass.

Bai, F.W.; Anderson, W.A.; Moo-Young, M. (2008). "Ethanol fermentation technologies from sugar and starch feedstocks." *Biotechnology Advances* 26: 89–105.

Balat, M. (2005). "Current alternative engine fuels." *Energy Sources* 27: 569–577.

Balat, M.; Balat, H.; Öz, C. (2008). "Progress in bioethanol processing." *Progress in Energy and Combustion Science* 34: 551–573.

Banerjee, S.; Mudliar, S.; Sen, R.; Giri, B. (2010). "Commercializing lignocellulosic bioethanol: Technology bottlenecks and possible remedies." *Biofuels, Bioproducts and Biorefining* 4: 77–93.

Basso, L.C.; de Amorim, H.V.; de Oliveira, A.J.; Lopes, M.L. (2008). "Yeast selection for fuel ethanol production in Brazil." *Federation of European Microbiological Societies (FEMS) Yeast Research* 8: 1155–1163.

Basso, L.C.; Basso, T.O.; Rocha, S.N. (2011). "Ethanol production in Brazil: The industrial process and its impact on yeast fermentation." In dos Santos Bernardes, M.A. (ed.) *Biofuel Production—Recent Developments and Prospects*. InTech Europe, Rijeka, Croatia.

Beckner, M.; Ivey, M.L.; Phister, T.G. (2011). "Microbial contaminations of fuel ethanol fermentations." *Letters in Applied Microbiology* 53: 387–394.

Binot, P.; Sindhu, R.; Singhania, R.R.; Vikram, S.; Devi, L.; Nagalakshmi, S.; Kurien, N.; Sukumaran, R.K.; Pandey, A. (2010). "Bioethanol production from rice straw: An overview." *Bioresource Technology* 101: 4767–4774.

Biofuel Database (East Asia), http://www.asiabiomass.jp/biofuelDB/japan/ (Accessed October 2012).

BioGasol, http://www.biogasol.com/ (Accessed October 2012).

BioWanze, http://www.biowanze.be/ (Accessed October 2012).

Blue Sugars, http://bluesugars.com/ (Accessed October 2012).

Bonin, C.; Lal, R. (2012). "Bioethanol potentials and life-cycle assessments of biofuel feedstocks." *Critical Reviews in Plant Science* 31: 271–289.

Borregaard, http://www.borregaard.com/ (Accessed October 2012).

Bothast, R.J.; Schlicher, M.A. (2005). "Biotechnological processes for conversion of corn into ethanol." *Applied Microbiology and Biotechnology* 67: 19–25.

BP, http://www.bp.com/ (Accessed December 2012).

Cardona, C.A.; Sánchez, O.J. (2007). "Fuel ethanol production: Process design trends and integration opportunities." *Bioresource Technology* 98: 2415–2457.

Cardona, C.A.; Sánchez, O.J.; Gutiérrez, L.F. (2009). Chapter 7 "Ethanolic fermentation technologies." In *Process Synthesis for Fuel Ethanol Production*. CRC Press, Taylor & Francis Group, Boca Raton, FL, USA.

Cardona, C.A.; Quintero, J.A.; Paz, I.C. (2010). "Production of bioethanol from sugarcane bagasse: Status and perspectives." *Bioresource Technology* 101: 4754–4766.

Cargill, www.cargill.com/ (Accessed October 2012).

Çaylak, B. (1998). "Comparison of different production processes for bioethanol." *Turkish Journal of Chemistry* 22: 351–359.

Chandel, A.K.; Chan, E.S.; Rudrvaram, R.; Narasu, M.L.; Roa, V.; Ravindra, P. (2007). "Economics and environmental impact of bioethanol production technologies: An appraisal." *Biotechnology and Molecular Biology Review* 2: 14–35.

Chandel, A.K.; Chandrasekhar, G.; Radhika, K.; Ravinder, R.; Ravindra, P. (2011). "Bioconversion of pentose sugars into ethanol: A review and future directions." *Biotechnology and Microbiology Review* **6**: 8–20.

Chandel, A.K.; Chandrasekhar, G.; Silva, M.B.; da Silva, S.S. (2012). "The realm of cellulases in biorefinery development." *Critical Reviews in Biotechnology* **32**: 187–202.

Chemtex, http://www.chemtex.com/ (Accessed October 2012).

Colorado, http://www.colorado.com.br/ (Accessed October 2012).

Copersucar, http://www.copersucar.com.br/ (Accessed October 2012).

Cosan, http://cosan.com.br/ (Accessed October 2012).

CropEnergies, http://www.cropenergies.com/ (Accessed October 2012).

DDCE (DuPont Danisco Cellulosic Ethanol), http://www.ddce.com/ (Accessed October 2012).

Dedini, http: www.dedini.com.br/ (Accessed October 2012).

Dien, B.S.; Cotta, M.A.; Jeffries, T.W. (2003). "Bacteria engineered for fuel ethanol production: Current status." *Applied Microbiology and Biotechnology* **63**: 258–266.

Drapcho, C.M.; Nhuan, N.P.; Walker, T.H. (2008). Chapter 5 "Ethanol production." In *Biofuels Engineering Process Technology*. MacGraw Hill Companies, Inc, New York, USA.

Elkins, J.G.; Raman, B.; Keller, M. (2010). "Engineered microbial systems for enhanced conversion of lignocellulosic biomass." *Current Opinion in Biotechnology* **21**: 657–662.

Ensus, http://ensusgroup.com/ (Accessed October 2012).

Environment Canada Renewable Fuel Regulations, http://www.ec.gc.ca/energie-energy/default.asp?lang=Enandn=0AA71ED2-1 (Accessed October 2012).

EPA Renewable Fuel Standard, http://www.epa.gov/otaq/fuels/renewablefuels/index.htm (Accessed October 2012).

EPure Statistics, http://www.epure.org/theindustry/statistics/ (Accessed October 2012).

Ethanol Producer Magazine, http://www.ethanolproducer.com/plants/listplants/USA/ (Accessed October 2012).

Flach, B.; Lieberz, S.; Bandz, K.; Dahlbacka, B. (2011). "EU-27 Annual Biofuels Report." USDA Foreign Agricultural Service. http://gain.fas.usda.gov/Recent%20 GAIN%20Publications/Biofuels%20Annual_The%20Hague_EU-27_6-22-2011. pdf (Accessed October, 2012).

Gibbons, W.; Hughes, S. (2011). Chapter 14 "Integrated biorefineries with engineered microbes and high-value co-products for profitable biofuels production." In *Biofuels, Global Impact on Renewable Energy, Production Agriculture, and Technological Advancements*.

Gnansounou, E. (2010). "Production and use of lignocellulosic bioethanol in Europe: Current situation and perspectives." *Bioresource Technology* **101**: 4842–4850.

Goldemberg, J. (2008). "The Brazilian biofuels industry." *Biotechnology for Biofuels* **1**: 6.

Gosh, T.K.; Prelas, M.A. (2011). Chapter 7 "Ethanol." In *Energy Resources and Systems*, Volume 2: Renewable Resources. Springer.

GraalBio, http://graalbio.com/ (Accessed October 2012).

Hahn-Hägerdal, B.; Karhumaa, K.; Fonseca, C.; Spencer-Martins, I.; Gorwa-Grauslund, M.F. (2007). "Towards industrial pentose fermenting yeast strains." *Applied Microbiology and Biotechnology* **74**: 937–953.

Hamelinck, C.N.; van Hooijdonk, G.; Faaij, A.P.C. (2005). "Ethanol from lignocellulosic biomass: Techno-economic performance in the short-, middle-, and long-term." *Biomass and Bioenergy* **28**: 384–410.

Harada, Y.; Sakata, K.; Sato, S.; Takayama, S. (1996). Chapter 1 "Fermentation pilot plant." In Vogel, H.C.; Todaro, C.L. (eds.) *Fermentation and Biochemical Engineering Handbook: Principles, Process Design, and Equipment*, 2nd Edition. Notes Publication, New Jersey, USA.

Hasunuma, T.; Kondo, A. (2012). "Consolidated bioprocessing and simultaneous saccharification and fermentation of lignocellulose to ethanol with thermotolerant yeast strains." *Process Biochemistry* **47**: 1287–1294.

Hu, F.; Ragauskas, A. (2012). "Pretreatment and lignocellulosic chemistry." *Bioenergy Research* **5**: 1043–1066.

Huang, H.-J.; Ramaswamy, S.; Tschirner, U.W.; Ramarao, B.V. (2008). "A review of separation technologies in current and future biorefineries." *Separation and Purification Technology* **62**: 1–21.

IEA (2008). "From 1st to 2nd generation biofuel technologies: An overview of current industry and RandD activities." Sims, R.; Taylor, M.; International Energy Agency, France.

Inbicon, http://www.inbicon.com/ (Accessed October 2012).

Ingledew, W.M. (2003). "Continuous fermentation in the fuel alcohol industry: How does the technology affect yeast?" In Jacques, K.A.; Lyons, T.P.; Kelsall, D.R. (eds.) *The Alcohol Textbook*, 4th Edition. Nottingham University Press, Nottingham, UK.

Inui, M.; Vertes, A.A.; Yukawa, H. (2009). Chapter 15 "Advanced fermentation technologies." In Vertes, A.; Quereshi, N.; Yukawa, H.; Blaschek, H.P. (eds.) *Biomass to Biofuel: Strategies for Global Industries.* Wiley, United Kingdom.

Iogen, http://www.iogen.ca/ (Accessed October 2012).

Itamarati, http://www.usinasitamarati.com.br/ (Accessed October 2012).

Jang, Y.-S.; Park, J.M.; Choi, S.; Choi, Y.J.; Seung, D.Y.; Cho, J.H.; Lee, S.Y. (2012). "Engineering of microorganisms for the production of biofuels and perspectives based systems metabolic engineering approaches." *Biotechnology Advances* **30**: 989–1000.

Jeffries, T.W. (2006). "Engineering yeasts for xylose metabolism." *Current Opinion in Biotechnology* **17**: 320–326.

Jenkins, R.; Alles, C. (2011). "Field to fuel: Developing sustainable biorefineries." *Ecological Applications* **21**: 1096–1104.

John, R.P.; Anisha, G.S.; Nampoothiri, K.M.; Pandey, A. (2011). "Micro and macroalgal biomass: A renewable source for bioethanol." *Bioresource Technology* **102**: 186–193.

Jones, C.S.; Mayfield, S.P. (2012). "Algae biofuels: Versatility for the future of bioenergy." *Current Opinion in Biotechnology* **23**: 345–351.

Jordan, B.D.; Bowman, M.; Braker, J.D.; Dien, B.S.; Hector, R.E.; Lee, C.C.; Mertens, J.A.; Wagschal, K. (2012). "Plant cell walls to ethanol." *Biochemical Journal* **442**: 241–252.

Kosaric, N.; Velikonja, J. (1995). "Liquid and gaseous fuels from biotechnology: Challenge and opportunities." *FEMS Microbiology Reviews* **16**: 111–142.

Kuhad, R.C.; Gupta, R.; Khasa, P.Y.; Singh, A.; Zhang, Y.H.P. (2011). "Bioethanol production from pentose sugars: Current status and future prospects." *Renewable and Sustainable Energy Reviews* **15**: 4950–4962.

Laluce, C.; Schenberg, A.C.G.; Gallardo, J.C.M.; Coradello, L.F.C.; Pombeiro-Sponchiado, S.R. (2012). "Advances and developments in strategies to improve strains of *Saccharomyces cerevisiae* and process to obtain the lignocellulosic ethanol—A review." *Applied Biochemistry and Biotechnology* **166**: 1908–1926.

Larsen, E.D. (2008). "Biofuel production technologies: Status. Prospects and implications for trade and development." *UNCTAD Biofuels Initiative*, United Nations Conference on Trade and Development.

Larsen, J.; Ostergaard Petersen, M.; Thirup, L.; Li, H.W.; Iversen, F.K. (2008). "The IBUS process—Lignocellulosic bioethanol close to a commercial reality." *Chemical Engineering and Technology* 31: 765–772.

Limayem, A.; Ricke, S.C. (2012). "Lignocellulosic biomass for bioethanol production: Current perspectives, potential issues and future prospects." *Progress in Energy and Combustion Science* 38: 449–467.

Lin, Y.; Tanaka, S. (2006). "Ethanol fermentation from biomass resources: Current state and prospects." *Applied Microbiology and Biotechnology* 69: 627–642.

Luis Dreyfus Commodities, http://www.ldcommodities.com/ (Accessed October 2012).

Lynd, L.R.; van Zyl, W.H.; McBride, J.E.; Laser, M. (2005). "Consolidated bioprocessing of cellulosic biomass: An update." *Current Opinion in Biotechnology* 16: 577–583.

Madhavan, A.; Srivastava, A.; Kondo, A.; Bisaria, V.S. (2012). "Bioconversion of lignocellulose-derived sugars to ethanol by engineered *Saccharomyces cerevisiae*." *Critical Reviews in Biotechnology* 32: 22–48.

Madson, P.W.; Monceaux, D.A. (1995). Chapter 16 "Fuel ethanol production." In Lyons, T.P.; Kelsall, D.R.; Murtagh, J.E. (eds.) *The Alcohol Textbook*. Nottingham University Press, Nottingham, UK.

Marquis, http://www.marquisenergy.com/ (Accessed October 2012).

Mascoma, http://www.mascoma.com/ (Accessed October 2012).

Menon, V.; Rao, M. (2012). "Trends in bioconversion of lignocellulose: Biofuels, platform chemicals and biorefinery concepts." *Progress in Energy and Combustion Science* 38: 522–550.

Merino, S.T.; Cherry, J. (2007). "Progress and challenges in enzyme development for biomass utilization." *Advances in Biochemical Engineering/Biotechnology* 108: 95–120.

Mosier, N.; Wyman, C.; Dale, B.; Elander, R.; Lee, Y.Y.; Holtzapple, M.; Ladisch, M. (2005). "Features of promising technologies for pretreatment of lignocellulosic biomass." *Bioresource Technology* 96: 673–686.

Mousdale, D.M. (2008). "Biofuels: Biotechnology, chemistry, and sustainable development." CRC Press, Taylor & Francis Group, Boca Raton, FL, USA.

Mussatto, S.I.; Dragone, G.; Guimaraes, P.M.R.; Silva, J.P.A.; Carneiro, L.M.; Roberto, I.C.; Vicente, A.; Domingues, L.; Teixeira, J.A. (2010). "Technological trends, global market, and challenges of bio-ethanol production." *Biotechnology Advances* 28: 817–830.

Nigam, P.S.; Singh, A. (2011). "Production of liquid biofuels from renewable resources." *Progress in Energy and Combustion Science* 37: 52–68.

O'Brien, D. (2010). "Updated trends in U.S. wet and dry corn milling production." Extension Agricultural Economists. http://www.agmanager.info/energy/CornRefining_01-19-10.pdf.

Ojeda, K.; Sanchez, E.; El-Halwagi, M.; Kafarov, V. (2011). "Exergy analysis and process integration of bioethanol production from acid pre-treated biomass: Comparison of SHF, SSF, and SSCF pathways." *Chemical Engineering Journal* 176–177: 195–201.

Olofsson, K.; Bertilsson, M.; Liden, G. (2008). "A short review on SSF—An interesting process option for ethanol production from lignocellulosic feedstocks." *Biotechnology for Biofuels* 1: 7.

Olson, D.G.; McBride, J.E.; Shaw, A.J.; Lynd, L.R. (2012). "Recent progress in consolidated bioprocessing." *Current Opinion in Biotechnology* **23**: 396–405.

POET, http://www.poet.com/plants (Accessed October 2012).

POET-DSM, http://www.poetdsm.com/ (Accessed October 2012).

Puligundla, P.; Smogrovicova, D.; Obulam, V.S.R.; Ko, S. (2011). "Very High Gravity (VHG) ethanolic brewing and fermentations: A research update." *Journal of Industrial Microbiology and Biotechnology* **38**: 1133–1144.

Rajagopal, D.; Sexton, S.E.; Roland-Holst, D.; Zolberman, D. (2007). "Challenge of biofuels: Filling the tank without emptying the stomach." *Environmental Research Letters* **2**: 1–9.

Rao, R.P.; Dufour, N.; Swana, J. (2011). "Using microorganisms to brew biofuels." *In Vitro Cellular and Developmental Biology—Plant* **47**: 637–649.

Renuka do Brasil, http://www.renukadobrasil.com.br/ (Accessed October 2012).

RFA (2012). "World fuel ethanol production." Renewable Fuel Association. http://ethanolrfa.org/ (Accessed October 29, 2012).

Rothman, H.; Greenshields, R.; Calle, F.R. (1983). "The alcohol economy: Fuel ethanol and the Brazilian experience." Francis Printer, London.

Ruiz, E.; Romero, I.; Moya, M.; Sánchez, S.; Bravo, V.; Castro, E. (2007). "Sugar fermentation by *Fusarium oxysporum* to produce ethanol." *World Journal of Microbiology and Biotechnology* **23**: 259–267.

Sánchez, O.J.; Cardona, C.A. (2008). "Trends in biotechnological production of fuel ethanol from different feedstocks." *Bioresource Technology* **99**: 5270–5295.

Sao Martinho, http://www.saomartinho.ind.br/ (Accessed October 2012).

Schurig, M.C. (2008). "Sugarcane and ethanol in Brazil: A literature review." Case study for the Sugar Ethanol Campaign (SEC) of Solidaridad, Aidenvironment, Amsterdam, The Netherlands.

Scragg, A.H. (2009). Chapter 6 "Liquid biofuels to replace petrol." In *Biofuels: Production, Application and Development*. CAB International, United Kingdom.

SEKAB, http://www.sekab.com/ (Accessed October 2012).

Sims, R.E.H.; Mabee, W.; Saddler, J.N.; Taylor, M. (2010). "An overview of second generation biofuel technologies." *Bioresource Technology* **101**: 1570–1580.

Singh, A.; Kumar, P.K.R. (1991). "*Fusarium oxysporum*: Status in bioethanol production." *Critical Reviews in Biotechnology* **11**: 129–147.

Singh, N.K.; Dhar, W.W. (2011). "Microalgae as second generation biofuel. A review." *Agronomy and Sustainable Development* **31**: 605–639.

Singh, V. (2008). Chapter 13 "Emerging technologies in dry grind ethanol production." In *Biocatalysis and Bioenergy*. Wiley, New Jersey.

Singh, V.; Johnston, D.B.; Rausch, K.D.; Tumbleson, M.E. (2010). Chapter 9 "Improvements in corn to ethanol production technology using *Saccharomyces cerevisiae*." *Biomass to Biofuels, Strategies for Global Industries*. John Wiley & Sons Ltd, Chichester, West Sussex, UK.

Sivakumar, G.; Vail, D.R.; Xu, J.; Burner, D.M.; Lay Jr., J.O.; Ge, X.; Weathers, P.J. (2010). "Bioethanol and biodiesel: Alternative liquid fuels for future generations." *Engineering in Life Sciences* **10**: 8–18.

Soccol, C.R.; Vandenberghe, L.P.S.; Costa, B.; Woiciechowski, A.L.; de Carvalho, J.C.; Medeiros, A.B.P.; Francisco, A.M.; Bonomi, L.J. (2005). "Brazilian biofuel program: An overview." *Journal of Industrial and Scientific Research* **64**: 897–904.

Solomon, B.D. (2010). "Biofuels and sustainability." *Annuals of the New York Academy of Science* **1185**: 119–134.

Taherzadeh, M.J.; Karimi, K. (2008). Chapter 3 "Bioethanol: Market and production processes." In Nag, A. (ed.) *Biofuels Refining and Performance*. MacGraw Hill Companies Inc., New York, USA.

Tereos, http://www.tereos.com/ (Accessed October 2012).

Tharaldson, http://www.tharaldsonethanol.com/ (Accessed October 2012).

União da Indústria de Cana de Açúcar (Brazilian Sugarcane Industry Association) (UNICA) (2012). "Company production ratings for sugarcane, sugar and ethanol." Sugarcane Industry Association. http://english.unica.com.br/ (Accessed October 29, 2012).

U.S. Department of Energy (2010). "Current state of the U.S. ethanol industry." Prepared by Cardno ENTRIX, New Castle, DE. http://www1.eere.energy.gov/biomass/pdfs/current_state_of_the_us_ethanol_industry.pdf (Accessed October 2012).

Valdes, C. (2011). "Brazil's ethanol industry: Looking forward." United States Department of Agriculture, Economic Research Service. http://www.ers.usda.gov/publications/bio-bioenergy/bio-02.aspx (Accessed October 2012).

van Zyl, W.H.; Lynd, L.R.; den Haan, R.; McBride, J.E. (2007). "Consolidated bioprocessing for bioethanol production using Saccharomyces cerevisiae." *Advances in Biochemical Engineering/Biotechnology* **108**: 205–235.

Verbelen, P.J.; De Schutter, D.P.; Delvaux, F.; Verstrepen, K.J.; Delvaux, F.R. (2006). "Immobilized yeast cell systems for continuous fermentation applications." *Biotechnology Letters* **28**: 1515–1525.

Verenium, http://www.verenium.com/ (Accessed October 2012).

Walker, M.G. (2010). "Bioethanol: Science and technology of fuel ethanol." Ventus Publishing ApS. Frederiksberg, Denmark.

Walter, A.; Rosillo-Calle, F.; Dolzan, P.; Piacente, E.; Borges da Cunha, K. (2008). "Perspectives on fuel ethanol consumption and trade." *Biomass and Bioenergy* **32**: 730–748.

Wang, P.; Singh, V.; Xue, H.; Johnston, D.B.; Rausch, K.D.; Tumbleson, M.E. (2007). "Comparison of raw starch hydrolyzing enzyme with conventional liquefaction and saccharification enzymes in dry grind corn processing." *Cereal Chemistry* **84**: 10–14.

Weber, C.; Farwick, A.; Benisch, F.; Brat, D.; Dietz, H.; Subtil, T.; Boles, E. (2010). "Trends and challenges in the microbial production of lignocellulosic bioalcohol fuels." *Applied Microbiology and Biotechnology* **87**: 1303–1315.

Wyman, C.E. (2007). "What is (and is not) vital to advancing cellulosic ethanol." *Trends in Biotechnology* **25**: 153–157.

Xu, Q.; Singh, A.; Himmel, M.E. (2009). "Perspectives and new directions for the production of bioethanol using consolidated bioprocessing of lignocellulose." *Current Opinion in Biotechnology* **20**: 364–371.

Young, E.; Lee, S.-M.; Alper, H. (2010). "Optimizing pentose utilization in yeast: The need for novel tools and approaches." *Biotechnology for Biofuels* **3**: 24.

Zhao, X.-Q.; Zi, L.-H.; Bai, F.-W.; Lin, H.-L.; Hao, X.-M.; Yue, G.-J.; Ho, N.W.Y. (2012). "Bioethanol from Lignocellulosic Biomass." *Advances in Biochemical Engineering/Biotechnology* **128**: 25–51.

Zilor, http://www.zilor.com.br/ (Accessed October 2012).

10

Fischer–Tropsch Synthesis from Biosyngas

Katrin Thommes and Vladimir Strezov

CONTENTS

10.1 Introduction

Transportation fuels are predominantly produced from crude oil. To reduce the dependence on this fossil resource and to help address associated environmental issues, transportation fuels derived from biomass have been increasingly investigated.

Biofuels can be divided into two categories—first generation and second generation fuels. First generation fuels include biodiesel derived from vegetable oils and bioethanol obtained from the fermentation of sugar- or starch-containing materials such as sugarcane or corn. These are produced on a commercial scale using well-established technologies (Sanchez and Cardona 2008). First generation fuel feedstocks, however, are limited and therefore costly. An alternative, which has received increasing interest, is the use of second generation biofuels produced from lignocellulosic biomass materials including forest and agricultural wastes.

There are two main pathways to achieve the transformation from carbon-containing lignocellulosic biomass to liquid transportation fuels—the thermochemical and biochemical pathways (Figure 10.1). Synthetic liquid fuels can be produced via the thermochemical pathway, which includes, for example, the gasification of biomass followed by Fischer–Tropsch (FT) synthesis (Damartzis and Zabaniotou 2011).

FT synthesis is used to convert carbon monoxide and hydrogen (synthesis gas or syngas) into liquid hydrocarbon products. The reaction was discovered in the 1920s by the German chemists, Franz Fischer and Hans Tropsch. The technology was first applied in Germany in the 1930s with the aim of converting coal into liquid transportation fuels to reduce petroleum dependence. The FT process has undergone many developments since then. FT products compete with similar products obtained from crude oil. The economic viability of the FT industry is therefore strongly influenced by oil prices and availability. Historically, the development and application of FT processes have often been a result of political and strategic planning (Schulz 1999; Steynberg and Dry 2004).

FT synthesis can be used to produce a range of hydrocarbons including gasoline and diesel fuels. The reaction takes place through heterogeneous

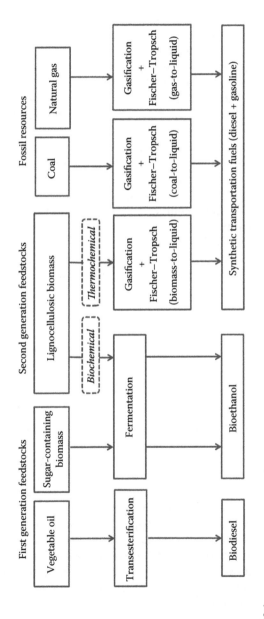

FIGURE 10.1
Selected processes for the production of liquid fuels from first and second generation feedstocks and fossil resources.

catalysis. Mainly iron- and cobalt-based catalysts are used for the commercial production of longer chain hydrocarbons and other chemicals (e.g. olefins). FT technology was first used to convert coal-to-liquid (CTL) fuels but is recently receiving increasing interest due to its potential for gas-to-liquid (GLT) and biomass-to-liquid (BTL) applications (Steynberg and Dry 2004; van Steen and Claeys 2008). It can be used to convert natural gas into transportable liquid fuels, which can then more easily enter global markets. FT synthesis is also of great interest for the production of sustainable second generation biofuels such as synthetic diesel.

Synthetic diesel produced via the FT pathway displays several advantages over conventional crude oil–derived diesel. Because it is mostly free of aromatics and sulphur impurities, fewer particles and pollutants are released through exhaust fumes. It also has a high cetane number of approximately 70, meaning that it displays very good ignition properties.

FT industries utilising coal and natural gas have reached commercial scale and are expected to grow in the coming years. As of 2013, however, BTL processes, which convert lignocellulosic biomass to biofuels, are still under investigation and have not yet progressed past the pilot plant scale. Well-established technologies such as gasification and FT synthesis still need to be optimised and tailored toward the processing of biomass materials. Process design and integration are challenges in developing an economically viable BTL system.

10.2 FT Synthesis: Concepts

10.2.1 FT Reaction

FT synthesis is not a recently developed reaction. Its discovery dates back to the 1920s when Franz Fischer and Hans Tropsch demonstrated the synthesis of various hydrocarbons from coal using a catalyst and high pressure (Fischer and Tropsch 1923). The first commercial plant using this technology was built in Germany in the 1930s. Interest in FT processes has often been linked to a limited access to crude oil resources, and hence the need to convert other resources such as coal and gas into transportable liquid fuels as well as other chemicals. This was the case in Germany in the 1940s and in South Africa in the 1950s and 1960s. These two countries still remain amongst the leaders in FT technology today. Development of FT technology has been strongly influenced by crude oil prices. The oil crisis in the 1970s, and a growing concern about the security of oil resources and supply, led to a renewed interest in FT technology. In addition to coal, natural gas and especially 'stranded' gas reserves (which are often remote and therefore not economically viable) became a valuable feedstock for FT processes. Coal-based and gas-based FT synthesis has been commercialised and several plants operate around the world (Steynberg and Dry 2004). In recent years, the use of biomass as a sustainable feedstock for FT processes has received increased attention, and research and development efforts have been undertaken to scale up BTL FT processes (Evans and Smith 2012; Hu et al. 2012).

Various feedstocks and drivers are associated with the development of CTL, GTL and BTL systems, but the heart of all these processes remains the FT synthesis with its long history of catalyst and reactor development.

In FT synthesis, a mixture of carbon monoxide and hydrogen (syngas) is converted into long-chain hydrocarbons through catalytic hydrogenation (Figure 10.2).

Next to this predominating reaction, other transformations can take place in the FT reactor. The chemical reactions involved are complex but can be simplified into the reactions shown in Table 10.1. In addition to alkanes and alkenes (olefins), alcohols may be formed or undesirable side reactions, such as methane formation or the Boudouard reaction, could occur (Guettel et al. 2008).

FT synthesis is based on the use of a heterogeneous catalyst. Iron and cobalt compounds are the most widely used in industrial applications. The reactions are usually carried out at temperatures between 190°C and 350°C, with high pressures (15–40 bar; Demirbas 2007; Hu et al. 2012). There are two operation modes: low-temperature FT (LTFT) operating between 190°C and

$$nCO + 2nH_2 \longrightarrow (-CH_2-)_n + nH_2O \qquad \Delta H = -165 \text{ kJ/mol}$$

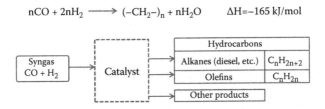

FIGURE 10.2

FT synthesis.

TABLE 10.1

Reactions That Can Take Place in an FT Reactor

	Reaction/Formation	Equation	H_2/CO ratio
Main/desired reaction	Alkanes (branched, linear)	$nCO + (2n + 1)H_2 \rightarrow C_nH_{2n+2} + nH_2O$	$(2n + 1)/n$
	Alkenes	$nCO + 2nH_2 \rightarrow C_nH_{2n} + nH_2O$	2
Side/undesired reaction	Alcohols	$nCO + 2nH_2 \rightarrow C_nH_{2n+2}O + (n - 1)H_2O$	2
	Methane	$CO + 3H_2 \rightarrow CH_4 + H_2O$	3
	WGS	$CO + H_2O \rightleftharpoons CO_2 + H_2$	
	Boudoir	$2CO \rightleftharpoons CO_2 + C$	

240°C, and high-temperature FT (HTFT), with temperatures from 300°C to
350°C. HTFT is usually employed with an iron-based catalyst to produce
gasoline or low molecular olefins, and LTFT uses Co- or Fe-based catalysts
for waxes and diesel synthesis (Dry 2002).

To obtain the desired long-chain hydrocarbons, a series of reactions including several intermediates is necessary. Many studies have been carried out to
gain an insight into reaction orders and the details and structures of intermediates, whereas numerous mechanisms have been suggested and reviewed
(Schulz 1999; van der Laan et al. 1999; Davis 2001; Maitlis and Zanotti 2009).
Generally, the FT chain growth can be regarded as a surface-catalysed polymerisation reaction with a repeating sequence of steps. Through adsorption,
transfer and desorption reactions that take place on the surface of the catalyst, the C–O bond is broken, hydrogen atoms are transferred (to carbon and
oxygen) and a new C–C bond is formed (Schulz 1999). The detailed mechanism and the number of C–C bonds that are formed (the growth of the carbon chain) predominantly depend on the catalyst properties.

10.2.2 Process Parameters and Product Distribution

The reactions in FT synthesis are mostly exothermic, and the FT products
are a mixture of different length hydrocarbons and other compounds (e.g.
alcohols). The selectivity of the FT synthesis reactions in influenced by various parameters and an overview is given in Table 10.2. The distribution of
the hydrocarbon products can be described with the Anderson–Schulz–
Flory (ASF) kinetics model represented by the equation shown in Figure 10.3
(Friedel and Anderson 1950; Patzlaff et al. 1999).

The chain growth probability (α) is defined by the reaction rates for propagation and termination of the carbon chain. It is influenced by the nature
of the catalyst, the ratio of CO and H_2 in the syngas and the temperature
and pressure in the reactor (Gupta and Demirbas 2010). The chain growth
probability (α) generally increases with increasing pressure and decreasing

TABLE 10.2

General Influence of Process Conditions on the Selectivity in FT Reactions

Parameter	Chain Length	Chain Branching	Olefin Selection	Alcohol Selection	Methane Selection	Carbon Deposition
Temperature	↓	↑	Complex	↓	↑	↑
Pressure	↑	↓	Complex	↑	↓	Complex
H_2/CO	↓	↑	↓	↓	↑	↓
Conversion	Complex	Complex	↓	↓	↑	↑

Source: van der Laan, G.P., and Beenackers, A.A.C.M., *Catalysis Reviews: Science and Engineering* 41: 255–318, 1999; Röper, M. Fischer–Tropsch synthesis. In *Catalysis in C1 Chemistry*, Reidel Dordrecht, The Netherlands, 1983.
Note: ↑ = increasing; ↓ = decreasing.

$$M_n = (1-\alpha)^2 \alpha^{n-1}$$

M_n = molar fraction of the hydrocarbon with n carbon atoms

α = chain growth probability

FIGURE 10.3
ASF equation.

temperature (Table 10.2), and is usually higher with Co-based than Fe-based catalysts (Hamelinck et al. 2004).

The higher the α value, the higher the molecular weight of the product. In the ASF plot, the log (M_n/n) is plotted against the carbon number. If the reaction follows an ASF distribution, this plot should give a straight line with α as the slope. In practice, however, the distributions often differ from the ideal ASF equation, with C_1 (methane) often being a larger fraction than anticipated (Patzlaff et al. 1999; Zwart and van Ree 2009).

In industry, an α value of greater than 0.9 is usually desired. If predicted by the ASF equation, the maximum direct yield of diesel (C_{11}–C_{20}) would be approximately 40% (Figure 10.4). Therefore, FT processes are often designed for a maximum α value targeting the production of waxes that can then be hydrocracked to obtain the desired fuel (in most cases, diesel).

The chain growth probability (α), and therefore the nature of the products, also depend on the composition of the feed gas. A low H_2/CO ratio is usually favourable for the selectivity toward longer chain hydrocarbons but is not favourable for an efficient conversion. For high conversion, a H_2/CO ratio of two or slightly higher is needed. The water–gas shift (WGS) reaction (see Table 10.1) can be used to adjust the value. Fe-based FT catalysts also act

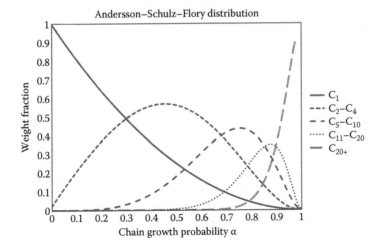

FIGURE 10.4
Weight distribution of FT products as predicted by the ASF equation.

as catalysts for the WGS reaction. FT synthesis and the WGS reaction can therefore take place in the same reactor. Co-based FT catalysts, however, are mostly inactive for the WGS reaction, and treatment of the feed gas prior to FT synthesis may be necessary to achieve the ideal H_2/CO ratio.

The catalyst support used in FT reactions can also have an influence on reaction rates and selectivities. These effects, however, have not yet been fully understood (Iglesia 1997). Another subject that has been investigated in many studies is the effect of water (one of the main products of the FT reaction) on the catalyst (Dalai and Davis 2008). It has been suggested that small amounts of water are favourable for reaction rates as well as selectivities (C_{5+}), but that large amounts of water would decrease the rates. The catalyst support was also found to play an important role in the extent of the water effect (Bertole et al. 2002; Dalai and Davis 2008).

For FT process design, a major consideration has to be given to the choice of catalyst as well as the type of reactor. The desired product (e.g. diesel) and the process conditions (temperature, pressure, feed gas composition and contact time) play important roles in the reactor and catalyst selection process.

10.3 Existing Reactor and Catalyst Designs for FT Synthesis

10.3.1 Catalysts for FT Synthesis

The properties of the catalyst are very important for the success of an FT process. The FT reaction can be regarded as the hydrogenation of carbon monoxide, and there are only four metals that show sufficient catalytic activity for this reaction: iron (Fe), cobalt (Co), nickel (Ni) and ruthenium (Ru).

Although ruthenium is the most active of these catalysts, and can be successfully used at low temperatures (<190°C), its lack of availability and high price prevent industrial application (Schulz 1999; Zhang et al. 2010). Nickel is also not considered suitable for larger scale applications due to a change of selectivity at higher temperatures (toward producing methane; Schulz 1999; Enger and Holmen 2013). Iron-based and cobalt-based catalysts were first applied by Franz Fischer and Hans Tropsch and remain the two catalysts used in industrial-scale FT synthesis. There are several differences between the performances of these two catalysts that must be considered in a FT process. An overview of the general advantages and disadvantages of Fe- and Co-based catalysts is shown in Table 10.3.

Several factors relating to the catalytic properties play an important role (Davis 2007; Jacobs and Davis 2010):

- Activity of the catalyst — refers to the conversion of substrate per gram/volume/area of catalyst

- Chain growth probability (α) — influences the product distribution and higher numbers are more favourable for longer chain hydrocarbons
- Product selectivity — refers to how selective the catalyst is for certain products (e.g. olefins)
- Stability and robustness (against deactivation) — operating conditions and costs are influenced by how long the catalyst can stay in its active form
- Activity of the FT catalyst for the WGS reaction — determines which ratio of CO and H_2 in the syngas can be fed into the FT reactor or which conditioning measures have to be undertaken

Because the composition of the feed gas and the levels of impurities depend on the material used for its production, FT process designs including the choice of catalyst vary depending on the feedstock used. Syngas from coal (CTL) or from biomass (BTL) usually displays low H_2/CO ratios, but syngas

TABLE 10.3

Characteristics of Fe-Based and Co-Based FT Catalysts

Properties	Cobalt-Based (Co)	Iron-Based (Fe)
Cost	Medium to high	Low to medium
Activity at low CO conversion	High	High
Productivity at high CO conversion	High	Lower (due to water inhibition)
Chain growth probability	Medium to high (maximum 0.94)	Low to high (maximum 0.95)
Activity for WGS reaction	Very low	Medium to high
Operation temperature	Low (LTFT)	Low to high
Temperature sensitivity	High (increased methane production at higher T)	Low (can be used in HTFT and LTFT)
Possible H_2/CO ratio	~2	0.5–2.5
Sulphur tolerance	Low (maximum S content of <0.1 ppm)	Medium (maximum S content of <0.2 ppm)
Robustness	Very high	Very low (not very resistant to water deactivation and attrition)
Selectivity for olefins	Low	High
Selectivity for methane	Medium	Low

Sources: Luo, M. et al., Fischer–Tropsch Synthesis: A Comparison of Iron and Cobalt Catalysts. AIChE Fall National Meeting, 2006; Khodakov, A.Y. et al., *Chemical Reviews* 107: 1692–1744, 2007; Jacobs, G., and Davis, B.H. Conversion of Biomass to Liquid Fuels and Chemicals via the Fischer–Tropsch Synthesis Route. Chapter 10 in *Thermochemical Conversion of Biomass to Liquid Fuels and Chemicals, RSC Energy and Environment Series* 1: 95, 2010.

from biomass has a lower ash and sulphur content (Luque et al. 2012). Syngas derived from natural gas (GTL) is usually rich in H_2, which can make the WGS reaction unnecessary or even undesirable (Zhang et al. 2010).

Catalyst supports and promoters can be of great importance to enhance catalyst activity and selectivity or to prevent sintering and deactivation of the catalyst. Alumina, silica and titania (Al_2O_3, SiO_2 and TiO_2) are commonly used as support materials. Promoters such as alkali metal ions, noble metals or transition metal oxides can be useful or even required to optimise the performance of the catalyst (Zhang et al. 2010).

The catalyst preparation and composition (e.g. the quantities of promoters) can have a considerable influence on the properties of the catalyst. Ongoing research efforts have been undertaken on the preparation methods and the effects of promoters, supports and additives (see Section 10.6.1; Iglesia 1997; van Steen and Claeys 2008; Luque et al. 2012).

Deactivation of the catalyst, which leads to a decrease in productivity, is a major problem and has been the subject of many research activities (see Section 10.6.1; Iglesia 1997; Dry 2002; Jun et al. 2004).

10.3.1.1 Fe-Based Catalysts for FT Synthesis

Compared with Ni, Co and Ru, Fe-based catalysts are the least expensive. They can also be employed under a wide range of temperatures and are therefore suitable for both LTFT and HTFT (Luque et al. 2012). The catalytic activity of iron for the WGS reaction allows for the use of feedgas with low H_2/CO ratios.

There are two broad classes of Fe-based catalyst that are used in commercial applications; fused iron catalysts and precipitated iron catalysts (Steynberg and Dry 2004). Fused iron catalysts are mainly used in HTFT synthesis for the production of olefins for the petrochemical industry. They are prepared from a molten magnetite (iron oxide) bath. Additives (usually K_2O) and promoters (Al_2O_3, MgO) are added and, after cooling, the magnetite is converted into a powder using microemulsion or spray drying methods. The magnetite is reduced with hydrogen before it is used in the FT reactor (Dry 2002; Steynberg and Dry 2004; Luque et al. 2012).

Precipitated iron catalysts are applied in LTFT synthesis to obtain higher molecular weight waxes from syngas, which can be converted into diesel. They are usually prepared from metallic iron, which is dissolved in an acidic solution where promoters (K_2O, Cu, SiO_2) are added. The catalyst is then precipitated by the addition of a basic solution. Further treatment requirements depend on the reactor type used in the process (Steynberg and Dry 2004).

A major challenge for Fe-based FT catalysts is their relatively short lifetime in industrial operations due to deactivation. Numerous investigations have been undertaken to obtain information on deactivation mechanisms and reasons. They include sintering, surface carbon formation, mechanical deactivation through attrition, oxidation and operational factors such as

TABLE 10.4

Commercially Applied Fe-Based and Co-Based FT Catalysts

Main Metal	Catalyst	Main Product	Reactors	Processes Type
Fe	Fe/K, Fe/Mn, Fe/Mn, Ce, Fe/K/S, Fe₂O₃Cₓ, Fe/C	Olefins (C₂–C₄)	Slurry bed, fluidised bed	HTFT
	Fused Fe/K, Fe/K, ZSM-5, Fe/Cu/K and ZSM-5	Gasoline	Fluidised bed, fixed bed, slurry/fixed bed	HFFT
	Fe/K	Diesel fuel	Fixed bed	LTFT
	Fe/K, Fe/Cu/K	Wax	Slurry bed	LTFT
Co	Co/ThO₂/Al₂O₃/Silicalite, Co-ZSM-5	Gasoline	Fixed bed, slurry fixed bed	LTFT
	Co/Zr, Ti or Cr/Al₂O₃, Co/Zr/TiO₂, Co/Ru/TiO2	Diesel fuel	Fixed bed, slurry bed	LTFT
	Co/Zr, Ti or Cr/Al₂O₃, Co/Ru/TiO₂	Wax	Fixed bed	LTFT

Sources: Bartholomew, C.H., *Catalysis Letters* 7: 303–316, 1990; Luque, R. et al., *Energy and Environmental Science* 5: 5186, 2012.

poisoning, the type of reactor and operation conditions (Dry 2002; Jun et al. 2003; van Steen and Claeys 2008; Luque et al. 2012).

Fe-based catalysts are widely used in FT processes, especially with coal-derived syngas due to their low price, flexibility (temperature and product range) and relatively low sensitivity toward sulphur impurities in the syngas. Selected commercially applied Fe catalysts are listed in Table 10.4. The South African petrochemical company Sasol uses Fe catalysts in their LTFT and HTFT processes (Steynberg and Dry 2004).

10.3.1.2 Co-Based Catalysts for FT Synthesis

Cobalt-based catalysts are more expensive than iron, but are also more selective for long-chain linear hydrocarbons. They are therefore the preferred catalyst in LTFT synthesis to produce waxes and diesel fuels. However, they can only be used in a narrow (low) temperature and pressure range. An increase in temperature results in a significant undesirable increase in methane production (Dry 2002; Khodakov et al. 2007).

Cobalt-based catalysts are generally less prone to deactivation by water than Fe-based catalysts. Their activity is comparable at low CO conversion rates. At higher CO conversion rates, however, cobalt-based catalysts show a higher activity because Fe-based catalysts are generally slowed down by the water formation of the FT reaction (Khodakov et al. 2007).

Due to the high price of cobalt, it is desirable to maximise the surface area of the catalyst to minimise the quantity required (Dry 2002). To achieve this, cobalt-based catalysts are usually dispersed on a support such as Al₂O₃, TiO₂, or SiO_2. The cobalt is impregnated on the support (using a cobalt salt), usually together with promoter metals (e.g. lanthanum, platinum and ruthenium) that facilitate the reduction step (Dry and Steynberg 2004). Because the cobalt crystallite size on the support is important for the catalyst activity and selectivity, various preparation methods have been investigated (Khodakov et al. 2007). Some of the commercially applied FT catalysts are listed in Table 10.4.

Due to their high activity at higher CO conversion rates even in the presence of water, Co-based catalysts are interesting for BTL processes. If the quality of the syngas is high, Co-based compounds are typically the catalyst of choice (van Steen and Claeys 2008). Because it displays very low or no activity for the WGS reaction, treatment of the syngas (if the H_2/CO ratio is low) may be necessary prior to the FT synthesis.

10.3.2 Reactors for FT Synthesis

In addition to catalyst selection, the type of reactor also plays a very important role in the industrial FT process. Since the FT synthesis first reached commercial scale, reactor designs have undergone many developments (Davis 2005). Due to the exothermic nature of the FT synthesis, heat removal and temperature control are of great importance in reactor designs to minimise catalyst damage and optimise product selectivity (Gupta and Demirbas 2010).

There are three main categories for commercial FT reactors: (i) fixed-bed reactors, (ii) slurry-bed reactors and (iii) fluidised-bed reactors (Dry 2002; Davis 2007). Over the years of development, four types of FT reactors have

TABLE 10.5

Overview of the Main Reactor Categories for FT Synthesis

Reactor Category	Operation Temperature	Catalyst	Reactor Design	Process
Fluidised bed	HTFT: 320°C–350°C	Fused Fe	CFB with circulating solids, gas recycling, cooling in recycling loop	Synthol
			FFB	SAS process
Fixed bed	LTFT: 220°C–260°C	Precipitated Fe or Co	Multitubular fixed-bed with internal cooling	ARGE process (Sasol), SMDS
Slurry bed	LTFT: 220°C–250°C	Precipitated Fe or Co	Slurry bubble column	Sasol slurry-bed process (SSBP), HTFSTP process (Synfuel China)

Sources: Steynberg, A.P., and Dry, M., *Studies in Surface Science and Catalysis* 152, 2004; Gupta, R.B., and Demirbas, A. Diesel from biomass gasification followed by Fischer–Tropsch synthesis. Chapter 8 in *Gasoline, Diesel and Ethanol Biofuels from Grasses and Plants*, Cambridge University Press, 2010; Yong-Wang, L., Xu, J., and Yang, Y.: Diesel from syngas. Chapter 6 in *Biomass to Biofuels: Strategies for Global Industries*. 2010. Copyright Wiley-VCH Verlag GmbH & Co. KGaA. Reproduced with permission.

been predominantly applied in large industrial processes. An overview is given in Table 10.5.

Fluidised-bed reactors are typically used for HTFT processes that operate at 300°C to 340°C, whereas fixed-bed and slurry-bed reactors are typically employed in LTFT processes (220°C–260°C). In Table 10.6, the main characteristics, advantages and disadvantages of the reactors are listed.

TABLE 10.6

Comparison between the Four Commercially Used Reactor Types for FT Processes

Feature	HTFT		LTFT	
	CFB	**FFB**	**Fixed Bed**	**Slurry**
Temperature control	Medium	Good	Poor	Good
Cost	Higher than FFB	Lower than CFB	Higher than slurry	Lower than fixed bed
Product	Low molecular weight (mainly olefins)		Full range (mainly wax/diesel)	Full range (mainly wax/diesel)
CH_4 formation	High	High	Low	Low
C_{5+} selectivity	Low	Low	High (>90% possible, but influenced by inert gases)	High (>90% possible, lower influence of inert gases)
Catalyst consumption	High due to severe conditions (lower bulk density and only part of catalyst used)	Lower than CFB (all of catalyst participates)	Medium (but high resistance to contaminants, e.g. H_2S)	Low (but contaminants spread instantly, higher sulphur poisoning than fixed bed)
Maintenance	High (high gas velocities/erosion and temperatures/carbon deposition)	Low (due to lower velocity and pressure drops across the reactor)	High (complicated catalyst replacement, longer downtime)	Low (online catalyst replacement, little downtime, lower catalyst consumption)
Flexibility	Little	Higher than CFB	Medium	High
Once-through conversion	High	High	Medium to high	Medium to high
Wax/catalyst separation	No wax production	No wax production	Easy, low cost	Difficult (higher downstream processing cost)

Sources: Tijmensen, M.J.A. et al., *Biomass and Energy* 23: 129–152, 2002; Guettel, R. et al., *Chemical Engineering and Technology* 37: 746–754, 2008; Hu, J. et al., *Catalysts* 2: 303–326, 2012.

10.3.2.1 Fluidised-Bed Reactors

Fluidised-bed reactors are used in HTFT processes, usually with a fused iron catalyst. The desired products are mainly low molecular weight hydrocarbons (e.g. olefins). These types of reactors are two-phase (gas and solid) systems and are based on the fluidisation of the catalyst when the gas stream is passed through the solid (Dry 2002). A simplified design is shown in Figure 10.5.

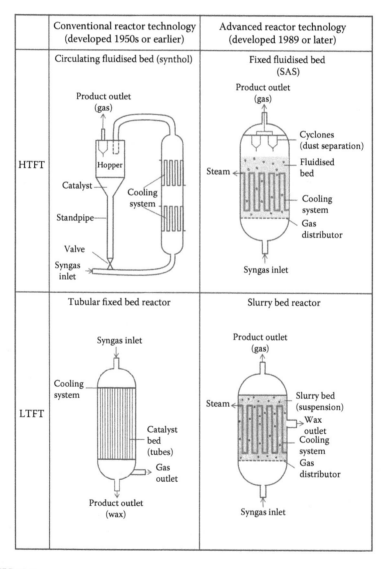

FIGURE 10.5
Different types of FT reactors.

There are two types of fluidised-bed reactors: circulating fluidised-bed (CFB) and fixed fluidised-bed (FFB) reactors.

The CFB reactor was first developed and commercially used in the 1950s by Sasol (Davis 2005). They were named Synthol reactors (Steynberg and Dry 2004). There are two phases of fluidised catalyst in CFB reactors; the dense phase, before the catalyst is added to the syngas feed, and the lean phase, when the fluidised catalyst is being carried up the reaction phase by the feedgas. Therefore, only a portion of the circulating catalyst is used for substrate conversion (Dry 2002; Steynberg and Dry 2004). A settling hopper separates product gas from the catalyst, which returns to the standpipe. Common challenges of the CFB include erosion of reactor sections due to high gas velocities and carbon depositions on the iron catalyst (leading to loss of bulk density of catalyst in the standpipe) due to high operating temperature (Dry 2002; Jager 2003).

The FFB reactor came into use in the late 1980s (it was called the Sasol advanced synthol [SAS] reactor) and has mainly replaced the CFB reactor. Its capital cost is much (40%) lower than that of the CFB reactor. The FFB also uses a fused iron catalyst, but the fluidised catalyst is not circulated. The gas stream is bubbled through the fluidised catalyst bed and the gas (products) leave the system through a cyclone, which retains the catalyst. Due to the absence of the catalyst recycling loop, maintenance is easier and the catalyst consumption is lower (all of the catalyst is used) than in the CFB reactor. The wider reaction zone in the FFB reactor also allows for more cooling coils and hence for a larger reactor capacity (Dry 2002; Jager 2003; Steynberg and Dry 2004).

10.3.2.2 Fixed-Bed Reactors

The multitubular fixed-bed reactor is one of the earliest FT reactor designs and has been used since World War II (Jager 2003). The ARGE reactor (used in the ARGE process) is used by Sasol in its commercial facility in South Africa. Fixed-bed reactors are used in LTFT processes to produce higher molecular weight hydrocarbons. Either Fe-based or Co-based catalysts can be used, depending on the composition and quality of the feed gas. The catalyst is packed into tubes that are surrounded by water (Figure 10.5). The heat exchange takes place through the wall of the tubes. Most heat is usually produced in the first section of the reactor because the highest conversion rates are found there. Achieving a uniform temperature profile along the reactor through effective heat removal and a manageable pressure drop across the catalyst bed are therefore challenging (Guettel et al. 2008; Yong-Wang et al. 2010). Furthermore, the catalyst removal can be quite complicated. Operated on smaller scales, however, the fixed-bed reactor has advantages such as robustness and resistance to contaminants (only the top catalyst layer is deactivated). Through high gas velocities, a turbulent flow can be created, which improves the heat exchange. In addition, the separation of wax (~50% of the products) and catalyst is not a problem due to the fixed location of the catalyst tubes (Spath and Dyton 2003; Steynberg and Dry 2004).

10.3.2.3 Slurry-Bed Reactors

The concept of a slurry-bed reactor was developed and investigated in the 1950s and the improved slurry-bed reactors have been used by numerous companies in recent years (Steynberg and Dry 2004; Guettel et al. 2008). Slurry-bed reactors are used in LTFT processes with high wax production and both iron-based and cobalt-based catalysts are used. The three-phase reactor contains slurry, which consists of liquid waxes (FT products) and a suspended catalyst. The syngas is bubbled through this slurry bed and the heat exchange takes place through cooling coils in the suspension (Figure 10.5; Jager 2003). Because the slurry can be well-mixed, an almost uniform temperature profile can be obtained and higher operation temperatures are possible (Yong-Wang et al. 2010). The hydrocarbon products (wax) are mixed with the catalyst in the slurry and must be separated before removal. This solid/liquid separation is one of the major challenges of slurry reactors. The advantages include, for example, a lower catalyst loading than fixed-bed reactors, online removal and addition of the catalyst resulting in longer runs and lower capital costs. Because poisonous substances such as H_2S spread instantly through the system, low levels of contaminants are required in the feed gas (Dry 2002; Jager 2003).

10.3.2.4 Microchannel Reactors

Compared with the reactor types listed above, FT microchannel reactors are amongst the newest reactor developments. Microchannel reactors consist of parallel arrays of microchannels, with a diameter of 0.1 to 0.5 mm each. These microchannels (often metallic) contain the catalyst, usually in the form of a thin layer on the inner walls (Gumuslu and Avci 2011). The reactor contains a large number (thousands) of these arrays adding up to a reactor diameter of approximately 0.6 m (Atkinson 2010; Evans and Smith 2012). This microchannel structure increases the surface areas and therefore enhances mass and heat transfer. A comparison of characteristics of conventional commercially applied LTFT (fixed bed, slurry bed) and microchannel reactors is shown in Table 10.7. For microchannel reactors, high productivities and high once-through conversion efficiencies have been observed. This might make them a valuable option for BTL FT plants to economically produce biofuels at smaller scales (200–2000 bpd, ~10,000–100,000 tpa; Evans and Smith 2012; Kolb 2013).

TABLE 10.7

Comparison of Microchannel Reactors with Tubular Fixed-Bed and Slurry-Bed Reactors

Reactor Type	Dimensions	Capacity (bpd)	CO Conversion Per Pass (%) [Dependent on Catalysts]	Productivity (FT Product Per Tonne of Reactor Mass) [bpd/tonne]
Tubular fixed-bed (e.g. Shell GTL plant, Bintulu)	~3–7 m diameter, 12 m and more long	4000–6000	30–35	3–5
Slurry bed (Sasol Oryx GTL plant, Qatar)	~9 m diameter, up to 60 m long	12,000–25,000	50–70	8
Microchannel	0.6–1.5 m diameter, up to 8 m long	300–500	65–75	12

Source: Steynberg, A.P., and Dry, M., *Studies in Surface Science and Catalysis* 152, 2004; Atkinson, D., *Biofuels, Bioproducts and Biorefining* 4: 12–16, 2010.

10.4 FT Process for the Production of Synthetic Fuels

The main purpose of the FT process is to convert a carbon-containing energy source, such as coal, natural gas or biomass, into a variety of liquid fuels that can be easily transported and distributed. The FT process dates back to the 1930s, and in the early years of synthetic FT fuel production, coal was mainly of interest as a feedstock to reduce dependence on oil.

Due to environmental concerns and the depletion of crude oil reserves, FT technology has received renewed interest in recent years (Tijmensen et al. 2002; Luque et al. 2012). In addition to coal, natural gas and biomass have now been added to the list of feedstocks for liquid fuel production. The processes are named according to the feedstock used: coal-to-liquid (CTL), gas-to-liquid (GTL) or biomass-to-liquid (BTL). Synthetic diesel fuels produced via FT synthesis have the advantage of being sulphur-free and aromatics-free, whilst still being compatible with normal vehicle engines and hence blendable with conventional fuels (Gill et al. 2011).

FT technology has been investigated over several decades. Higher crude oil prices and large reserves of coal and natural gas have fuelled research and development. Processes utilising both coal and natural gas have been commercialised. Plants operated by companies such as Sasol and Shell use well-developed process designs to produce fuels and chemicals from coal and gas (Steynberg and Dry 2004).

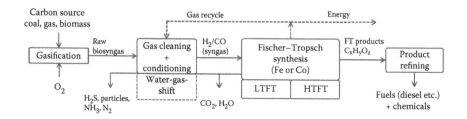

FIGURE 10.6
Simplified flow diagram of an FT process.

Although interest in renewable FT feedstocks such as biomass has increased, as of 2013, the BTL FT processes have not yet reached commercial scale (Kim et al. 2013). The economic viability of the BTL process has been subject to numerous studies (Spath and Dyton 2003; Hamelink et al. 2004; van Vliet et al. 2009). Design and integration of the various process units (especially gasification) in the BTL FT process has been a challenge (Swain et al. 2011).

Generally, the FT process contains three basic steps: (i) syngas preparation and cleaning/conditioning, (ii) FT synthesis and (iii) product upgrading (Steynberg and Dry 2004; Figure 10.6). During syngas production (gasification), the carbon source is reacted with oxygen and converted into a mixture of (mainly) carbon monoxide (CO) and hydrogen (H_2). After the raw syngas is cleaned and conditioned, it is used in FT synthesis, resulting in the production of a range of liquid hydrocarbons and other products. The variety of products undergoes refining to obtain the desired fuels.

These steps are found in all three (CTL, GTL, BTL) processes. In principle, the basic FT technology is the same or very similar for biomass as for coal and gas, but different designs and integration of units (e.g. of gasifiers, cleaning operations and FT conditions and catalysts) are required.

10.4.1 FT Synthesis in Commercial CTL and GTL Processes

Commercial operations exist for both CTL and GTL FT processes using the reactors described in Table 10.8. The historical development of processes and reactors has been subject to several reviews (Dry 2002; Steynberg and Dry 2004; Davis 2005; Guettel et al. 2008).

The design of an FT process involves more than only the FT reactor and the catalyst. Efficiency can be reached by the integration of process units and by using gas recycling. A gas loop is used in all commercial CTL and GTL operations (Steynberg and Dry 2004).

10.4.1.1 CTL: SAS Process

Sasol operates several CTL plants that use high-temperature syngas conversion technology in the SAS process. Figure 10.7 shows a simplified process diagram of the Secunda plant in South Africa. First, the coal is processed in

TABLE 10.8

Selected Existing Commercial Processes

Type	Catalyst	Reactor Type	FT Technology	Operator and Commercial Operation
HTFT	Fused Fe	CFB	Sasol Synthol	Petro SA, Mossel Bay, South Africa
	Fused Fe	FFB	SAS	Sasol, Secunda, South Africa
LTFT	Precipitated Fe	Fixed bed	ARGE	Sasol, Sasolburg, South Africa
	Precipitated Fe	Slurry bed	Sasol SPD Process	Sasol, Sasolburg, South Africa
	Co-SiO$_2$	Fixed bed	SMDS	Shell, Bintulu, Malaysia
	Co-Al$_2$O$_3$	Slurry Bed	SPD	Oryx GTL (Qatar Petroleum and Sasol) Ras Laffan, Qatar

Source: de Klerk, A., *Green Chemistry* 10: 1249–1279, 2008; Leckel, D., and Phillips, T., *Biofuels* 2: 109–113, 2011; Luque, R. et al., *Energy and Environmental Science* 5: 5186, 2012.

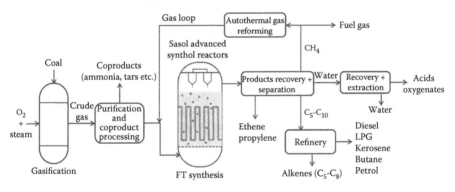

FIGURE 10.7
Simplified flowchart of the SAS process in the Secunda plant.

a gasifier (Lurgi gasifier) with the addition of steam and oxygen. The reaction product is raw syngas, which is cleaned and conditioned. The purified syngas is then transported to a series of SAS reactors that operate at high temperatures (350°C) and pressures (24 bar). A fused iron-based catalyst is used for the FT synthesis. The methane that is formed is converted to syngas by gas reforming. The hydrocarbons are cooled, separated and converted into a range of products (Steynberg and Dry 2004; Sasol 2013).

10.4.1.2 GTL: Shell Middle Distillate Synthesis (SMDS) FT Process

Shell's middle distillate synthesis (SMDS) plant, based on natural gas is located in Bintulu, Malaysia, and uses an LTFT process to produce (predominantly)

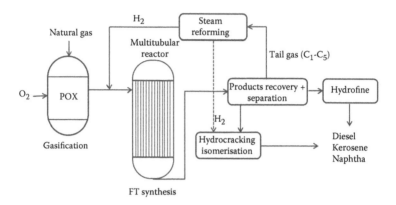

FIGURE 10.8
Simplified flowchart of the SMDS.

waxes (Figure 10.8). The methane is reacted at high temperatures in a partial oxidation process (POX) to produce syngas. The H_2/CO ratio (1.7) of the syngas is slightly less than the required usage ratio (slightly more than 2) for the cobalt-based catalyst in the FT reactor. Hydrogen gas from a steam reformer is therefore added. The steam reforming is based on the tail gas separated from the FT reactor. Multitubular fixed-bed reactors operate within a temperature range of 200°C to 230°C and a pressure of 30 bar. With the cobalt-based catalyst, a conversion of approximately 80% and a selectivity of more than 85% can be reached. The C_1 to C_5 products are recycled to the catalytic steam reformer. The other products undergo refining (e.g. hydrocracking) to obtain diesel, kerosene and other products (Steynberg and Dry 2004; Shell 2013).

10.4.1.3 GTL: Sasol Slurry Phase Distillate Process

The Sasol Slurry Phase Distillate (SPD) process was developed in the 1980s and uses natural gas as feedstock. Natural gas is reacted with oxygen in an autothermal reformer (Haldor Topsøe) to produce syngas. The FT synthesis is carried out in a slurry-bed reactor with a cobalt-based catalyst. After the reaction, the wax is separated from the catalyst particles using a proprietary Sasol process. The gases that leave the reactor at the top are cooled and processed. The hydrocarbons from the wax are then refined (Chevron Isocracking) to obtain diesel, naphtha and liquefied petroleum gas (LPG; Sasol 2013).

10.4.2 BTL Process with FT Synthesis

Although the basic FT technology is well known and developed, as of 2013, BTL FT processes have not yet been commercialised. There are a large number of configurations that can be used in BTL production processes, depending on the choice of biomass gasification type, FT reactor and catalysts and desired product.

Many studies have investigated and analysed the configurations, energy, process efficiency and economics of FT processes using biomass-derived syngas (Tijmesen et al. 2002; Hamelink et al. 2004; Prins et al. 2004; van Vliet et al. 2009; Heinrich et al. 2009; Damartzis and Zabaniotou 2011; Leibbrandt et al. 2013). However, there remain large uncertainties concerning the viability of commercial BTL FT synfuel facilities. Two very challenging steps on the way to a commercial-scale BTL FT process are the gasification of biomass and the cleaning of the syngas. Another major challenge is the feedstock supply network of BTL plants because the transportation of biomass is expensive and limited. These issues concern the first steps in the BTL process. Once the syngas is produced, cleaned and conditioned, the remaining steps (including FT synthesis) are similar to already established commercial CTL or GTL processes (Heinrich et al. 2009).

Two main concepts are usually considered in process analyses: (i) the 'once-through' FT process, which aims to maximise energy efficiency by using all tail gas for electricity generation and (ii) the full conversion FT process, which uses recycling of the tail gas to maximise liquid hydrocarbon yield. In both cases, there are several well-defined steps in the BTL FT process that have to be integrated to optimise yields, energy and costs (Evans and Smith 2012). An overview of these steps is shown in Figure 10.10.

10.4.2.1 BTL FT Process Steps

10.4.2.1.1 Syngas Production, Cleaning and Conditioning

Unlike coal or natural gas, the physical properties of the BTL feedstock vary and therefore affect the processing conditions. Numerous biomass materials can be used as feedstock, with wood and agricultural wastes being amongst the most common. The preparation of biomass usually includes size reduction and drying. In addition, pretreatment, such as pelletising, is an option to facilitate transport and storage (Evans and Smith 2012; Hu et al. 2012).

In the next step, the biomass needs to be converted into syngas, which can then be used in the FT synthesis. This is achieved by gasification (see Chapter 4). Under high temperatures and with the addition of oxygen, the carbon source is transformed into CO and H_2. Gasification technologies are well-known in coal-based FT processes. They have also been applied to biomass, but the resulting syngas has mainly been used for energy and heat applications (Evans and Smith 2012). The choice, optimisation and integration of the gasifier system for BTL applications therefore remain a challenge. The gasification process, gasifier types and the current status are reviewed in Chapter 4.

$$CO + H_2O \leftrightarrow CO_2 + H_2$$

FIGURE 10.9
WGS reaction.

The syngas for FT synthesis needs to be of high quality with a well-defined H_2/CO ratio. This is a challenge for the gasification mode, and for the subsequent gas cleaning and conditioning. Typical impurities that are found in biosyngas include tars, inorganic substances such as H_2S, NH_3, HCl and particulates. Several techniques can be used for the removal of contaminants, for example, tar cracking and wet and dry gas cleaning (cyclones, filters, scrubbers, etc.; Tijmensen et al. 2002; Boerrigter et al. 2004; Hamelinck et al. 2004; Hu et al. 2012). High levels of contaminants can lead to catalyst poisoning, resulting in lower activity and productivity. The gas-cleaning step is therefore of importance for the overall efficiency of the FT synthesis.

Ideally, the syngas should also not contain more than a certain percentage (~15%) of inert gas such as CH_4 or CO_2 (Boerrigter 2006). If the methane content is significant, autothermal reforming is an option. As mentioned earlier in this chapter, the ratio of H_2 and CO also plays a very important role for the success and efficiency of the FT synthesis. A conditioning step using the WGS reaction (Figure 10.9) might be necessary to achieve the optimal ratio. The CO_2 content present after the gasifier increases with the WGS reaction and the inert gas is usually removed before entering the FT reactor (e.g. with an amine treatment process; Tijmensen et al. 2002).

10.4.2.1.2 FT Synthesis

After cleaning and conditioning, the syngas is compressed and then fed to the FT reactor. As described earlier, there are two catalyst types, iron-based and cobalt-based, and two temperature modes, HTFT and LTFT, that are currently commercially applied in FT processes. They are used in large-scale CTL and GTL operations. These large-scale operations may not be appropriate for BTL applications, in which smaller scale operations seem to be more favourable (van Steen and Claeys 2008; Evans and Smith 2012).

To produce valuable biofuels from biomass, long-chain hydrocarbons should be the main products in FT processes because they can be used for diesel production. A high CO conversion and a high C_{5+} selectivity (high α value) are required (van Steen and Claeys 2008). Because cobalt-based catalysts are considered to be more active than iron-based catalysts, and have a good selectivity for longer chain hydrocarbons, they were chosen as BTL FT catalysts in most studies and investigations (Tijmensen et al. 2002; Hamelink et al. 2004; Prins et al. 2004). It has been debated though, whether cobalt is really the better choice for BTL processes (van Steen and Claeys 2008). The advantages of using an iron-based catalyst, such as activity in the WGS reaction, lower price and a slightly higher tolerance for sulphur contaminants, should be considered.

TABLE 10.9

Product Distribution in the Syncrude of LTFT and HTFT

Hydrocarbon	Mass % in Syncrude		
	HTFT–Fe	LTFT–Fe	LTFT–Co
C_1 — methane	13	4	5
C_2	10	2	1
C_3-C_4 — LPG, olefins	25	8	5
C_5-C_{10} — naphta/gasoline	33	12	20
C_{11}-C_{22} — distillate/diesel	7	20	22
C_{22+} wax	3	50	45
Aqueous products	9	4	2
Paraffins (saturated hydrocarbons)	10	68	79
Olefins (unsaturated hydrocarbons)	53	20	12
Aromatics	3	Very low	Very low
Oxygenates	11	8	2

Source: de Klerk, A., *Energy and Environmental Science* 4: 1177–1205, 2011.

The deactivation of the catalyst has been a major concern in larger scale operations because it leads to loss of activity (productivity) and lifetime. It is therefore of interest to study the reasons for deactivation and find ways to avoid it. The design of a BTL process and the development and improvement of the FT catalyst should not be isolated and both iron-based and cobalt-based catalysts should be considered for BTL FT operations (van Steen and Claeys 2008; Hu et al. 2012).

If the desired product is a liquid transportation fuel, such as diesel, LTFT (180°C–250°C) synthesis is the mode of choice for BTL due to the higher selectivity for long-chain hydrocarbons in this temperature range (Table 10.9). Either fixed-bed or slurry-bed reactors can be used. Both have advantages and disadvantages (Section 10.3.2). Slurry-bed reactors seem to be less sensitive to inert gases (CH_4, CO_2) being present, but wax/catalyst separation is more complex than for a fixed-bed reactor (Geerlings et al. 1999; Tijmensen et al. 2002).

10.4.2.1.3 Refining/Upgrading

The products in the FT reactor after FT synthesis depend on the conversion of the syngas and on the distribution of the products. Often, unreacted CO and H_2 remain, and low molecular weight hydrocarbons (C_1–C_4) are found in addition to the (mostly) desired C_{5+} products. The latter are separated by condensation and then sent to the refining and upgrading unit. The major products of LTFT are waxes, diesel and naphta (see Table 10.9; de Klerk 2008). The common refining for waxes to obtain diesel is hydrocracking. Olefins (double bonds) are converted to paraffins by the addition of hydrogen and then the hydrocarbons are catalytically cracked, often using a platinum-based or palladium-based catalyst (de Klerk 2008; Lappas and Heracleous 2011). If gasoline is the desired product, fluid catalytic cracking (FCC) might be of interest. In BTL FT processes, naphtha is a by-product with a low octane number. Upgrading options exist to increase the octane number for it to be blendable with gasoline fuels, but it is questionable whether they are feasible for commercial BTL FT processes (Kreutz et al. 2008).

10.4.2.2 Once-Through and Full Conversion FT Process

Most large-scale CTL and GTL processes have been developed and improved based on industrial data and experiences, and they usually use some form of gas recycling (gas loop). Because only pilot and demonstration facilities currently exist for BTL processes, most analyses and process designs are based on concepts and calculations. The two main categories considered in process analysis are the once-through and the full conversion FT processes.

The full conversion FT process is aimed at maximising the production of FT liquids. Therefore, the off-gas, which usually contains unreacted CO and H_2, as well as lower molecular weight hydrocarbons (C_1–C_4) can be recycled back to the FT reactor. Reforming (mostly autothermal reforming) can be used to convert the C_1 to C_4 gases into syngas, and the WGS reaction can adjust H_2/CO ratios.

In the once-through FT concept, the production of both FT fuels and electricity is targeted. Instead of recycling the off-gas back to the gasifier or the FT reactor, it is used completely for electricity generation. The tail gas is combusted in a gas turbine to produce electricity that can be used in units of the

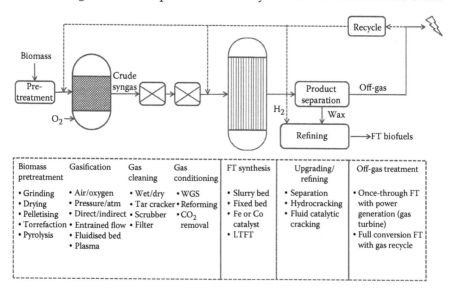

Biomass pretreatment	Gasification	Gas cleaning	Gas conditioning	FT synthesis	Upgrading/refining	Off-gas treatment
• Grinding • Drying • Pelletising • Torrefaction • Pyrolysis	• Air/oxygen • Pressure/atm • Direct/indirect • Entrained flow • Fluidised bed • Plasma	• Wet/dry • Tar cracker • Scrubber • Filter	• WGS • Reforming • CO_2 removal	• Slurry bed • Fixed bed • Fe or Co catalyst • LTFT	• Separation • Hydrocracking • Fluid catalytic cracking	• Once-through FT with power generation (gas turbine) • Full conversion FT with gas recycle

FIGURE 10.10
Concept of a BTL FT process.

FT process. The aim of this particular concept is a process that is as energy efficient as possible rather than aiming for maximal conversion of biomass to FT fuels (Tijmensen et al. 2002; Hamelink et al. 2004).

The concepts, shown in Figure 10.10, still need to be transferred to large-scale BTL operations to collect valuable data. The calculations revealed that pretreatment of the biomass, gasification and gas cleaning account for the majority of the capital cost (~75%; Tijmensen et al. 2002). Almost all pilot or demonstration projects focus on the integration and improvement of these steps and mainly use well-established FT technologies, such as those used in commercial CTL and GTL facilities (Figures 10.7 and 10.8; Boerrigter 2006; Kim et al. 2013). Choren Industries in Germany, for example, developed Carbo-V technology for biomass gasification, but applies the Shell-developed SMDS technology in FT synthesis (fixed-bed reactor and cocatalyst; European Biofuels Technology Platform [EBTP] 2013).

10.5 Current State of FT Fuel Production from Biosyngas

Coal-based and gas-based FT processes have been operated on a commercial scale for many years. Large facilities with capacities of up to 150,000 bpd (more than 5 million tonnes per year) can be found in South Africa, as well as in Malaysia and Qatar (Table 10.8; Luque et al. 2012).

Although biomass-based FT fuel production uses very similar FT technology, the feedstock and hence the gasification step are significantly different. This requires the development of an integrated gasification/FT process to make BTL operations viable. No BTL process using FT technology has been commercialised yet, but there are numerous institutes and companies that have focussed on the development of an integrated gasification/FT process to produce liquid biofuels. The scale of the operation varies. Depending on the technology provider or the company using the provided technology, operation sizes range from laboratory to pilot/demonstration scales. Universities and other research-focussed organisations may use small-scale processes whereas commercial companies have already reached pilot or demonstration scale. Integrated gasifier/FT technologies are expected to soon be used in larger scale operations. It has been suggested, however, that the trend will go to medium sized, more distributed facilities to reduce costs associated with logistics and supply of the biomass feedstock (Atkinson 2010; Evans and Smith 2012).

10.5.1 Current and Future FT Facilities

Most of the ongoing FT projects to produce liquid fuels (mainly diesel) are located in the United States or Europe. Research activities have been aimed at the development and optimisation of an integrated gasification/FT process. The status of plants and projects has been subject to constant change. More biomass gasification/FT processes are expected to soon be operational. With more data available, an assessment of the viability of these processes will become more accurate. Most technologies can work at a small scale, but the scaling-up of facilities remains a considerable challenge (Yeh 2011).

The raw material used as the biomass feedstock in these facilities varies depending on availability and technology. The main type of biomass used is woody material, for example, forest residues and wood chips. However, other feedstock materials such as straw-like crops, and agricultural and municipal waste have also been utilised (Kavalov and Peteves 2005; Bacovsky et al. 2013). The major projects and BTL FT facilities are listed in Table 10.10 (for Europe) and Table 10.11 (for the United States), and are described in more detail in the next section.

10.5.2 Technology Providers and Projects

10.5.2.1 Europe

In Europe, the research and development of BTL technologies has been supported by the European Commission with funding and projects (e.g. NER300), and by initiatives such as the RENEW project (RENEW 2013; NER300 2013). The following companies and research institutes have been involved in the development and application of BTL FT processes.

10.5.2.1.1 CEA (Atomic and Alternative Energy Commission)/GTL.F1

In 2009, the Bure Saudron project was announced, in which CEA, in collaboration with AirLiquide, would build a pilot plant in northeast France to convert forestry and agricultural residues into liquid biofuels. The FT technology will be provided by the Swiss-registered company GTL.F1, which is focussed on the commercial development and marketing of FT technologies and catalysts. The plant in Bure Saudron will use a slurry-bed reactor and a cobalt-based catalyst. The plant construction is expected to be completed in 2015 (AirLiquide 2013).

The CEA is also involved in the joint project BioTfueL, which was launched in 2010. This BTL project in France will use Uhde's gasification technology, PRENFLO and Gasel FT technology with slurry-bed reactors. The project includes the construction of two pilot plant facilities in France, followed by a scale-up planned for 2020 (IFP Energies Nouvelles 2013).

10.5.2.1.2 Choren Industries

One of the most important European BTL process developers has been Choren Industries, a German company, which developed the Carbo-V gasification process to produce diesel from biomass (called SunDiesel). The first FT liquids using this technology were produced in the alpha plant in Freiberg

TABLE 10.10

FT BTL Facilities in Europe

Company/Institute	Location	Input Material/Biomass Feedstock	Process Technology			Output Biofuels (t/a)	Type/Scale	Status/Start-Up
			Gasification	FT Reactor Type	FT Catalyst			
Choren/Shell	Freiberg, Germany	Wood chips, waste wood	Carbo-V, three-stage gasifier, entrained flow	Fixed bed (Shell process, SunDiesel)	Co-catalyst	13,500	Demonstration	Under commissioning
CUTEC	Clausthal-Zellerfeld, Germany	Straw	CFB	Fixed bed (ArtFuel process)	Co-catalyst, or fused Fe catalyst	~3	Pilot/Lab	Operational, 2010
Forest BTL Ltd	Ajos, Finland	Woody biomass	Carbo-V, three-stage gasifier, entrained flow	Slurry bubble column (Gasel)	Co based (Gasel)	115,000	Commercial	Planned, 2015
NSE Biofuels/Stora Enso/Neste Oil	Varkaus, Finland	Forest residues	CFB	Fixed bed or slurry bed	n/a	650	Pilot	Operation stopped (after trials)
TUBITAK	Gebze, Turkey	Hazelnut shell, olive cake, wood chips, lignite blends	CFB, pressurised FB	Multi tubular fixed bed	Fe-based catalyst	250	Pilot	Under construction
UPM	Stracel, France	Logging residues, bark	Oxygen blown	n/a	n/a	105,000	Commercial	Planned
Vienna University of Technology (TUV)	Güssing, Austria	Syngas from gasifier	Dual fluidised bed (DFB)	Slurry bed	Co or Fe based	0.2	Pilot	Operational, 2005
Velocys/SGS Energia	Güssing, Austria	Wood chips	DFB, steam blown (TUV)	Microchannel reactor	Oxford catalysts, Co based	40	Demonstration	Operational, 2010

Note: n/a = no information found at the time of writing.

TABLE 10.11
FT BTL Facilities in the United States

Company/ Institute	Location	Input Material/ Biomass Feedstock	Process Technology			Output Biofuels (t/a)	Type/Scale	Status/Start-Up
			Gasification	FT Reactor Type	FT Catalyst			
Clearfuels/ Rentech/ SilvaGas	Commerce City, Colorado	Woody materials	HEHTR (entrained flow)	Slurry bubble column (RenDiesel)	Fe catalyst	500	Demonstration	Closed 2013
Gas Technology Institute	Des Plaines, Illinois	Forest residues	Andritz Carbona, fluidised bed	n/a	n/a	880	Pilot	Operational, 2004
Iowa State University	Boone, Iowa	Grains, oilseeds	Fluidised bed	Slurry reactor	Co-Zr/ Al₂O₃	200 (including ethanol)	Pilot	Operational, 2009
Flambeau River Biofuels, Inc.	Park Falls, Wisconsin	Forest residuals, wood	Steam reforming (TRI)	n/a	n/a	51,000	Demonstration	Plans stopped
Renewable Energy Institute International/ Synterra	Gridley, California	Waste	Solids steam reforming process (SSRP)	Syntrex process (designed by SynTerra)	Syntrex process (designed by SynTerra)	Up to 130,000	Commercial	Planned

Research Triangle Institute	Research Triangle Park, North Carolina	Lignocellulosics	DFB	Slurry bubble column	Fe catalyst	20	Pilot	Under construction
Southern Research Institute	Durham, North Carolina	Cellulosics, municipal waste	Fluidised bed	n/a	n/a	n/a	Pilot	Operational, 2007
Thermochem Recovery International/ Emerging Fuel Technology	Durham, North Carolina	Woody material	Bubbling fluidised-bed (BFB; two-stage), steam blown	Fixed bed	Co catalyst	25 t/y	Pilot	Operational, 2009
SynTerra Energy, Inc. (Red Lion Bioenergy/ Pacific Renewable Fuels)	Toledo, Ohio	Municipal waste, crops, wood	BFB (two-stage), steam reforming with pyrolysis	Syntrex process (designed by SynTerra)	Syntrex process (designed by SynTerra)	n/a	Pilot/ demonstration	2008/2010

in 2003. The beta demonstration plant in Freiberg was built in 2008, and the construction of a commercial plant was planned in Schwedt, Germany. The FT synthesis was carried out using the Shell middle distillate process (multitubular fixed-bed reactor, cocatalyst, see Section 10.4.1.2). In 2011, however, Choren Industries filed for insolvency; and in 2012, the Carbo-V gasification technology was sold to Linde Engineering Dresden (EBTP 2013).

10.5.2.1.3 CUTEC

CUTEC (Clausthal Umwelttechnik Institut) is a research facility in Germany that has developed a small-scale integrated gasifier/FT system called ArtFuel. The construction of a pilot plant was initiated in 2009 and completed in 2012. It uses a CFB gasifier, and the syngas is converted in a fixed-bed reactor using a cobalt-based catalyst. Various types of woody biomass as well as straw and other agricultural residues have been used as feedstocks (CUTEC News 2012).

10.5.2.1.4 Forest BtL Oy

The Finnish company Forest BtL Oy is a joint venture of Metsä and Vapo, providing expertise in the integration of second generation biofuels to enable large-scale projects. In 2012, their Ajos Project received funding under the NER300 call to build a BTL plant to produce biodiesel and bionaphtha. The plant, with an annual output of 115,000 tonnes, will be located in Ajos near Kimi, Finland. The gasification process will use Choren's Carbo-V technology. The FT process step will use Gasel technology, licensed by Axens, which includes slurry bubble column reactors and a proprietary cobalt-based catalyst for the FT process step, and an upgrading section for refining of the paraffin products. The production is planned to start in 2016 (Axens 2013; Forest BtL 2013).

10.5.2.1.5 NSE Biofuels Oy (Stora Enso/Neste)

NSE Biofuels Oy is a joint venture between the Finnish companies Neste Oil and Stora Enso, which was formed in 2009 with the aim of producing liquid fuels from biomass. A demonstration plant was installed at the Stora Enso paper mill in Varkaus. The feedstock consisted of wood waste provided by Stora Enso. The refining of the crude FT products (e.g. wax) was provided by Neste Oil. The project was also supported by the VTT Technical Research Centre of Finland. With an output of 656 tonnes per year, the plant provided valuable data. The gas produced from the wood waste also served as fuel in the pulp mill's lime kiln, replacing oil. A commercial plant with a capacity of 100,000 tonnes per year was being planned, but in 2012, it was announced that further plans were cancelled because the project did not receive the expected funding from the European Commission (EBTP 2013; NER300 2013).

10.5.2.1.6 Technical University of Vienna

In the Austrian town of Güssing, a biomass gasifier has been operated since 2002 to supply the town with heat and energy using local wood feedstocks.

In 2005, the Technical University of Vienna (TUV), part of the competence centre BIOENERGY2010+, added a laboratory/pilot scale-FT system (BioFit) with a tubular slurry-bed reactor that uses part of the syngas coming from the gasifier. Both iron and cobalt catalysts have been tested in the facility. The results show that with iron-based catalysts, more alkenes and oxygenates are produced whereas with cobalt-based catalysts, *n*-alkane products are favoured. The output capacity of the integrated system is 0.2 tonnes per year (Yeh 2011; Bacovsky et al. 2013) The BioFit system uses a syngas stream from the same gasifier as the FT pilot plant developed by Velocys (see Section 10.5.2.1.8).

10.5.2.1.7 UPM

UPM is a Finnish forestry industry company whose business is based around products obtained from fibre and biomass. In 2012, the UPM Stracel received a large grant from the European Commission (NER 300) for the construction of a BTL plant in Stracel, France. Biodiesel will be obtained from logging residues, bark and woodchips. The integrated technology that will be used was tested in the United States in collaboration with Andritz Carbona and the Gas Technology Institute (GTI; see Section 10.5.2.2.2). The plant is planned to have an annual output of 105,000 tonnes of biofuel (EBTP 2013; UPM 2013).

10.5.2.1.8 Velocys

Velocys, now part of Oxford Catalysts Ltd., provides FT technology based on the use of microchannel reactors. The company also conducts FT catalyst development. Mainly cobalt-based catalysts are used in the FT BTL processes. In 2010, a pilot plant commenced operation in Güssing, Austria, which is the first integrated FT system using the microchannel reactors. The plant is managed by SGS Energia, which also provided the gas cleaning technology. The capacity of the FT system in the pilot plant is more than 100 kg/day, and can achieve a CO conversion of 70% (single pass-through).

In 2012, it was announced that Velocys was selected by Solena Fuels Corporation as the supplier of FT technology for the Green Sky London waste/biomass to jet fuel project. The aim of the project is to build a sustainable jet fuel plant to supply fuel to part of the British Airways fleet from 2015 (Velocys 2013).

10.5.2.2 United States

In the United States, BTL developments can be supported by the U.S. Department of Energy and its Bioenergy Technology office. The programme's aim is to work with and support companies and other partners to develop and apply technologies for biofuel production from renewable biomass (U.S. DOE 2013). A number of companies have focussed on BTL FT developments,

10.5.2.2.1 Clearfuels/Rentech

In this collaboration, with the goal of producing liquid fuels from biomass, Clearfuels provides the gasification technology and Rentech provides the FT technology. The Clearfuels gasifier is referred to as the high-efficiency hydrothermal reformer (HEHR; entrained flow) and consists of a multitubular steam reformer. For the FT process (Rentech process), Rentech uses a slurry bubble column reactor and an iron-based catalyst. Their developments have focussed on improving catalyst composition and reactor design. The iron-based catalyst is nontoxic and can be used with various syngas compositions (Yeh 2011; Rentech 2013).

A pilot/demonstration-scale facility was setup in Commerce City, Colorado in 2008, which first used syngas from a natural gas reformer, but then later changed to syngas from biomass feedstocks (waste wood). In 2013, however, it was announced that operations would cease and research and development would be stopped at the product demonstration unit in Commerce City. The technology is believed to have commercial value, but due to current energy prices and a lack of government incentives, Rentech decided to focus on profitable nearer-term opportunities (Rentech 2013).

10.5.2.2.2 Gas Technology Institute

GTI's research facilities have focussed on the development and testing of gasifiers and gas cleaning to produce syngas. A gasifier/FT system was planned in collaboration with UPM Kymmene, providing the feed of logging residues, and Andritz Carbona, developing a gas-cleaning system. A pilot testing facility has been operating in Des Plaines, Illinois since 2004. The FT unit was added later and the testing of the integrated gasifier/FT operation resulted in valuable data for the construction of commercial facilities planned in Finland and France (see Sections 10.5.2.1.4 and 10.5.2.1.7).

A new project has been funded that does not use conventional FT technology, but employs the Haldor Topsøe TIGAS process to convert the syngas to liquid fuels through a methanol intermediate. GTI's research activities have also focussed on the IH^2 process, which is new technology to directly convert biomass into transportation fuels using catalytic hydropyrolysis and hydroconversion. A pilot plant in Des Plaines, Illinois commenced operation in 2012 using wood, corn stover and algae as feedstocks (Bacovsky et al. 2013).

10.5.2.2.3 SynTerra (Red Lion/Pacific Renewable Fuels)

In 2009, Pacific Renewable Fuels and Red Lion Bioenergy merged as a new company called SynTerra Energy. Red Lion Bioenergy was the provider of the gasification technology whereas Pacific Renewable Fuels employed its FT technology. The approach to convert biomass into liquid fuels is now called the Syntrex platform, which includes a solid steam reforming process followed by a one-step hydrocarbon production. A Syntrex designer catalyst is employed for the direct conversion of syngas to the desired hydrocarbon mixture. The company claims that the Syntrex process does not need expensive procedures such as refining or upgrading of products (SynTerra 2013). Red Lion's pilot plant is located close to the University of Toledo, Ohio but a larger synthetic diesel fuel plant is planned near the Port of Toledo.

10.5.2.2.4 Research Triangle Institute

The Research Triangle Institute (RTI) is a nonprofit research organisation based in North Carolina, which has developed a syngas cleaning system, called Therminator. The system has been tested at a pilot-scale gasification facility at the University of Utah. In the coming years, a FT system will be put in place to convert the clean biomass-derived syngas into liquid transportation fuels (Bacovsky et al. 2013).

10.5.2.2.5 Thermochem Recovery International/Emerging Fuels Technology

Thermochem Recovery International (TRI) has been involved in the development of gasification technology, especially for the pulp and paper industry. The company has built a pilot demonstration unit at the Southern Research Institute in Durham, North Carolina. Emerging Fuels Technology, provided the FT technology with a fixed-bed reactor and cobalt-based catalyst (Emfuels 2013; TRI 2013). The facility commenced operation in 2009 and the data obtained was intended as support for the scale-up projects of New Page and Flambeau Rivers (paper mill). These projects, however, which received awards from the Department of Energy, were mutually terminated in 2012 and the projects were stopped (U.S. DOE 2013).

10.6 Research Trends and Challenges

There are several challenges associated with BTL FT processes, including the overall efficiency, integration of technologies and problems associated with supply and distribution of the biomass feedstock. The main areas for research include the FT catalyst, FT reactors, the integration of processes and the reduction of environmental effects.

10.6.1 FT Catalysts

Many research activities have focussed on improving the heart of the FT synthesis—the FT catalyst. Areas for potential improvement include catalyst activity, selectivity and stability toward deactivation. Understanding reaction details, such as size and promoter effects, and enhancing catalyst characteristics for FT synthesis has been a task for more than a few decades (Glasser et al. 2012; Zhang et al. 2013). Product selectivity and catalyst deactivation, however, still remain major limitations on the way to commercialising FT processes (Calderone et al. 2011).

10.6.1.1 Catalyst Deactivation

Table 10.12 lists and explains the main types of catalyst deactivation. Understanding deactivation mechanisms and how to avoid them is crucial to develop methods to avoid deactivation or initiate regeneration of the active phase (Bartholomew 2001; de Smit and Weckhuysen 2008; van Steen and Claeys 2008; Luque et al. 2012). Most investigations focus on deactivation

TABLE 10.12

Types of Catalyst Deactivation

Deactivation Type	Description	Co-Based	Fe-Based
Attrition	Mechanical deactivation, abrasion leading to loss of catalyst, crushing of catalyst particles leading to loss of surface area	Higher/important for slurry phase industrial processes	
Poisoning	Chemical deactivation, chemisorption of poisonous species (e.g. H_2S and NH_3) on active sites of catalyst, blocking of FT reaction	Co-based catalysts are generally more sensitive to sulphur poisoning than Fe catalysts	More sulphur resistant, but levels should be less than $0.02 \ mg/m^3$
Carbon formation and deposition; carbide formation	Chemical and mechanical deactivation, formation of carbonaceous species that can block the surface, inhibit diffusion, chemisorb on active sites; formation of carbides through diffusion of carbon into catalyst crystals	Gradual deposition of polymeric carbon; carbide formation rare and not taken into consideration	Increases with increasing temperature (important for HTFT); carbide formation common, active carbide species might be transformed to less active species
Sintering (aging)	Crystallite growth and transformations or loss of support area can lead to reduction of active surface area, occurs at higher temperatures	Sintering of metal nanoparticles is one of the main reasons for deactivation for Co catalysts	Loss of catalytic surface area is one of the main problems

Sources: Bartholomew, C.H., *Applied Catalysis A: General* 212: 17–60, 2001; van Steen, E., and Claeys, M., *Chemical Engineering and Technology* 31: 655, 2008; Luque, R. et al., *Energy & Environmental Science* 5: 5186, 2012.

mechanisms associated with Co-based catalysts (Saib et al. 2010; Tsakoumis et al. 2010).

10.6.1.2 Catalyst Promoters

Catalyst activity is usually enhanced by the addition of a promoter. The activity of Fe-based and Co-based catalysts can be influenced by alkali metals, transition metals and noble metals. These promoters can have a structural effect (changing structure of active phase) or an electronic effect (by electron transfer or interaction; Zhang et al. 2010). Different promoters were found to have different effects for Fe-based and Co-based catalyst.

For Fe catalysts, the addition of potassium (K^+) and sodium (Na^+) was generally found to enhance the FT and WGS activity. They are believed to change the electronic properties and therefore enhance chemisorption of CO (Zhang et al. 2010; Hu et al. 2012). Potassium was also found to enhance the product selectivity (toward C_5–C_{11}). A high content of alkali metals, however, can cause deactivation of the catalyst. Transition metals such as Cr, Zr and Mn were also found to enhance catalyst activity, but did not change product selectivity (Lohitharn et al. 2008; Hu et al. 2012). The reduction of Fe can be facilitated by the addition of noble metals such as Ru or Cu. This can lead to higher activities, but without changing selectivities (Zhang et al. 2010).

For Co catalysts, promoters such as noble metals and transition metal oxides (e.g. ZrO_2 and MnO_x) were found to have a positive effect on catalyst activity. Pt, Ru and Pd help with the reduction of cobalt oxides and therefore increase activities (Diel and Khodakov 2009). Zirconium oxide (ZrO_2) was shown to enhance activities through structural effects that improve CO conversion and C_{5+} selectivity (Zhang et al. 2010). Rhenium (Re) is also widely used as a promoter for Co-based catalysts (Iglesia 1997).

10.6.1.3 Catalyst Supports (Nanopourous Materials, Zeolites and Carbon Materials)

Supports play an important role for the activity, selectivity and lifetime of the catalyst. They can increase the surface area and stabilise the active phase (increase resistance to attrition), and can also help to enhance mass and heat transfer. A range of supports have been investigated for Co-based and Fe-based FT catalyst with silica (SiO_2), alumina (Al_2O_3) and titania (TiO_2) being amongst the most commonly applied (Storsæter et al. 2005).

Mesoporous materials, such as mesoporous silica, have become increasingly popular in recent years. They display a high surface area and channels with defined diameters. These channels can influence the product selectivity (control chain length) by acting as a 'nanoreactor' with the catalyst particles inside. They have been mainly investigated in combination with Co-based FT catalysts. The pore size of these supports was found to have an influence on the catalyst performance (Martínez and Prieto 2009).

Zeolites as supports for FT synthesis have also been increasingly investigated. These microporous solids (aluminosilicate minerals) have cavities and channels and hence display shape-selective features (Zhang et al. 2010). They can also be acidic, which may catalyse secondary reactions such as cracking and isomerisation. The amount of liquid fuel (middle distillate) that can be obtained from FT synthesis generally follows the ASF distribution and hence heavier waxes usually have to undergo a refinement step afterward. These bifunctional catalysts, composed of the active metal and the acidic zeolite, have been investigated to control product selectivity and overcome ASF distribution limits (Bessell 1995; Abelló and Montané 2011). For example, a zeolite-supported Co catalyst (Co-H-ZSM5) was used to directly produce gasoline with selectivities close to 60% (Sartipi et al. 2013).

Other materials that have been of interest as supports for FT synthesis include carbon nanotubes and carbon nanofibres. They display high strength and stability as well as a high surface area. Several carbon-supported Co and Fe catalysts have been investigated with promising results (Yang et al. 2011; Zhang et al. 2013).

10.6.1.4 Bimetallic Catalysts

Cobalt is widely used as a FT catalyst, especially in middle distillate operations. The cost of cobalt, however, is high and with large quantities of catalyst used in FT facilities, it becomes an economic problem. Some research has therefore focussed on bimetallic catalysts with the goal of developing a cheaper substitute for Co-based catalysts with the same or better activity and selectivity. The combinations of metals include Co, Ni, Fe and Ru, but with a main focus on the most widely used metals Fe and Co (Calderone et al. 2011). A catalyst with an iron core and a cobalt shell, for example, has been successfully synthesised and tested. However, many results in this field remain contradictory (Calderone et al. 2013).

10.6.2 FT Reactors

In addition to the catalyst, the FT reactor and the reaction medium are of great importance. A good heat transfer and a low pressure drop can significantly influence the outcome of the reaction. Aims of research activities include the investigation of FT reaction kinetics to develop more accurate models for industrial applications, and increasing the efficiency of reactors by using novel designs and conditions.

10.6.2.1 Microstructured Reactors

Microstructured and, in particular, microchannel reactors have received increasing attention in recent years. These reactors, described in Section 10.3.2.4, display some advantages over the conventional slurry phase or fixed-bed reactors (Lerou et al. 2010). A better heat and mass transfer can lead to higher productivities, which is favourable for economics at smaller scales. Microchannel reactors with highly efficient catalysts could therefore provide an option for medium-scale decentralised biomass processing units (Atkinson 2010; Kolb 2013). Several studies on microchannel reactors have been undertaken (Myrstad et al. 2009; Deshmukh et al. 2010), and commercial applications are being investigated by Velocys (Atkinson 2010). A challenge of microchannel reactors could be their cost and the difficulties associated with catalyst removal/change.

Membrane reactors have also been subject to research activities. They may have potential for small-scale and medium-scale facilities. The FT reactants are forced through a membrane, which can result in a high gas–liquid mass transfer rates and also influences product distribution (Rohde et al. 2005).

10.6.2.2 Supercritical Fluid Reactors

For LTFT, both fixed bed and slurry phase reactors have certain disadvantages (see Table 10.6). The use of supercritical fluids has been investigated as a way to combine the advantages of both reactors. Supercritical fluid FT (SF-FT) usually involves the addition of a hydrocarbon solvent (C_3–C_7) and the increase of reactor pressure (Durham et al. 2013). These operation conditions can have several benefits including decreased methane selectivity, enhanced diesel and wax selectivity, increased catalyst activity and increased *in situ* extraction of heavy hydrocarbons (Elbashir et al. 2009; Durham et al. 2013).

10.6.3 Economical and Environmental Challenges

Process integration remains one of the major challenges for BTL FT processes (Damartzis and Zabaniotou 2011). Cogeneration of heat/power (electricity) and fuel has been studied as one method to improve the overall efficiency of BTL FT facilities (Larson et al. 2009; Baliban et al. 2011, 2013). Wastewater production and use of oxygen and hydrogen during the process has also been of concern for the overall environmental effect. Challenges therefore include the reduction of wastewater generation and oxygen introduction (Noureldin et al. 2012). In addition, the logistics of feedstock supply and the utilisation of carbon in the biomass have been identified as hurdles toward economically feasible BTL FT facilities (Unruh et al. 2010; Leckel and Phillips 2011).

10.6.3.1 Cofeedstocks (with Coal or Gas)

Driven by the high feedstock cost for biomass-derived syngas and the unfavourable economics for scale-ups, there has been an interest in hybrid processes that use a combination of feedstocks (cofeedstocks) for FT synthesis (Baliban et al. 2011). This can be a combination of coal and biomass (CBTL; Kreutz et al. 2008), or coal, gas and biomass (CBGTL; Elia et al. 2010). When coal and biomass are used as cofeedstocks, there are several gasification configurations that can be used. The gasification can either take place in the same gasifier, the feedstocks can be fed to different gasifiers, or a hybrid between the two can be used. Each option has advantages and drawbacks (Kreutz et al. 2008). CBTL has been of interest to decrease the carbon footprint of CTL processes. Although cogasification of coal and biomass has been explored at the bench and pilot scales (McLendon et al. 2004; Meerman et al. 2013), only (mainly theoretical) studies have been undertaken for CBFT processes (Leckel and Phillips 2011; Liu et al. 2011).

10.6.3.2 Carbon/CO_2 Utilisation

As well as CO and H_2, the gasification step produces CO_2, which is usually separated before the syngas is converted to hydrocarbon in the FT synthesis. This, however, decreases the overall carbon utilisation from the biomass because the carbon in the CO_2 is lost. Research interests therefore also include the hydrogenation of CO_2 in the syngas mixture to decrease CO_2 emissions and increase overall carbon utilisation (Dorner et al. 2010; James et al. 2010; Hu et al. 2012). The WGS reaction plays an important role in improving carbon utilisation because it can convert CO_2 to CO. Although using Co-based FT catalyst in CO_2 hydrogenation has been found to significantly increase the production of methane (Zhang et al. 2002), Fe-based FT catalysts have been of interest due to their ability to catalyse the WGS reaction (Dorner et al. 2010). Biomass-based syngas, however, usually has a low H_2/CO ratio, and to maximise carbon utilisation, the addition of H_2 would be required (which ideally has to come from a carbon-neutral source). Improvements in FT systems (e.g. catalysts) would be needed to make CO_2 hydrogenation feasible.

Overall, as shown in Table 10.13, a range of technologies (catalysts and reactors) is available for FT processes due to historical and current developments. The interest in FT synthesis using biomass feedstocks has significantly increased in recent years, with ongoing research and development activities in various areas. However, several challenges and limitations (listed in Table 10.14) still have to be addressed, and a combination of scientific research and changes of economical and political factors may be required to make BTL FT facilities a viable option for transportation fuel supply.

TABLE 10.13

Overview and Comparison of Catalyst and Reactor Types

		Temperature	Example Process	Cost	Products/ Characteristics	Advantages	Disadvantages
Catalysts	Fused iron	HTFT	Synthol, SAS	Low	Mainly olefins	Low methane selectivity, can operate at lower H_2/CO ratios (good for biomass)	Less resistant to deactivation, lower activity at higher conversion rates
	Precipitated iron	LTFT	ARGE, SPD	Low	Mainly waxes (and branched liquid hydrocarbons)	Low methane selectivity, can operate at lower H_2/CO ratios (good for biomass), less sensitive to sulphur poisoning	Less resistant to deactivation (e.g. by water), lower activity at higher conversion rates
	Co based	LTFT	SMDS SPD	Medium–high	Straight-chain heavy hydrocarbons	More resistant to deactivation, higher productivities at higher conversion, more resistant to attrition (suitable for slurry reactors)	Not active for WGS, less flexible (significant influence of temperature and pressure on selectivity), cannot operate at low H_2/CO ratios
	Ru based	Can be low (<150°C)	Laboratory scale	Very high	Long-chain hydrocarbons	Very high activity, can work without promoters	High cost, limited reserves—industrial-scale application hindered
	Ni based	Low	Laboratory scale	Medium	Shorter hydrocarbons, methane	Cheaper than cobalt	Selectivity changes to methane at higher temperatures

(continued)

TABLE 10.13 (CONTINUED)

Overview and Comparison of Catalyst and Reactor Types

	Temperature	Example Process	Cost	Products/Characteristics	Advantages	Disadvantages
Reactors						
CFB reactor	HTFT	Synthol	High (higher than FFB)	Only good for low molecular weight products	High catalyst affectivity, high once-through conversion	High catalyst consumption, high CH_4 formation, low flexibility
FFB reactor	HTFT	SAS	Lower than FFB	Only good for low molecular weight products	Good temperature control, high once-through conversion, lower maintenance and catalyst consumption	High CH_4 formation
Multitubular fixed-bed reactor	LTFT	ARGE, SMDS	Higher than slurry bed	High C_{5+} selectivity, full range of products	Easy wax separation, low CH_4 formation	Poor temperature control, high maintenance
Slurry-bed reactor	LTFT	Sasol slurry bed (SSBP)	Medium	Large-scale, mainly used with Co based catalysts, high C_{5+} selectivity	Good temperature control, simple construction, high flexibility, low maintenance	Wax separation difficult, high sulphur poisoning (through instant spreading)
Microchannel reactor	LTFT	Velocys BTL FT	High	Small capacity, full range, mainly wax/diesel	High CO conversion per pass, high productivity, good heat transfer properties	Small capacity, relatively high capital cost

TABLE 10.14

Challenges and Research Activities Associated with FT BTL

	Challenges and Limitations	Research and Development
FT synthesis	Integration of units (gasification, gas cleaning, FT, heat/energy production)	Modelling of processes Integration of gasifier and FT synthesis Cogeneration
	Product selectivity and catalyst activity	Promoters Bifunctional catalysts Nanoporous materials and carbon nanomaterials as supports
	Efficiency, cost and stability of the FT catalyst	Bimetallic catalysts Studying of mechanisms
	Efficiency of the reactor	Microctructured reactors Thermally coupled reactors Supercritical media
Other	Logistics, supply of biomass	Medium-sized, scattered facilities Cofeedstocks
	Environmental factors (GHGs)	Reduction of oxygen and hydrogen input Reduction of wastewater generation
	Energy intensity, carbon efficiency	Mass and energy integration techniques CO_2 feed
	Cost, economical feasibility	Scale-up to economically viable size but not going to large scale Cofeedstock (coal, gas) Increasing oil price

References

Abelló, S., and Montané, D. (2011). Exploring iron-based multifunctional catalysts for Fischer–Tropsch synthesis: A review. *Chem Sus Chem* **4**: 1538–1556.

AirLiquide, http://www.airliquide.com/. Accessed May 2013.

Atkinson, D. (2010). Fischer–Tropsch reactors for biofuels production: New technology needed! *Biofuels, Bioproducts and Biorefining* **4**: 12–16.

Axens, http://www.axens.net/. Accessed May 2013.

Bacovsky, D.; Ludwiczek, N.; Ognissanto, M.; Wörgetter, M. (2013). Status of Advanced Biofuels Demonstration Facilities in 2012. Report to IEA Bioenergy Task 39, T39-P1b.

Baliban, R.C.; Elia, J.A.; Floudas, C.A. (2011). Optimization framework for the simultaneous process synthesis, heat and power integration of a thermochemical hybrid biomass, coal and natural gas facility. *Computers and Chemical Engineering* **35**: 1647–1690.

Baliban, R.C.; Elia, J.A.; Floudas, C.A. (2013). Biomass to liquid transportation fuels (BTL) system: Process synthesis and global optimization framework. *Energy and Environmental Science* **6**: 267–289.

Bartholomew, C.H. (1990). Recent technological developments in Fischer–Tropsch catalysis. *Catalysis Letters* **7**: 303–316.

Bartholomew, C.H. (2001). Mechanisms of catalyst deactivation. *Applied Catalysis A: General* 212: 17–60.

Bertole, C.J.; Mims, A.C.; Kiss, G. (2002). The effect of water on the cobalt-catalyzed Fischer–Tropsch synthesis. *Journal of Catalysis* 210: 84–96.

Bessell, S. (1995). Investigation of bifunctional zeolite supported cobalt Fischer–Tropsch catalysts. *Applied Catalysis A: General* 126: 235–244.

Boerrigter, H. (2006). Economy of Biomass-To-Liquids (BTL) plants. Energy Research Centre of the Netherlands (ECN) Report, ECN-C-06-019.

Boerrrigter, H.; Calis, H.P.; Slort, D.J.; Bodenstaff, H.; Kaandorf, A.J.; den Uil, H.; Rabou, L.P.L.M. (2004). Gas Cleaning for Integrated Biomass Gasification (BG) and Fischer–Tropsch Systems. Energy and Research Centre of the Netherland (ECN). Report, ECN-C-04-056.

Calderone, R.V.; Shiju, N.R.; Curulla-Ferré, D.; Rothenberg, G. (2011). Bimetallic catalysts for the Fischer–Tropsch reaction. *Green Chemistry* 13: 1950–1959.

Calderone, R.V.; Shiju, N.R.; Curulla-Ferré, D.; Chambrey, S.; Khodakov, A.; Rose, A.; Thiessen, J.; Jess, A.; Rothenberg, G. (2013). De novo design of nanostructured iron-cobalt Fischer–Tropsch catalysts. *Angewandte Chemie International Edition* 52: 4397–4401.

CUTEC News (2012). Issue 2, May 2012, available at http://www.cutec.de/. Accessed May 2013.

Damartzis, T., and Zabaniotou, A. (2011). Thermochemical conversion of biomass to second generation fuels through integrated process design—A review. *Renewable and Sustainable Energy Reviews* 15: 366–378.

Dalai, A.K., and Davis, B.H. (2008). Fischer–Tropsch synthesis: A review of water effects on the performances of unsupported and supported Co catalysts. *Applied Catalysis A: General* 348: 1–15.

Davis, B.H. (2001). Fischer–Tropsch synthesis: Current mechanism and futuristic needs. *Fuel Processing Technology* 71: 175–166.

Davis, B.H. (2005). Fischer–Tropsch synthesis: Overview of reactor development and future potentialities. *Topics in Catalysis* 32: 143–168.

Davis, B.H. (2007). Fischer–Tropsch synthesis: Comparison of performances of iron and cobalt catalyst. *Industrial and Engineering Chemistry Research* 46: 8938–8945.

Demirbas, A. (2007). Converting biomass derived synthetic gas to fuels via Fischer–Tropsch synthesis. Energy sources Part A: Recovery. *Utilization and Environmental Effects* 29: 1507–1512.

de Klerk, A. (2008). Fischer–Tropsch refining: Technology selection to match molecules. *Green Chemistry* 10: 1249–1279.

de Klerk, A. (2011). Fischer–Tropsch fuels refinery design. *Energy and Environmental Science* 4: 1177–1205.

de Smit, E., and Weckhuysen, B.M. (2008). The renaissance of iron-based Fischer–Tropsch synthesis: On the multifaceted catalyst deactivation behavior. *Chemical Society Reviews* 37: 2758–2681.

Deshmukh, S.R.; Tonkovich, A.L.Y.; Jarosch, K.T.; Schrader, L.; Fritzgerlad, S.P.; Kilanowski, D.R.; Lerou, J.J.; Mazanec, T.J. (2010). Scale-up of microchannel reactors for Fischer–Tropsch synthesis. *Industrial and Engineering Chemistry Research* 49: 10883–10888.

Diel, F., and Khodakov, A.J. (2009). Promotion of cobalt Fischer–Tropsch catalysts with noble metals: A review. *Oil and Gas Science and Technology* 64: 11–24.

Dorner, R.W.; Hardy, D.R.; Williams, F.W.; Willauer, H.D. (2010). Heterogeneous CO_2 conversion to value-added hydrocarbons. *Energy and Environmental Science* 3: 884–890.

Dry, M.E. (2002). The Fischer–Tropsch process: 1950–2000. *Catalysis Today* 71: 227–241.

Durham, E.; Xu, R.; Zhang, S.; Eden, M.R.; Roberts, C.B. (2013). Supercritical adiabatic reactors for Fischer–Tropsch synthesis. *Industrial and Engineering Chemistry Research* 52: 3133–3136.

European Biofuels Technology Platform (EBTP), http://www.biofuelstp.eu/. Accessed May 2013.

Elia, J.A.; Baliban, R.C.; Floudas, C.A. (2010). Toward novel hybrid biomass, coal, and natural gas processes for satisfying current transportation fuel demands, 2: Simultaneous heat and power integration. *Industrial and Engineering Chemical Research* 49: 7371–7388.

Elbashir, N.O.; Bukur, D.-B.; Durham, E.; Roberts, C.B. (2009). Advancements of Fischer–Tropsch synthesis via utilization of supercritical fluid reaction media. *American Institute of Chemical Engineers* 56: 997–1015.

Emfuels, Emerging Fuels Technology, http://emfuelstech.com/. Accessed May 2013.

Enger, B.C., and Holmen, A. (2013). Nickel and Fischer–Tropsch synthesis. *Catalysis Reviews: Science and Engineering* 54: 437–488.

Evans, G., and Smith, C. (2012). Biomass to liquids technology. *Comprehensive Renewable Energy* 5: 155–204.

Fischer, F., and Tropsch, H. (1923). Über die Herstellung synthetischer Ölgemische (Synthol) durch Aufbau aus Kohlenoxyd und Wasserstoff. *Brennstoff Chemie* 4: 276–285.

Forest Btl, http://forestbtl.com/2nd-generation-btl-technology/. Accessed May 2013.

Friedel, R.A., and Anderson, R.B. (1950). Composition of synthetic liquid fuels. I. Product distribution and analysis of C_5–C_8 paraffin isomers from cobalt catalyst. *Journal of the American Chemical Society* 72: 1212–1215.

Geerlings, J.J.C.; Wilson, J.H.; Kramer, J.G.; Kuipers, H.P.C.E.; Hoek, A.; Huisman, H.M. (1999). Fischer–Tropsch technology—From active site to commercial process. *Applied Catalysis A: General* 186: 27–40.

Gill, S.S.; Tsolakis, A.; Dearn, K.D.; Rodríguez-Fernández, J. (2011). Combustion characteristics and emissions of Fischer–Tropsch diesel fuels in IC engines. *Progress in Energy and Combustion Science* 37: 503–523.

Glasser, D.; Hildebrandt, D.; Liu, X.; Lu, X.; Masuku, C.M. (2012). Recent advances in understanding the Fischer–Tropsch synthesis (FTS) reaction. *Current Opinion in Chemical Engineering* 1: 296–302.

Guettel, R.; Kunz, U.; Turek, T. (2008). Reactors for Fischer–Tropsch synthesis. *Chemical Engineering and Technology* 37: 746–754.

Gumuslu, G., and Avci, A.K. (2011). Parametric analysis of Fischer–Tropsch synthesis in a catalytic microchannel reactor. *American Institute of Chemical Engineers Journal* 54: 227–235.

Gupta, R.B., and Demirbas, A. (2010). Diesel from Biomass Gasification followed by Fischer–Tropsch Synthesis. Chapter 8 in *Gasoline, Diesel and Ethanol Biofuels from Grasses and Plants*, Cambridge University Press, New York.

Hamelinck, C.A.; Faaij, A.P.C.; den Uil, H.; Boerrigter, H. (2004). Production of FT transportation fuels from biomass, technical options, process analysis and optimization, and development and potential. *Energy* 29: 1743–1771.

Heinrich, E.; Dahmen, N.; Dinjus, E. (2009). Cost estimate for biosynfuel production via biosyncrude gasification. *Biofuels, Bioproducts and Biorefining* **3**: 28–41.

Hu, J.; Yu, F.; Lu, Y. (2012). Application of Fischer–Tropsch synthesis in biomass to liquid conversion. *Catalysts* **2**: 303–326.

IFP Energies Nouvelles, http://www.ifpenergiesnouvelles.com/. Accessed May 2013.

Iglesia, E. (1997). Design, synthesis and use of Co-based Fischer–Tropsch synthesis catalysts. *Applied Catalysis A: General* **161**: 59–78.

Jacobs, G., and Davis, B.H. (2010). Conversion of Biomass to Liquid Fuels and Chemicals via the Fischer–Tropsch Synthesis Route. Chapter 10 in Thermochemical Conversion of Biomass to Liquid Fuels and Chemicals. *RSC Energy and Environment Series* **1**: 95.

Jager, B. (2003). Development of Fischer–Tropsch Reactors. AIChE Spring Meeting, New Orleans.

James, O.O.; Mesubi, A.M.; Ako, T.C.; Maity, A. (2010). Increasing carbon utilization in Fischer–Tropsch synthesis using H_2-deficient or CO_2-rich syngas feed. *Fuel Processing Technology* **91**: 136–144.

Jun, K.-W.; Roh, H.-S.; Kim, K.-S.; Ryu, J.-S.; Lee, K.-W. (2004). Catalytic investigation for Fischer–Tropsch synthesis from bio-mass derived syngas. *Applied Catalysis: General* **259**: 221–226.

Kavalov, B., and Peteves, S.D. (2005). Status and Perspectives of Biomass-to-Liquid Fuels in the European Union. Joint Research Center, European Comission, EU 21745 EN.

Khodakov, A.Y.; Chu, W.; Fongarland, P. (2007). Advances in the development of novel cobalt Fischer–Tropsch catalysts for synthesis of long-chain hydrocarbon and clean fuels. *Chemical Reviews* **107**: 1692–1744.

Kim, K.; Kim, Y.; Yang, C.; Moon, J.; Lee, J.; Lee, U.; Lee, S.; Kim, J.; Eom, W.; Lee, S.; Kang, M.; Lee, Y. (2013). Long-term operation of biomass-to-liquid systems coupled to gasification and Fischer–Tropsch processes for biofuel production. *Bioresource Technology* **127**: 391–399.

Kolb, G. (2013). Review: Microchannel reactors for distributed and renewable production of fuels and electrical energy. *Chemical Engineering and Processing: Process Intensification* **65**: 1–44.

Kreutz, T.G.; Larson, E.D.; Liu, G.; Williams, R.H. (2008). Fischer–Tropsch Fuels from Coal and Biomass. 25th Annual International Pittsburgh Coal Conference.

Lappas, A., and Heracleous, E. (2011). Production of biofuels via Fischer–Tropsch synthesis: Biomass-to-liquids. Chapter 19 in *Handbook of Biofuels Production: Processes and Technologies*, Woodhead Publishing Ltd, Cambridge, UK.

Larson, E.D.; Jin, H.; Celik, F.E. (2009). Large-scale gasification-based coproduction of fuels and energy from switchgrass. *Biofuels, Bioproducts and Biorefining* **3**: 174–194.

Leckel, D., and Phillips, T. (2011). Fischer–Tropsch: Extending the biofuels toolbox? *Biofuels* **2**: 109–113.

Leibbrandt, N.H.; Aboyade, A.O.; Knoetze, J.H.; Gérgens, J.F. (2013). Process efficiency of biofuel production via gasification and Fischer–Tropsch synthesis. *Fuel* **109**: 484–492.

Lerou, J.J.; Tonkovich, A.L.; Silva, L.; Pery, S.; McDaniel, J. (2010). Microchannel architecture enables greener processes. *Chemical Engineering Science* **65**: 380–385.

Liu, G.; Larson, E.D.; Williams, R.H.; Kreutz, T.G.; Gua, X. (2011). Making Fischer–Tropsch fuels and electricity from coal and biomass: Performance and cost analysis. *Energy Fuels* **25**: 415–437.

Lohitharn, N.; Goodwin Jr., J.G.; Lotero, E. (2008). Fe-based Fischer–Tropsch synthesis catalysts containing carbide-forming transition metal promoters. *Journal of Catalysis* **255**: 104–113.

Luo, M.; Bao, S.; Keogh, R.S.; Sarkar, A.; Jacobs, G.; Davis, B.H. (2006). Fischer–Tropsch Synthesis: A Comparison of Iron and Cobalt Catalysts. AIChE Fall National Meeting.

Luque, R.; de la Osa, A.R.; Campelo, J.M.; Romero, A.A.; Valverde, J.L.; Sanchez, P. (2012). Design and development of catalysts for Biomass-To-Liquid-Fischer–Tropsch (BTL-FT) processes for biofuels production. *Energy and Environmental Science* **5**: 5186.

Maitlis, P.M., and Zanotti, V. (2009). The role of electrophilic species in the Fischer–Tropsch reaction. *Chemical Communications* **13**: 1619–1643.

Martínez, A., and Prieto, G. (2009). The application of zeolites and periodic mesoporous silicas in the catalytic conversion synthesis gas. *Topics in Catalysis* **52**: 75–90.

McLendon, T.R.; Lui, A.P.; Pienault, R.L.; Beer, S.K.; Richerdson, S.W. (2004). High-pressure co-gasification of coal and biomass in a fluidized bed. *Biomass and Bioenergy* **26**: 377–388.

Meerman, J.C.; Knoope, M.M.J.; Ramírez, A.; Turkenburg, W.C.; Faaij, A.P.C. (2013). Technical and economical prospects of coal- and biomass-fired integrated gasification facilities equipped with CCS over time. *International Journal of Greenhouse Gas Control* **16**: 311–323.

Myrstad, R.; Eri, S.; Pfeifer, P.; Rytter, E.; Holmen, A. (2009). Fischer–Tropsch synthesis in a microstructured reactor. *Catalysis Today* **147S**: S301–S304.

NER300, http://www.ner300.com/. Accessed May 2013.

Noureldin, M.M.B.; Bao, B.; Elbashir, N.O.; El-Halwagi, M.M. (2012). Benchmarking, insights, and potential for improvement of Fischer–Tropsch-based biomass-to-liquid technology. Clean Technologies and Environmental Policy.

Patzlaff, J.; Liu, Y.; Gaube, G.J. (1999). Studies on product distributions of iron and cobalt catalyzed Fischer–Tropsch synthesis. *Applied Catalysis A: General* **186**: 109–119.

Prins, M.J.; Ptasinski, K.J.; Janssen, F.J.J.G. (2004). Exergetic optimisation of a production process of Fischer–Tropsch fuels from biomass. *Fuel Processing Technology* **86**: 375–389.

RENEW, http://www.renew-fuel.com/. Accessed May 2013.

Rentech, www.rentechinc.com/. Accessed May 2013.

Rohde, M.P.; Unruh, D.; Schaub, G. (2005). Membrane application in Fischer–Tropsch synthesis reactors: Overview of concepts. *Catalysis Today* **106**: 143–148.

Röper, M. (1983). Fischer–Tropsch Synthesis. In *Catalysis in C1 chemistry*, Reidel Dordrecht, The Netherlands.

Saib, A.M.; Moodley, D.J.; Ciobîca, I.M.; Hauman, M.M.; Sigwebela, B.H.; Weststrate C.J.; Niemantsverdriet, J.W.; van de Loosdrecht, J. (2010). Fundamental understanding of deactivation and regeneration of cobalt Fischer–Tropsch synthesis catalysts. *Catalysis Today* **154**: 271–282.

Sanchez, O.J., and Cardona, C.A. (2008). Trends in biotechnological production of fuel ethanol form different feedstocks. *Bioresource Technology* **99**: 5270–5295.

Sasol, http://www.sasol.com, Accessed May 2013.

Sartipi, S.; Parashar, K.; Makkee, M.; Gascon, J.; Kapteijn, F. (2013). Breaking the Fischer–Tropsch synthesis selectivity: Direct conversion of syngas to gasoline over hierarchical Co/H-ZSM-5 catalyst. *Catalysis Science and Technology* **3**: 572–575.

Schulz, H. (1999). Short history and present trends of Fischer–Tropsch synthesis. *Applied Catalysis A: General* **186**: 3–12.

Shell, www.shell.com/Accessed May 2013.

Spath, P.L., and Dyton, D.C. (2003). Preliminary Screening—Technical and Economical Assessment of Synthesis Gas to Fuels and Chemicals with Emphasis on the Potential for Biomass-Derived Syngas. National Renewable Energy Laboratory, NREL/TP-510-34929.

Steynberg, A.P., and Dry, M. (2004). Fischer–Tropsch technology. *Studies in Surface Science and Catalysis* **152**.

Storsæter, S.; Tøtdal, B.; Walmsley, J.C.; Steinar Tanem, B.; Hilmen, A. (2005). Characterization of alumina-, silia-, and titania-supported cobalt Fischer–Tropsch catalyst. *Journal of Catalysis* **236**: 139–152.

Swain, P.K.; Das, L.M.; Naik, S.N. (2011). Biomass-to-liquid: A prospective challenge to research and development in 21st century. *Renewable and Sustainable Energy Reviews* **15**: 4917–4933.

SynTerra Energy, http://www.synterraenergy.com/Accessed May 2013.

Tijmensen, M.J.A.; Faaij, A.P.C.; Hamelick, C.N.; van Hardeveld, M.R.M. (2002). Exploration of the possibilities for production of Fischer–Tropsch liquids and power via biomass gasification. *Biomass and Energy* **23**: 129–152.

TRI, http://www.tri-inc.net/Accessed May 2013.

Tsakoumis, N.E.; Ronning, M.; Borg, O.; Rytter, E.; Holmen, A. (2010). Deactivation of cobalt based Fischer–Tropsch catalysts: A review. *Catalysis Today* **154**: 162–182.

Unruh, D.; Pabst, K.; Schaub, G. (2010). Fischer–Tropsch synfuels from biomass: Maximizing carbon efficiency and hydrocarbon yield. *Energy and Fuels* **24**: 2634–2641.

UPM, http://www.upm.com/. Accessed May 2013.

US Department of Energy, BioenergyTechnology Office, http://www1.eere.energy.gov/biomass/. Accessed May 2013.

van der Laan, G.P., and Beenackers, A.A.C.M. (1999). Kinetics and selectivity of the Fischer–Tropsch synthesis: A literature review. *Catalysis Reviews: Science and Engineering* **41**: 255–318.

van Steen, E., and Claeys, M. (2008). Fischer–Tropsch catalysts for the biomass-to-liquid process. *Chemical Engineering and Technology* **31**: 655.

van Vliet, O.P.R.; Faaij, A.P.C.; Turkenburg, W.C. (2009). Fischer–Tropsch diesel production in a well-to-wheel perspective: A carbon, energy flow and cost analysis. *Energy Conversion and Management* **50**: 855–876.

Velocys, http://www.velocys.com/. Accessed May 2013.

Yang, Y.; Chiang, K.; Burke, N. (2011). Porous carbon-supported catalysts for energy and environmental application: A short review. *Catalysis Today* **178**: 197–205.

Yeh, B. (2011). Independent Assessment of Technology Characterizations to Support the Biomass Program Annual State-of-Technology Assessments. National Renewable Energy Laboratory, Subcontract Report NREL/SR-6A10-50441.

Yong-Wang, L.; Xu, J.; Yang, Y. (2010). Diesel from Syngas. Chapter 6 in *Biomass to Biofuels: Strategies for Global Industries*, John Wiley and Sons Ltd, Chichester, West Sussex, UK.

Zhang, Y.; Jacobs, G.; Sparks, D.E.; Dry, M.E.; Davis, B.H. (2002). CO and CO$_2$ hydrogenation study on supported cobalt Fischer–Tropsch synthesis catalysts. *Catalysis Today* **71**: 411–418.

Zhang, Q.; Kang, J.; Wang, Y. (2010). Development of novel catalysts for Fischer–Tropsch synthesis: Tuning the product selectivity. *ChemCatChem* **2**: 1030–1058.

Zhang, Q.; Deng, W.; Wang, Y. (2013). Recent advances in understanding the key factors for Fischer–Tropsch synthesis. *Journal of Energy Chemistry* **22**: 27–38.

Zwart, R., and van Ree, R. (2009). Bio-based Fischer–Tropsch Diesel Production Technologies. Chapter 6 in *Biofuels*, Wiley Series in Renewable Resources, John Wiley and Sons Ltd, Chichester, West Sussex, UK.

11

Bio-Oil Applications and Processing

Annette Evans, Vladimir Strezov and Tim J. Evans

CONTENTS

11.1 Introduction

When biomass is heated in the absence of oxygen, it produces a pyrolysis liquid (bio-oil or biocrude), char (biocharcoal or biochar) and noncondensable gases (synthetic gas [syngas] or biogas) in various proportions. The resultant bio-oil is a complex and unique mixture of organic compounds and water, closely resembling the elemental composition of the parent biomass. It is a brown, free-flowing, highly oxygenated, dense and viscous polar liquid (Bridgwater 2011). It has a distinctive acrid and smoky odour due to the presence of low molecular weight aldehydes and acids, and can irritate the eyes upon prolonged exposure (Bridgwater 2012). Bio-oil can be considered as a microemulsion, with a continuous phase of an aqueous solution of holocellulose decomposition products that stabilise the discontinuous phase of pyrolytic lignin macromolecules through mechanisms including hydrogen bonding (Bridgwater 2012). Ageing and instability seen in bio-oil is thought to result from the breakdown of this microemulsion (Meier et al. 2013).

Due to the high oxygen content, the energy content of bio-oil is lower than most fossil fuels with a heating value approximately half that of petroleum-derived fuels such as heavy heating oil; however, bio-oil contains fewer trace metals and sulphur, making it an attractive low-emission fuel. Also, the high yield and high concentration of oxygenated hydrocarbons, including aromatic compounds, make pyrolysis oil a promising route for the production of large quantities of fungible biopetroleum and biodiesel (Boateng 2011).

The viscosity of bio-oil can vary greatly, from 25 to 1000 m^2/s (measured at 40°C) or more depending on the feedstock, water content of bio-oil, amount of light ends collected and extent of bio-oil ageing. Pyrolysis liquids cannot be completely vaporised again once collected. If heated to more than 100°C to remove water or distil lighter fractions, it reacts rapidly and forms a solid residue (Meier et al. 2013).

The density of bio-oil is very high at 1.2 kg/L, compared with light fuel oil at 0.85 kg/L. This means that bio-oil has 42% of the energy of light fuel oil on a weight basis, but 61% on a volumetric basis. This has important implications for the design and specification of pumps and atomisers in boilers and engines (Bridgwater 2011).

11.2 Bio-Crude Production

Rapid heating rates favour liquid formation, whereas slow pyrolysis maximises char yield. As much as 50 to 75 wt% of the biomass can be converted into bio-oil using fast pyrolysis wherein biomass is heated rapidly (>1000°C/s) to 450°C to 550°C (Boateng 2011). Vapours and aerosols from fast pyrolysis must be rapidly cooled and condensed to form bio-oil, a complex mixture of oxygenated organic compounds with a water content between 15 and 30 wt%. Because bio-oil is an intermediate product of incomplete combustion, it is highly unstable. It is also highly acidic, with a pH of around 2.3, making it highly corrosive. It contains hundreds of individual organic compounds and water. Liquid organics and oxygenated hydrocarbons present in the biomass include acids, alcohols, aldehydes, esters, furans, ketones, sugars, phenols and many multifunctional compounds. On an elemental basis, the compositional analysis of bio-oil is similar to the parental biomass pyrolysed. Although bio-oil has the appearance of crude petroleum, it is not miscible with petroleum-derived fuels, but instead is miscible with polar solvents including methanol, ethanol and acetone (Boateng 2011).

Pyrolysis reactions are complex because biomass is a mixture of hemicellulose, cellulose, lignin and other minor components, each degrading at different rates, mechanisms and pathways. Lignin decomposes over a wide temperature range, whereas cellulose and hemicellulose degrade rapidly over much narrower temperature ranges. Careful optimisation of the multiple reactions produces a higher quantity and quality bio-oil. Maximum yields are obtained at high heating rates, reaction temperatures of approximately 500°C and with short vapour residence times to reduce secondary reactions (Bridgwater 1999).

The advantage of liquid fuel production is that the fuel production is decoupled from fuel usage, allowing for decentralised pyrolysis of biomass, with transportation of liquids to a centralised bio-oil facility (Bridgwater 1999).

11.2.1 Bio-Crude Characteristics

Bio-crude is a corrosive, viscous, polar and thermally unstable product (Adjaye and Bakhshi 1995). Unfavourable characteristics of the biocrude also include acidity, high water and oxygen content, wide volatility distribution and the presence of char. Bio-oil is prone to ageing, which results from the breakdown of the microemulsion, with viscosity tending to increase over time. The presence of fine char in the oil accelerates the ageing process. Due to these complications, bio-oil is typically upgraded to form a less acidic, stable bio-oil of reduced water and oxygen content.

The most abundant compound in the biocrude, after water, is hydroxyacetaldehyde (up to 10%), followed by acetic acid (up to 5%) and formic acid (up to 3%), which lower the bio-oil pH to approximately 2 to 3 (Mohan et al. 2006).

Biomass contains very active catalysts within its structure, namely, the alkali metals that form ash. The most active of these is potassium, followed by sodium, causing secondary cracking of vapours and reducing the liquid yield and quality. Ash can be managed but not eliminated with crop selection and harvesttime management. Washing the biomass before pyrolysis reduces the ash content but the unwanted effects of washing are the loss of hemicellulose and cellulose through hydrolysis, reducing the liquid yield and quantity, which makes this preprocessing step not viable (Bridgwater 2012).

The water component of bio-oil cannot be easily separated because the effects of water on bio-oil are complex and important. If heated to more than 100°C, the oil reacts rapidly to eventually produce a solid residue. Large amounts of water in bio-oil are unavoidable, even with dry feed material (Adam et al. 2006).

The typical properties of a wood-derived bio-oil, as compared with petroleum, are summarised in Table 11.1. This table highlights the significant

TABLE 11.1

Typical Properties of Bio-Oil and Light and Heavy Fuel Oils

Analysis	Pyrolysis Liquids	Light Fuel Oil	Heavy Fuel Oil
Water, wt %	20–30	0.025	0.1
Solids, wt %	<0.5	0	0.2–1
Ash, wt %	<0.2	0.01	0.03
Carbon, wt %	32–48	86	85.6
Hydrogen, wt %	7–8.5	13.6	10.3
Nitrogen, wt %	<0.4	0.2	0.6
Oxygen, wt %	44–60	0	0.6
Sulphur, wt %	<0.05	<0.18	2.5
Vanadium, ppm	0.5	<0.05	100
Sodium, ppm	38	<0.01	20
Calcium, ppm	100	Not analysed	1
Potassium, ppm	220	<0.02	1
Chloride, ppm	80	Not analysed	3
Stability	Unstable	Stable	Stable
Viscosity, cSt	15–35 at 40°C	3–7.5 at 40°C	351 at 50°C
Density (at 15°C), kg/dm^3	1.1–1.3	0.89	0.94–0.96
Flash point, °C	40–110	60	100
Pour point, °C	−10 to −35	−15	21
Conradson carbon residue, wt %	14–23	9	12.2
LHV, MJ/kg	13–18	40.3	40.7
pH	2–3	Neutral	Not analysed
Distillability	Not distillable	160°C–400°C	

Source: Chiaramonti, D. et al., *Renewable and Sustainable Energy Reviews* 11, 1056–1086, 2007.

differences in the properties of bio-oil compared with traditional petroleum fuels. The primary differences are in the water and oxygen contents. Bio-oil has approximately 30% water whereas petroleum products have less than 1%; the oxygen content of bio-oil can be as high as 60% whereas there are very low amounts or none in petroleum oils. Other significant differences are seen in the density, in which bio-oil is up to 20% more dense, and lower heating value (LHV), in which bio-oil has less than half of petroleum oil's LHV.

The viscosity of bio-oil is a direct function of the oxygen content, with high oxygen content giving high viscosity. Therefore, only highly upgraded oils are suitable in product applications in which low viscosities are critical, such as in turbines (Elliott 2007). Product oil density approaches 1 kg/m^3 at relatively low oxygen content (~10%). Products with 10% to 15% oxygen and density of approximately 1 tend to form emulsions with by-product water, which cannot be easily separated.

Currently, there is no defined standard pyrolysis liquid. The definition of oil quality is a major uncertainty. The key properties needing definition

TABLE 11.2

Organic Components of Bio-Oils

Category	Chemicals
Acids	Formic, acetic, propanoic, hexanoic, benzoic, etc.
Esters	Methyl formate, methyl propionate, butyrolactone, methyl n-butyrate, velerolactone, etc.
Alcohols	Methanol, ethanol, 2-propene-1-ol, isobutnol, etc.
Ketones	Acetone, 2-butanone, 2-pentanone, 2-cyclopentanone, 2, 3-pentenedione, 2-hexanone, cyclo-hexanone, etc.
Aldehydes	Formaldehyde, acetaldehyde, 2-butenal, pentanal, ethanedial, etc.
Phenols	Phenol, methyl substituted phenols.
Alkenes	2-methyl propene, dimethylcyclopentene, alpha-pinene, etc.
Aromatics	Benzene, toluene, xylenes, naphthalenes, phenanthrene, fluoranthrene, chrysene, etc.
Nitrogen compounds	Ammonia, methylamine, pyridine, methylpyridine, etc.
Furans	Furan, 2-methyl furan, 2-furanone, furfural, furfural alcohol, etc.
Guiacols	2-methoxy phenol, 4-methyl guaiacol, ethyl guaiacol, eugenol, etc.
Syringols	Methyl syringol, 4-ethyl syringol, propyl syringol, etc.
Sugars	Levoglucosan, glucose, fructose, D-xylose, D-arabinose, etc.
Miscellaneous oxygenates	Hydroxyacetaldehyde, hydroxyacetone, dimethyl acetal, acetal, methyl cyclopentenolone, etc.

Source: Goyal, H. B. et al., *Renewable and Sustainable Energy Reviews* 12, 504–517, 2008.

to allow for standardisation include density, viscosity, surface tension and heating values; however, char level and ash content may also have a major effect and should be considered (Bridgwater 1999).

Pyrolysis bio-oil constituents include both organic and inorganic species. The organic components of pyrolysis-produced bio-oils are shown in Table 11.2. Many of these organic species can be separated for use as speciality chemicals. Inorganic compounds of the bio-oils are associated with counterions, connected to organic acids and related to various enzymatic compounds. Inorganics present in the bio-oil include Ca, Si, K, Fe, Al, Na, S, P Mg, Ni, Cr, Zn, Li, Ti, Mn, Ln, Ba, V, Cl, etc. (Goyal et al. 2008).

11.2.2 Product Applications

There are many possible applications for the bio-oils produced from the pyrolysis of biomass (Czernik and Bridgwater 2004). These include but are not limited to the following:

- Combustion fuel
- Power generation
- Production of chemicals and resins
- Transportation fuel

- Liquid smoke
- Acetic acid
- Production of anhydrosugars (e.g. levoglucosan)
- Binder for pelletising and briquetting combustible waste
- Preservatives (e.g. wood preservative)
- Blended with diesel oil to make diesel engine fuel
- Making adhesives and plastics
- In some instances, used directly in diesel-fuelled engines

Bio-oil can substitute for fuel oil or diesel in many static applications including boilers, furnaces, engines and turbines for electricity generation. The most valuable application of bio-oil is as a renewable transport fuel because other renewable technologies produce electrons for direct use as electricity. In the future, even with the further development of electric vehicles, there will continue to be a great need for liquid fuels in heavy transportation and aviation, and bio-oils are ideally suited to fill this market (Elliott Douglas 2010).

The conversion of biomass to bio-oil can act as a value-adding pretreatment method for an energy carrier, reducing transportation costs and densifying the product. Biomass is a widely dispersed, low-bulk density (150 kg/m^3) product, whereas bio-oil has a typical density of approximately 1200 kg/m^3 (Bridgwater 2011). Because the costs of harvesting, collecting and transporting raw biomass to large-scale processing facilities are high, the conversion to liquid fuels at or near the biomass source reduces transportation costs and environmental effects. Conversion to liquid also reduces handling costs because bio-oil can be pumped. This leads to a concept of small, decentralised fast pyrolysis plants of 100,000 to 300,000 t/year capability, sending the resultant bio-oil to a centralised processing plant. This is a concept supported by the company Envergent, which is making delocalised pyrolysis plants, followed by centralised upgrading using existing crude oil facilities or biorefineries (Butler et al. 2011).

Bio-oil can also be used in co-firing applications. This is potentially attractive because it enables full economies of scale to be achieved and reduces the problems associated with product quality and clean-up. Typically, current practice mixes approximately 5% total energy demand as bio-oil in the coal feed. Examples of co-firing fast pyrolysis liquids already underway include a 20 MW$_e$ coal-fired power station at Manitowac, Wisconsin in the United States using the by-product of liquid smoke production, and a 50 MW$_e$ combined cycle natural gas plant in Harculo in the Netherlands (San Miguel et al. 2011). Large-scale investigations of the combustion of bio-oil have shown that it is clean, with no adverse changes in the boiler operation or emissions levels (Bridgwater 2012). Investigations have also been made into the direct injection of bio-oil enriched with calcium into the postcombustion section of a coal-fired power station to desulphurise the flue gases (Yang et al. 2008).

There is some experience with direct combustion of bio-oil in purpose-built boilers for heat generation. A commercially operated unit owned by Red Arrow in Wisconsin (United States) produces 5 MWt in industrial boilers. Burners and boilers in contact with bio-oil need to be adapted to cope with the corrosivity, particle content and viscous nature of the product (San Miguel et al. 2011).

Pyrolysis oil has a dynamic viscosity of 18 to 25 cSt, which is similar to that of fuel oil. The viscosity can be lowered by heating just before injection, but must not be heated to more than 90°C to avoid chemical breakdown. The viscosity can also be reduced by blending with alcohol. A mixture of 80% pyrolysis bio-oil and 20% ethanol gives similar combustion performance to Jet Propellant 4 jet fuel. This fuel has reasonable heat of combustion as well as low sulphur, nitrogen and ash content (Gupta et al. 2010).

Bio-oil has been successfully combusted in a diesel testing engine in which the behaviour was similar to that of diesel with respect to engine parameters and emissions (Bridgwater 1999). The heating value of pyrolysis oil is approximately 59% that of diesel; however, the cost of pyrolysis oil is low, so the equivalent energy cost is still lower. A major concern with pyrolysis oils are contaminants such as alkali, ash, char and tar (Gupta et al. 2010).

Advantages of pyrolysis liquids as fuels include the following:

- Low-cost liquid biofuel
- Favourable CO_2 balance
- Possible use in small-scale electricity systems and large power stations (co-firing)
- Stability and transportability
- High energy density compared with atmospheric biomass gasification fuel gases
- Potential for use in existing power plants (Gupta et al. 2010)

There are many applications for separation and application of individual chemicals present in the bio-oil. Some examples are shown in Table 11.3. Levoglucosan (1,6-anhydro-β-D-glucopyranose, $C_6H_{10}O_5$) is a major component in bio-oil, with the potential to produce polymers, food additives, pharmaceuticals, pesticides, surfactants, bioethanol and more. It can be easily separated from the bio-oil via phase separation (Gupta et al. 2010; Bennett et al. 2009). The application of ethanol to the fuel chain is well-established and documented. Furfural (2-furaldehyde or furan-2-carboxaldehyde, $C_4H_4O_2$) has many application opportunities due to its unique ability to dissolve aromatics and unsaturated olefines, it is used as a solvent for refining lubricating oils, as a fungicide and as a weed killer. It is also treated to produce furan, methylfuran, acetylfuran, furfurylamine and furoic acid; however,

TABLE 11.3

Product Applications for Chemicals in Bio-Oil

Chemical in Bio-Oil	Uses
Levoglucosan	Food additive, pharmaceutical
Ethanol	Biofuel
Furfural	Pharmaceutical, pesticide
Acetic acid	Specialty chemical
Formic acid	Preservative, antispectic agent
Hydroxyacetaldehyde	Fragrance, pharmaceutical intermediates

Source: Gupta, K.K. et al., *Renewable and Sustainable Energy Reviews* 14, 2946–2955, 2010.

the primary market is hydrogenation to form tetrahydrofuran, a more important solvent then furfural itself (European Commission 2012; Wondu Business and Technology Services 2006). Acetic acid (ethanoic acid, $C_2H_4O_2$) is one of the world's most common chemicals, with applications in food and pharmaceuticals, and it is also used as an acidulant and a raw material in the production of vinyl acetate monomer, acetic anhydride and the acetate esters (BP 2006). Formic acid (methanoic acid, CH_2O_2) has primary applications as a preservative and antibacterial agent for animal feed. It is also used in dying textiles, tanning leather and electroplating (Bull 2010). Hydroxyacetaldehyde (glycolaldehyde, monomethylolformaldehyde, $C_2H_4O_2$) has uses in strengthening sausage casings and as a browning agent in foods (Majerski et al. 2006).

The removal of acids, such as formic and acetic acid, from the bio-oil has net positive effects on the refined product because, whilst delivering saleable chemical products, it also removes substances that have been linked with metal corrosion and instability in the bio-oil (Sukhbaatar et al. 2009).

11.3 Upgrading Technologies

Upgrading of bio-oil to biofuels requires fuel deoxygenation and conventional refining (hydrocracking) by either integrated catalytic pyrolysis or through a decoupled operation. There is also significant interest in partial upgrading to produce an oil compatible with refinery streams. The possibility of integrating bio-oil upgrading in conventional petroleum refineries is extremely attractive. The combined process of hydrotreating and hydrocracking is known as hydroprocessing.

There are many different routes to producing a stable bio-oil. Upgrading methods can be classified as physical, catalytic or chemical as outlined below.

- Physical
  - Filtration
  - Solvent addition
  - Emulsions
- Catalytic
  - Hydrotreating
  - Zeolite cracking
    - Integrated catalytic hydrolysis
    - Close-coupled vapour upgrading
    - Decoupled vapour upgrading
    - Decoupled liquid upgrading
- Chemical
  - Aqueous phase processing
  - Mild cracking
  - Esterification
  - Aqueous phase reforming
  - Hydrogen
  - Gasification for synfuels
  - Model compounds and model bio-oil

This work focuses on catalytic upgrading methods.

11.3.1 Catalytic Upgrading Technologies

The process of catalytic upgrading uses heterogeneous catalysts to increase selectivity to certain products. The primary upgrading mechanism is the rejection of oxygen in biomass as coke or gas (Butler et al. 2011). The liquid product is usually more viscous than bio-oils from noncatalytic processes and contains more aromatics (Butler et al. 2011).

The biorefinery processing route for fuel production from biomass is shown in Figure 11.1, in which the numbers represent fast pyrolysis (1), hydrotreating (2), hydrocracking and product separation (3) and steam reforming (4; Jones et al. 2009).

11.3.1.1 Hydrotreating

The process of hydrotreating rejects oxygen as water through a catalytic reaction with hydrogen. This is considered as a separate and distinct phase from fast pyrolysis, and can therefore be conducted remotely. Hydrotreating is

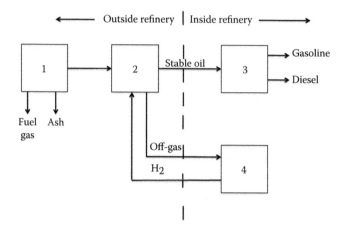

FIGURE 11.1
Biorefinery flows: (1) pyrolysis, (2) hydrotreating, (3) hydrocracking and product separation and (4) steam reforming.

considered to be the key process available to meet the quality specifications for refineries (Brown and Holmgren 2006).

Hydrotreating is usually conducted under high pressure (up to 20 MPa), moderate temperature (up to 400°C), and requires a hydrogen supply or source. Full hydrotreating produces a naptha-like product that requires orthodox refining to produce conventional transport fuels. The projected yield of naptha equivalent is approximately 25% by biomass weight or 55% by biomass energy, excluding hydrogen provision. Hydrogen inclusion reduces the yield down to approximately 15% by weight and 33% by energy. This reaction is depicted in Equation 11.1:

$$C_1H_{1.33}O_{0.43} + 0.77H_2 \rightarrow CH_2 + 0.43H_2O \qquad (11.1)$$

Other key reactions within hydrotreating remove sulphur, nitrogen, olefins and metals, whilst improving distillate fuel quality, such as polyaromatics, cetane and smoke point (Brown and Holmgren 2006).

The optimal conditions for hydroprocessing bio-oil are different from those for crude petroleum products. To address instability problems within the bio-oil, it has been necessary to develop a two-stage hydrotreatment process. Attempts at single-stage hydroprocessing have been unsuccessful because they produce a heavy, tar-like product (Jones et al. 2009). The first stage involves mild stabilisation, applying catalytic hydrotreatment at temperatures lower than 300°C with a nickel or sulphided cobalt molybdenum catalyst, producing viscous black oil with a density of around 1 kg/m³, approximately 25% oxygen, and a hydrogen-to-carbon atomic ratio of 1.5. The presence of a hydrogenation catalyst is critical to the process. The product is significantly upgraded after the first step, as shown by its thermal stability and elemental composition. The second step involves more intense upgrading, treating the phase 1 stable oil at around 350°C, 13.8 MPa over a sulphided cobalt/molybdenum catalyst to produce gasoline range hydrocarbons. This process shows a carbon conversion exceeding 80%, with liquid yields of around 77 L/L and hydrogen consumption of 728 L/L (Brown and Holmgren 2006). Overall, the bio-oil is almost completely deoxygenated by the combination of hydrodeoxygenation and decarboxylation, which are represented in Equations 11.2 and 11.3, respectively. The most common catalyst used in both phases is sulphided cobalt/molybdenum (CoMo). During the two-stage hydrothermal processing, less than 2% oxygen still remains in the treated, stable oil whereas water and off-gas are produced as by-products. The water phase contains some dissolved organics, whereas the off-gas contains light hydrocarbons, excess hydrogen and oxygen. Once stabilised, the oil can be further processed into conventional fuels or sent to a refinery (Jones et al. 2009).

$$C_n COOH \xrightarrow{\text{catalyst}/3H_2} C_{n+1} + 2H_2O \tag{11.2}$$

$$C_n COOH \xrightarrow{\text{catalyst}/H_2} C_n + CO_2 \tag{11.3}$$

An alternative process involves hydrotreatment coupled with catalytic cracking. Williams and Nugranad (2000) investigated the difference between pyrolysis oil and catalytic pyrolysis oil. It was found that catalytic pyrolysis reduced the oil yield, and the oxygen content of the oil was reduced with the formation of coke on the catalyst. Oxygen in the oil was converted by the catalyst to water at lower temperatures and largely to carbon monoxide and carbon dioxide at increased temperatures. The molecular weight distribution of the oils was reduced postcatalysis and further reduced with increasing temperature of catalysis. The catalysed oils showed markedly increased contents of single-ring polyaromatic hydrocarbons. Concentrations of aromatic and polycyclic aromatics increased with increasing temperature of the catalysis. Catalyst deactivation is a constant problem in bio-oil upgrading. It is typically believed to result from carbon deposition on the active catalyst; however, Pindoria et al. (1997) found that catalyst deactivation was primarily the result of volatile components blocking activated sites and not from carbon deposition.

Current research in this area is focusing on the optimisation of the two-stage hydrothermal process, reductions in hydrogen consumption and development of alternative catalysts in preference to modification of traditional hydroprocessing catalysts. Catalysts now being researched include palladium/carbon (for hydrotreating), nickel/molybdenum, ruthenium/

carbon (for hydrodeoxygenation), liquid phase ruthenium and bifunctional nonsulphided nickel–copper catalysts (Butler et al. 2011).

Recent findings in the field include the following:

- Bio-oils from different feedstocks and reactors are similar after hydroprocessing
- Noble metal catalysts on carbon achieve better deoxygenation than traditional catalysts
- Repeated use of the catalyst reduces liquid yield and the hydrogen-to-carbon ratio with increasing solids
- Upgraded oils contain lower quantities of organic acids, ketones and ethers and an increased quantity of phenolics, aromatics and alkanes
- Newly developed catalysts reduce the oxygen content with limited increases in mean cellular retention time and viscosity
- The lignin portion is not responsible for residue formation, it instead forms phenolics and alkanes
- The carbohydrate fraction of the bio-oils is very reactive (Butler et al. 2011)

Catalysts developed in the 1980s and 1990s were based on sulphided cobalt–molybdenum (CoMo) or nickel–molybdenum (Ni–Mo) catalysts supported on an alumina or aluminosilicate, with conditions similar to petroleum desulphurisation. Problems with the use of catalysts include unstable catalyst support in high water contents, and stripping of sulphur from the catalysts due to low sulphur concentrations in the bio-oil requiring constant catalyst resulphurisation (Bridgwater 2012). Recent attention has been given to precious metal catalysts on less susceptible supports. These catalysts are summarised in Table 11.4.

There is a substantial hydrogen requirement in all hydrotreating processes to hydrogenate organic constituents and remove the oxygen as water. The hydrogen can be provided by gasifying additional biomass. Approximately 80% surplus biomass in the feed is required for this, significantly reducing the efficiency of the process. If only the organic fraction of the bio-oil is hydrotreated after phase separation, the required hydrogen can be produced by steam reforming the aqueous phase. Phase separation of organic and aqueous phases will naturally occur if the bio-oil is left unagitated for some time or it may be readily achieved quickly by the addition of water (Teella 2011). The aqueous phase contains 80% to 95% water (Adjaye and Bakhshi 1995).

Major drawbacks to the hydrotreating process are the high cost from the need for high-pressure equipment and significant catalyst deactivation from coking due to the poor carbon-to-hydrogen ratio.

TABLE 11.4

Catalysts Used for Hydrothermal Upgrading of Bio-Oils

Al-MCM-41	Norwegian U. Sci. & Tech.; CPERI, Greece; SINTEF, Norway
Al/SBA-15	U. Sci & Tech. China, Anhui, China
clinoptlolite (natural zeolite, NZ)	Anadolu U., Turkey
CoMo-P sulfided	East China U. Sci & Tech Shanghai, China
CoMo/Al$_2$O$_3$	IRCELYON CNRS U. Lyon, France
CoMo/Y Al$_2$O$_3$	Mississippi State U., USA
FCC	Inst. Superior Tech., Portugal; KiOR, Inc. Pasadena, USA; SE U. Nanjing, China Petrobras, Brazil
H-γ	Anadolu U., Turkey; Georgis Inst. of Tech., USA; U. Sci & Tech of China, Anhui, China
HZSM-5	E China U. Sci & Tech, Shanghai, China; Virginia Tech, USA; U. Basque Country, Spain; U. Pisa, Italy
spent HZSM-5	U. Seoul, Korea; Kongju Nat. U., Korea; Kangwon Nat. U., Korea
MCM-41	CPERI, Greece
Na/γ zeolite	Sichuan U. China
Ni-HZSM-5	U. Basque Country, Spain
NiMo on Al$_2$O$_3$	Guagzhou Inst. Energy Conversion, China
NiMo/γ Al$_2$O$_3$	Mississippi State U., USA
Pd on C	Tech U. of Munich, Germany
Pd on carbon nanotubes	U. Oklahoma, USA
Pd on ZrO$_2$ with SBA1$_5$	East China U. Sci & Tech Shanghai, China
Pd, Ru	Pacific Northwest Laboratory, USA
Precious metal	Mississippi State U., USA; U. Twente, Netherlands; UOP, USA
Pt	U. Kentucky, USA
Ru and homogeneous Ru	Groningen U., Netherlands
Ru on C	U. Jyväskylä/VTT, Finland
SBA-15	U. Sci & Tech. China, Anhui, China
SUZ-4	Mississippi State U., USA
Zr based superacids	Virginia Tech, USA
ZrO$_2$ & TiO$_2$	U. Sci & Tech. China, Anhui, China
ZSM-5	Anadolu U., Turkey; Aston U., UK; U. Leeds, UK; U. Massachusetts, USA

11.3.1.2 Hydrocracking

Hydrotreated oil is stabilised by removing butane and lighter components in a light removal distillation column. The stable oil is then separated into heavy and light fractions. The heavy fraction (boiling temperature >350°C) is sent to a hydrocracker to completely convert the oil to gasoline and diesel blend components. The product is a mix of liquids spanning the gasoline

and diesel range and some by-product gas. The gasoline and diesel products
are separated by distillation. These end products are suitable for blending
into finished fuel (Jones et al. 2009).

11.3.2 Zeolite Cracking

The process of zeolite cracking rejects oxygen as carbon dioxide, which is
conceptually given in Equation 11.4

$$C_1H_{1.33}O_{0.43} + 0.26O_2 \rightarrow 0.65CH_{1.2} + 0.34CO_2 + 0.27H_2O \qquad (11.4)$$

Zeolite cracking can operate on the liquid or vapours within or closely
coupled to the pyrolysis process, or it can be decoupled to upgrade either
liquids or revaporised liquids. Biomass oils are best upgraded by the zeolite
catalysts HZSM-5 or ZSM-5 because these catalysts provide high yields of
liquid products and propylene. Challenges are presented by the propensity
of these liquids to coke, their high total acidic number and the generation of
undesirable by-product such as water and CO_2 (Bridgwater 2012).

11.3.2.1 Integrated Catalytic Pyrolysis

A number of recent developments integrate or combine catalysts with pyrolysis. The addition of a catalyst during pyrolysis produces a pyrolysis liquid
of increased stability and reduced oxygen content, with the aim of producing
biofuel products in a single step. The catalysts used are similar to those in
hydrothermal upgrading. Catalytic reactor problems that need to be overcome arise primarily from poisoning of the catalyst by sulphur and chlorine,
and coking within the reactor (Brown and Holmgren 2006).

11.3.2.2 Close Coupled Vapour Cracking

Catalytic vapour cracking over acidic zeolite catalysts provides deoxygenation by simultaneous dehydration–decarboxylation, producing mostly aromatic hydrocarbons at 450°C, and atmospheric pressure. Oxygen is rejected
as CO_2 or CO from a secondary oxidising reactor to burn off the coke depos-
ited on the catalyst, similar to the process of fluid catalytic cracking in a conventional refinery (Bridgwater 2012).

The low hydrogen-to-carbon ratio imposes a relatively low limit on the
hydrocarbon yield. A projected typical yield of aromatic hydrocarbons suitable for gasoline blending from biomass is approximately 20% by weight or
45% in energy terms (i.e. by calorific value). The crude aromatic hydrocarbon
products would be sent for refining in a conventional refinery (Bridgwater
2012).

The key features of close coupled vapour cracking are the absence of a
hydrogen requirement and the ability to operate at atmospheric pressure.

Catalyst deactivation remains a concern, although coking problems with zeolites can, in principle, be overcome by conventional fluid catalytic cracking arrangements with continual catalyst regeneration by oxidation of the coke. Some concerns remain over the poor control of molecular size and shape when using orthodox zeolites and the propensity for the formation of more noxious hydrocarbons. Processing costs are presently high and therefore products are not competitive with fossil fuels. This approach has only been studied at a basic research level and considerably more development is needed (Bridgwater 2012).

11.3.2.3 Decoupled Liquid Bio-Oil Upgrading

Decoupled liquid bio-oil upgrading has been studied in a pretreated fluid bed zeolite cracking reactor. The separation of thermal pretreatment from catalytic upgrading reduced coking; however, the proposal for secondary upgrading of thermally degraded products in the pretreatment stage suggests the potential for blockage (Bridgwater 2012).

11.4 Opportunities for Integration of Bio-Oils with Petroleum Refineries

11.4.1 Process of Petroleum Refining

Petroleum refining is a well-established process, with over 100 years of operational experience and more than 750 refineries worldwide. It is a complex but efficient process for converting crude petroleum into many valuable and useful products. Petroleum refining consists of the separation of crude oil into different fractions by distillation, followed by further treatment through cracking, reforming, alkylation, polymerisation and isomerisation. It is then separated using fractionation and solvent extraction. Impurities are removed by dehydration, desalting, sulphur removal and hydrotreating (Australian Institute of Petroleum 2013). Because crude oil is a mixture of hydrocarbons of different boiling points, it can be readily separated by distillation into groups of hydrocarbons that boil between two specified boiling points. This can occur at atmospheric pressure or under vacuum.

In the refining process, crude oil is heated and vaporised at or near atmospheric pressure. The evolved vapour is piped into the distilling columns passing through a series of perforated or sieve trays. Heavier hydrocarbons condense more quickly and settle on lower trays, whereas lighter hydrocarbons remain as vapour longer and condense on the upper trays. Liquid fractions are then drawn from trays and removed. Light gases with boiling points lower than 40°C, such as methane, ethane, propane and butane (C_1–C_4), pass through the top of the column. Petroleum fuel, with boiling points between 40°C and 200°C (C_5–C_{12}), is formed on the top trays; kerosene (C_{12}–C_{16}, boiling point 200°C–250°C) and gas oils (C_{15}–C_{18}, boiling point 250°C–300°C) form in the middle, with fuel oils (C_{19} up, boiling point 300°C–370°C) gathering on the lowest tray. The residue from the bottom (C_{25} up) may be burnt as fuel, processed to lubricating oils, waxes and bitumen, or used as a feedstock for cracking units (Elmhurst College 1998).

To recover heavy distillates from the residue, it can be piped to a second distillation column in which the process is repeated under vacuum. This allows heavy hydrocarbons with higher boiling points to be separated without partly cracking them to unwanted products such as coke and gas. These heavy distillates can be converted to lubricating oils in a variety of processes.

11.4.2 Applications for Refining Bio-Oil

Bio-oil upgrading was initially based on prior learning from petroleum refining technologies. Thus, it began with the aim of producing a product similar to petroleum, that is, liquid hydrocarbon fuel products by utilising the sulphided catalysts that had proved successful in petroleum refining. This gave a highly aromatic product with an associated high hydrogen consumption. Advancements since then have seen the refining process optimised for bio-oil products, using nonsulphided catalysts, production of liquid fuel and chemical products of mixed hydrocarbons, and targeted hydrogen consumption. It has been found that ruthenium and palladium are improved catalysts for hydrogenation (Elliott 2010). The need for modification of traditional refinery processing is highlighted by the differences between crude petroleum and biocrude, as shown in Table 11.1. Whereas petroleum is rich in paraffins, some napthenes and aromatics, with very few oxygen atoms, the bio-oil primarily consists of napthenes, with significant amounts of hydrodeoxygenation aromatics and straight chain and branched alkanes.

When processed through a fractionation column, the naptha fraction has a reduced octane content because it contains high levels of cyclic compounds, which require reforming before use in the gasoline pool. The diesel fraction has an increased density and reduced cetane content due to the increased aromatic content requiring hydrogenation to stabilise it. The vacuum gas oil meets the limits for Conradson carbon residue and metals content for hydrocracking. The residue constitutes a very small fraction, which might not be separated in conventional distillation. Corrosion problems arise due to the high levels of organic acids present in the bio-oil (Elliot 2007).

11.4.3 Biorefinery Concepts

The majority of chemicals in the world are made from petroleum feedstocks. The value of these chemicals is high, with comparable revenue to fuel and energy products. Therefore, there is an economic incentive to build such capabilities into the biomass market. Bio-crude is a better starting point than crude oil for chemical manufacture because it is more heterogeneous (Bridgwater 2012). The biorefinery is based on the multiprocess coproduction of fuels, chemicals and energy.

The empirical composition of biomass $\sim(CH_{1.3}O_{0.47})_n$ varies markedly from oil $(CH_2)_n$ (Mohan et al. 2006); therefore, the range of primary chemicals easily derived from biomass and oil are also quite different (Bridgwater 2012). Hence, the biomass chemical industry may need to be based on appropriate and simple chemicals different from the petroleum industry. The biomass composition may also vary geographically with the biomass type. Such a model should allow for biomass to substitute for more valuable feedstocks, such as vegetable oils, in biodiesel production (Bridgwater 2012).

A good biorefinery must be optimised for use of resources, with maximised profitability, maximised benefits and minimised wastes. This should include consideration of saleable chemicals as outlined in Table 11.3.

11.4.3.1 Solvent Fractionation of Bio-Oil

Fractional distillation of bio-oil cannot be achieved due to the prevalence of dimeric and tetragenic phenolic lignin decomposition products, high water content, plethora of compounds of many classes and a significant range of polarities, from nonpolar [e.g. pentane with a polarity index (PI) of 0], weakly polar (e.g. benzene with PI of 3), to strongly polar compounds (such as methanol with a PI of 6.6; Garcìa-Pérez et al. 2007; San Miguel et al. 2011). A separation technique is needed to generate fractions of similar polarity and remove undistillable compounds. Solvents that can be applied for this purpose include pentane, benzene, dichloromethane, ethylacetate, methanol, hexane, diethylether and sodium hydroxide (Mohan et al. 2006). More than 300 compounds have been identified within bio-oil, but only 40% to 50% of the bio-oil (excluding water) has been completely structurally characterised (Mohan et al. 2006).

11.5 Current Status of Bio-Oil

Recent years have seen significant activity in commercial and demonstration bio-oil production plants. Table 11.5 shows a summary of the large-scale projects developed, or that are under development. Canada is most heavily represented, with the Canadian Government having invested significantly in programmes to develop fast pyrolysis bio-oils.

TABLE 11.5

Commercial and Demonstration Bio-Oil Installations in IEA Bioenergy Member Countries

Company	Type of Process	Country	Demonstration or Commercial	Capacity and Products	Company	Commenced	Feedstock	Comments
UOP LLC	Integrated biorefinery	USA	Demonstration		UOP LLC	Due 2014		
GTI	Integrated biorefinery	USA	Demonstration	50 kg/day pilot plant	GTI	2012		
Envergent	Fast pyrolysis	USA	Commercial		Envergent	In design		4 plants in design worldwide
KiOR	Catalytic pyrolysis + hydrotreating	USA	Commercial	Hydrocarbon fuels	KiOR			
Domtar	Modified ABRI-Tech	Canada	Demonstration	100 t/day pilot plant; bio-crude + gas	Domtar		Wood waste	
Dynamotive	Bubbling fluidised bed	Canada	Demonstration	100 tpd delivering up to 2.5 MW$_e$	Dynamotive	2005		Went into recivership, disassembled
Dynamotive	MegaCity Recycling	Canada	Demonstration	200 t/day	Dynamotive	2006		Not currently operating
Ensyn	Fast pyrolysis	Canada	Commercial	Designed 75 tpd, Max demonstrated capacity 100 dtpd	Ensyn	2007		
Ensyn	RTP	Canada	Commercial		Ensyn			

Company	Process	Country	Status	Capacity/Description	Operator	Date	Feedstock	Notes
Ensyn	RTP	Canada	Commercial	400 dtpd	Ensyn	Proposed	Sawmill residues	
Manitoba Hydro	RCE	Canada	Commercial	Anticipate avg $3500–5000/kW electrical	Manitoba Hydro			Operated 200 h then mothballed
Manitoba Hydro	Bio-oil co-firing	Canada	Demonstration	Pyrolysis oil as replacement for heavy fuel oil	Manitoba Hydro			
Pyrovac	Vacuum-assisted pyrolysis	Canada	Demonstration	84 tpd	Pyrovac	1998	Bark	
KIT	Bioliq®	Germany	Demonstration	Produces synthetic fuels and chemicals	KIT	2007	Pyrolysis condensates and char	
PYTEC	BtO	Germany	Demonstration	4 t bio-oil production/day	PYTEC	2005	Wood	Bio-oil tested in CHP with Mercedes-Benz engine
Fortum	Integrated fast pyrolysis	Finland	Commercial	50,000 t bio-oil/yr + heat as CHP	Fortum	Due to commence	Forest residues + wood biomass	
Green Fuel Nordic	GFN process	Finland	Commercial	3 × 400 BDMTPD biorefineries	Green Fuel Nordic	Due 2014	Forest based materials	Total capacity 270,000 t bio-oil/yr
BTG Bioliquids BV	Fast pyrolysis	Netherlands	Demonstration	25 Mwth polygeneration	BTG Bioliquids BV	Under construction	Woody biomass	Producing steam, electricity and fuel oil

11.5.1 Economics

Fast pyrolysis plants for the production of liquid fuel have, on a small scale, been successfully demonstrated, with several demonstration and commercial plants now fully operational. However, the resultant bio-oil is still relatively expensive when compared with fossil energy (Bridgwater 2012).

References

Adam, J., Atonakou, E., Lappas, A., Stocker, M., Nilsen, M. H., Bouzga, A., Hustad, J. E. & Oye, G. 2006. In situ catalytic upgrading of biomass derived fast pyrolysis vapours in a fixed bed using mesopourous materials. *Micropourous and Mesopourous Materials*, 96, 93–101.

Adjaye, J. D. & Bakhshi, N. N. 1995. Production of hydrocarbons by catalytic upgrading of a fast pyrolysis bio-oil. Part 1: Conversion over various catalysts. *Fuel Processing Technology*, 45, 161–183.

Australian Institute of Petroleum. 2013. *Australian Institute of Petroleum.* Available: http://www.aip.com.au [Accessed 1/9/2013].

Bennett, N. M., Helle, S. S. & Duff, S. J. B. 2009. Extraction and hydrolysis of levoglucosan from pyrolysis oil. *Bioresource Technology*, 100, 6059–6063.

Boateng, A. 2011. Pyrolysis Oil—Overview of characteristics and utilization. *Distributed-scale pyrolysis of agricultural biomass for production of refinable crude bio-oil and valuable coproducts* [Online].

BP. 2006. *Acetic acid: End use applications.* Available: http://www.bp.com/liveassets/bp_internet/aromatics_acetyls/aromatics_acetyls_english/STAGING/local_assets/downloads_pdfs/a/aceticacidenduse2.pdf [Accessed 11/3/2014].

Bridgwater, A. V. 1999. Principles and practice of biomass fast pyrolysis processes for liquids. *Journal of Analytical and Applied Pyrolysis*, 51, 3–22.

Bridgwater, A. V. 2011. Upgrading Fast Pyrolysis Liquids. *Thermochemical Processing of Biomass.* John Wiley & Sons, Ltd.

Bridgwater, A. V. 2012. Review of fast pyrolysis of biomass and product upgrading. *Biomass and Bioenergy*, 38, 68–94.

Bridgwater, A. V. & Double, J. M. 1991. Production costs of liquid fuels from biomass. *Fuel*, 70, 1209–1224.

Brown, R. & Holmgren, J. 2006. Fast Pyrolysis and Bio-Oil Upgrading.

Bull, S. 2010. Formic acid—General information. Health protection agency (ed.).

Butler, E., Devlin, G., Meier, D. & Mcdonnell, K. 2011. A review of recent laboratory research and commercial developments in fast pyrolysis and upgrading. *Renewable and Sustainable Energy Reviews*, 15, 4171–4186.

Chiaramonti, D., Oasmaa, A. & Solantausta, Y. 2007. Power generation using fast pyrolysis liquids from biomass. *Renewable and Sustainable Energy Reviews*, 11, 1056–1086.

Czernik, S. & Bridgwater, A. V. 2004. Overview of applications of biomass fast pyrolysis oil. *Energy & Fuels*, 18, 590–598.

Elliott, D. C. 2007. Historical developments in hydroprocessing bio-oils. *Energy & Fuels*, 21, 1792–1815.

Elliott Douglas, C. 2010. Advancement of bio-oil utilization for refinery feedstock. *The Washington Bioenergy Research Symposium.*

Elmhurst College. 1998. *Fractional Distillation of Crude Oil* [Online]. Available: http://www.elmhurst.edu/~chm/onlcourse/chm110/outlines/distill.html.

European Commission. 2012. Scientific committee on consumer safety. Opinion on furfural.

Garcìa-Pérez, M., Chaala, A., Pakdel, H., Kretschmer, D. & Roy, C. 2007. Vacuum pyrolysis of softwood and hardwood biomass: Comparison between product yields and bio-oil properties. *Journal of Analytical and Applied Pyrolysis,* 78, 104–116.

Goyal, H. B., Seal, D. & Saxena, R. C. 2008. Bio-fuels from thermochemical conversion of renewable resources: A review. *Renewable and Sustainable Energy Reviews,* 12, 504–517.

Gupta, K. K., Rehman, A. & Sarviya, R. M. 2010. Bio-fuels for the gas turbine: A review. *Renewable and Sustainable Energy Reviews,* 14, 2946–2955.

Jones, S. B., Valkenburg, C., Walton, C. W., Elliott, D. C., Holladay, J. E., Stevens, D. J., Kinchin, C. & Czernik, S. 2009. Production of Gasoline and Diesel from Biomass via Fast Pyrolysis, Hydrotreating and Hydrocracking: A Design Case. *US Department of Energy.* (ed.). Pacific Northwest National Laboratory.

Majerski, P. A., Piskorz, J. K. & Radlein, D. S. a. G. 2006. *Production of glycolaldehyde by hydrous thermolysis of sugars.* Patent US 7,094,932 B2.

Meier, D., Van De Beld, B., Bridgwater, A. V., Elliott, D. C., Oasmaa, A. & Preto, F. 2013. State-of-the-art of fast pyrolysis in IEA bioenergy member countries. *Renewable and Sustainable Energy Reviews,* 20, 619–641.

Mohan, D., Pittman, C. U. & Steele, P. H. 2006. Pyrolysis of wood/biomass for bio-oil: A critical review. *Energy & Fuels,* 20, 848–889.

Pindoria, R. V., Lim, J. Y., Hawkes, J. E., Lazaro, M. J., Herod, A. A. & Kandiyoti, R. 1997. Structural characterization of biomass pyrolysis tars/oils from eucalyptus wood waste: Effect of H-2 pressure and sample configuration. *Fuel,* 76, 1013–1023.

San-Miguel, G., Makibar, J. & Fernandez-Akarregi, A. R. 2011. New advances in the fast pyrolysis of biomass. *In: Proceedings of the 12th International Conference on Environmental Science and Technology.* Rhodes, Greece: University of the Aegean.

Sukhbaatar, B., Steele, P. H., Ingram, L. L. & Kima, M. G. 2009. An exploratory study on the removal of acetic and formic acids from bio-oil. *BioResources,* 4, 1319–1329.

Teella, A. V. P. R. 2011. *Separation of Carboxylic Acids From Aqueous Fraction of Fast Pyrolysis Bio-Oils Using Nanofiltration and Reverse Osmosis Membranes.* PhD, University of Massachusetts - Amherst.

Williams, P. T. & Nugranad, N. 2000. Comparison of products from the pyrolysis and catalytic pyrolysis of rice husks. *Energy,* 25, 493–513.

Wondu Business and Technology Services 2006. Furfural chemicals and biofuels from agriculture. Australian Government Rural Research and Development Corporation.

Yang, X. L., Zhang, J. & Zhu, X. F. 2008. Decomposition and calcination characteristics of calcium-enriched bio-oil. *Energy & Fuels,* 22, 2598–2603.

Index

Page numbers followed by f and t indicate figures and tables, respectively.